THE

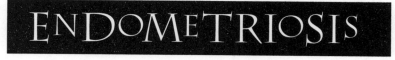

ENDOMETRIOSIS

SOURCEBOOK

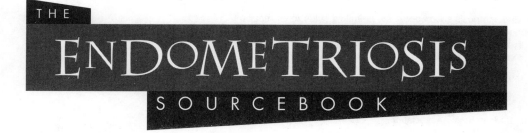

THE ENDOMETRIOSIS SOURCEBOOK

The definitive guide to current treatment
options, the latest research, common myths
about the disease, and coping strategies—
both physical and emotional

Mary Lou Ballweg
and the Endometriosis Association
Foreword by Dr. Dan Martin

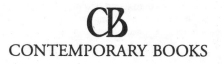

CONTEMPORARY BOOKS

Library of Congress Cataloging-in-Publication Data

The Endometriosis sourcebook: the definitive guide to current
    treatment options, the latest research, common myths about the
    disease, and coping strategies—both physical and emotional /
    [compiled by] Mary Lou Ballweg and the Endometriosis Association.
        p.   cm.
    Includes index.
    ISBN 0-8092-3263-4
    1. Endometriosis—Popular works.   I. Ballweg, Mary Lou.
II. Endometriosis Association.
RG483.E53E56   1995
618.1—dc20   95-24526
                                                            CIP

Cover design by Kim Bartko
Interior design and production by Susan H. Hartman

Acknowledgment of permissions on page 473

Dedicated to the Endometriosis Association leaders, staff, and members. Without their support this book would not exist, nor would the help that has been so vital to women with endometriosis around the world. We invite women and girls with endometriosis everywhere to join in our efforts to help each other and find the cause and cure for endometriosis.

Contents

◎◎

✸

Foreword

By Dan C. Martin, M.D.

One of the joys of being a physician is being asked to write what I enjoy writing. The invitation to contribute this foreword to *The Endometriosis Sourcebook* by Mary Lou Ballweg and the members and supporters of the Endometriosis Association is an honor and a privilege. The contributors are committed to the Endometriosis Association's mission of providing mutual support and help to those affected by endometriosis, educating the public and medical community about the disease, and promoting research related to endometriosis. The importance of this book is stated appropriately in the Endometriosis Association's basic "yellow" brochure: "Ending the feeling of being alone, sharing with others who understand what one is going through, counteracting lack of information and misinformation about endometriosis, and learning from each other are ways those affected by the disease help each other." The ability of the Endometriosis Association to achieve these ideals is manifest in the large number of women, their partners, and their families who thank the association for helping change their lives.

One of the difficulties for those who have endometriosis is understanding why it is a controllable problem in some women and a devastating disease in others. In this regard it is not unlike several diseases, such as the common cold or the flu. The majority of common cold or flu sufferers get well with rest and orange juice, yet a significant minority experience superinfection, pneumonia, or life-threatening debilitation. An additional concern is the potentiality of one disease process masking another, such as when meningitis causes flulike symptoms. Under these circumstances, if such symptoms remain misdiagnosed, improper response and treatment can not only cause frustration but also result in a worsening condition. Similarly, many diseases presenting the symptoms of endometriosis—pelvic inflammatory disease, pelvic chlamydia infections, tubal pregnancies, premenstrual syndrome, endosalpingosis, and splenosis, to mention a few—can coexist or be confused with endometriosis. The treatment of endometriosis is complicated because medical science has not ascertained whether endometriosis is a separate and distinct disease process or the result of some unidentified problem.

Despite significant increases in knowledge and awareness, a clinical understanding of endometriosis continues to be obscured by myths and misinformation. Many patients still say that their previous physicians told them their problem is frigidity, neuroticism, or drug addiction or that it is a normal condition. Other patients state their doctors believe endometriosis cannot occur after having children or a hysterectomy. Some African American women are still told they cannot get endometriosis because of their race. Some women with deep endometriosis report that they were first told that they did not have endometriosis because their laparoscopic results revealed no evidence of the disease. Experience continues to be an effective teacher even for the most skilled, whether understanding and knowledge come from observing correct or incorrect diagnostic methodology, self-care, or medical treatment. It is important that all individuals concerned with the issues regarding endometriosis recognize that health education and medical excellence are a never-ending challenge. This book adds to existing knowledge and data with sections devoted to treatment, coping, and new research.

The Endometriosis Association has also been diligent in areas of research. For example, when Mary Lou Ballweg heard that a dioxin-exposed rhesus monkey colony at the University of Wisconsin–Madison in which two monkeys had died of endometriosis was about to be sold, she saw the possibilities for research. After an emergency meeting of the association board, Ballweg raised funds to support research teams from three universities to examine the remaining monkeys. Subsequently, reviews on the adverse effects on the monkeys associated with dioxin exposure appeared in *Science* and *Scientific American*. This work has been used to help create a research program at Dartmouth Medical School under the direction of Sherry Rier, Ph.D., former vice president of research of the Endometriosis Association. Currently, studies prompted by this work are under way at the Environmental Protection Agency, the National Institute of Environmental Health Sciences, and other academic centers.

However, it is important to remember that research findings need confirmation and time for assessment, something at which the Endometriosis Association excels. This book seeks to balance, clarify, and resolve the issues within a cohesive framework. It reviews the various positions regarding endometriosis today and what an individual can and cannot expect in diagnosis and treatment. Consequently this approach should prove especially valuable as a resource for patients, their partners, their families and friends, practicing physicians, physicians in training, and researchers.

Medical treatment, conservative surgery, hysterectomy, and supportive care each has its place. The difficulty lies in keeping the options open so that an appropriate diagnosis and therapy for each patient can be determined. Establishing and maintaining a good doctor-patient relationship cannot be stressed enough. This relationship is a key factor in producing potentially better outcomes such as reducing confusing diagnoses and inadequate or delayed therapy with related complications. To this end I believe this publication excels because it increases awareness about the disease process and facilitates more effective care for endometriosis sufferers.

■ **Dan Martin**, *M.D., is a reproductive surgeon at Baptist Memorial Hospital and clinical associate professor in the Department of Obstetrics and Gynecology at the University of Tennessee, Memphis. He has been honored with a Picker Foundation fellowship in physics and radiology, two Codman surgical awards for medical education, the Endometriosis Association Recognition Award, and the Clinical Research Award of the Society of Reproductive Surgeons for his work in endometriosis. He has been a divisional director of medical education at the Johns Hopkins Hospital, president of the American Association of Gynecologic Laparoscopists, and president of the Gynecologic Surgery Society.*

Author's Note

The Endometriosis Association is an independent organization for those with the disease, governed primarily by those with the disease, and independent of vested interests. The contents of this book are not to be construed as medical advice, nor is the book a substitute for proper medical treatment. Unless clearly stated as such, treatment options are not recommended by the Endometriosis Association. The association does not promote any drugs, treatments, or specific theories about endometriosis unless clear evidence of their efficacy emerges.

Letters published reflect the experience and/or opinions of the writers. Publication in the text does not constitute endorsement of the letter writers' opinions or verification of their experiences. Likewise, articles published in the text reflect the research, experience, and opinions of the individual authors. The Endometriosis Association neither endorses nor disclaims specific theories or treatment recommendations in the articles unless such endorsement or disclaimer is specifically stated.

Acknowledgments

Many wonderful people have made this book possible. First, and foremost, without the thousands of members and supporters of the Endometriosis Association—members, donors, chapter and group leaders, board members, and advisors—the Endometriosis Association and all of its programs, including the production of this book, would not be possible. All of these wonderful people cannot be thanked individually, but please rest assured that you are deeply appreciated, and because of you, we have made huge strides in helping women with endometriosis and in unraveling the mysteries of this frustrating disease.

A particular debt of gratitude is owed to Mary Lou Ballweg, whose devotion to women with endo and the Endometriosis Association is legendary; to Tracy H. Dickinson, whose wonderful generosity has made our research program at Dartmouth Medical School possible; to Sherry E. Rier, Ph.D., who has put her whole heart and soul into our research; and to the staff of the Endometriosis Association, who have worked to assist women with endometriosis under often difficult conditions—less than ideal equipment and an overwhelming workload.

We'd like to take this moment to particularly recognize the many contributions of our advisors: G. David Adamson, M.D.; Michel Canis, M.D.; Donald L. Chatman, M.D.; Kiu-Kwong Chu, M.D.; W. Paul Dmowski, M.D., Ph.D.; Robert R. Franklin, M.D.; W. F. (Dub) Howard, M.D.; Robert B. Hunt, M.D.; Arnold J. Kresch, M.D.; Karen Lamb, Ph.D., R.N.; André Lemay, M.D., Ph.D.; Kay Lie, M.D.; Dan C. Martin, M.D.; Subbi Mathur, Ph.D.; Deborah Metzger, Ph.D., M.D.; Charles E. Miller, M.D.; Camran R. Nezhat, M.D.; David L. Olive, M.D.; David B. Redwine, M.D.; Michael W. Vernon, Ph.D.; and Robert A. Wild, M.D.

In the production of the book, many wonderful people were invaluable. First, the book would not exist without the ongoing efforts of Mary Lou Ballweg, who wrote many of the articles on weekends and evenings and worked under tight deadlines. We also appreciate her family, Jim Dorr and Aquene, who had to pick up the slack at home when Mary Lou was on deadline, and whose ongoing support is very much appreciated. In particular, we want to thank the writers who prepared articles especially for this book—again, often on tight deadlines. Thank you to Dr. David Olive; Mona Trempe Norcum, Ph.D.;

Cathy Corman (Cathy also helped with the Resource Listing); Lyse Tremblay; Karen Gould; Nicole Denison; Dr. Dan Martin; and Meri Lau, whose delightful artwork for "Joe with Endo" will again be enjoyed by readers. Thank you to Nancy Merrill, who assisted in the early planning of the book before health problems made it impossible to continue; Lynda Van Dien, who was a terrific help with the manuscript production and permissions; Lisa Rosbeck, our former secretary who helped with production; Chuck Shantz, who helped with copyediting; our advisors and reviewers; our agents, Margaret Russell and Jacqueline Simenauer; and all the folks at Contemporary Books, especially Nancy Crossman, Gigi Grajdura, and Maureen Musker.

THE

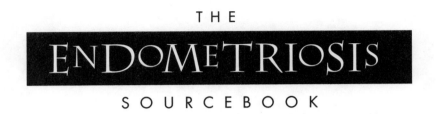

ENDOMETRIOSIS

SOURCEBOOK

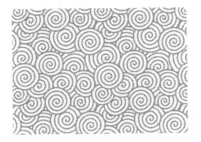

PART I

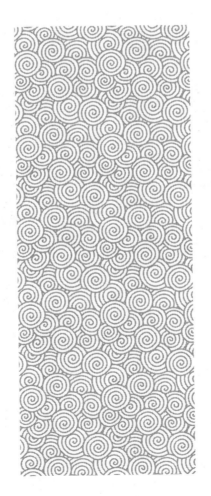

Introduction

Building a Sourcebook for Women with Endometriosis

By Mary Lou Ballweg

Sourcebook: an original writing as a document, record, or diary that supplies an authoritative basis for future writing, study, or evaluation etc.

Random House Unabridged Dictionary, second edition, 1993

Sourcebook is certainly an appropriate title for the Endometriosis Association's second book. First, it is full of *authoritative* information based on what we've learned by pulling together the experiences of hundreds of thousands of women with endometriosis as well as working with researchers, our advisors, and top medical professionals.

Second, this sourcebook provides a *document, record, or diary* of our endometriosis journey. Since we published our first book, *Overcoming Endometriosis* (now reprinted five times), in 1987, the number of research studies done has climbed to more than 5,000, and the association itself has been responsible for some truly breakthrough research. All these studies have added much to our knowledge, but they have also shown us how complex endometriosis is. Sharing this new knowledge is an important goal of this book.

Not that everything about endo is new. When I was showing my spouse, Jim, the "Joe with Endo" series for this book—the cartoon saga of our role-reversal hero continued from our first book—he said, "But Joe is going through the same things again—problems with sex due to his disease, problems with work due to the disease, problems getting good medical help." Yes, I said, Joe is still going through all these rotten experiences, variations on a theme—just as are the millions of women and girls with endometriosis. They repeat the endless cycles of denial, lack of help, difficulties in their relationships and at work as they wrestle with new aspects of the disease or its impact on their lives. How I wish I could give Joe a better outcome! (At least at the end of this series he is no longer alone and finds help through the support group, as so many women have through the association.)

I had the same feeling of déjà vu when I was working on many of the chapters in this book. It was a great pleasure to see how much we've learned in the eight years since *Overcoming Endometriosis* was published. But at the same time I kept thinking about how many women all over the world are still going through all the things I went through in the late seventies that led me to start the association. (After being bedridden with severe symptoms and experiencing great difficulty obtaining a diagnosis, I'd vowed to help other women with the disease. After several treatments and surgeries, a "miracle" baby, and being bedridden for months twice more, I'd had a hysterectomy and removal of my ovaries after all treatment options had been attempted. For the complete story, see the Introduction to *Overcoming Endometriosis*, available from the association and bookstores.) For that matter, I was still going through it, not only the disbelief and dismay when my disease reactivated in 1990 (see "Decision Making on Surgery" in Chapter 2) but also Hashimoto's thyroiditis, an autoimmune disease that appears to occur in women with endo, severe allergies and candidiasis (which my daughter also struggles with), and severe osteoporosis. With the support and information I've gleaned from the Endometriosis Association, I can now manage, with care and attention to my health, to stay functional and have not been bedridden since 1982. Like other women with endo, I have often asked myself: How can this be happening again? By *this* I mean not only that the disease comes back but also that some of the medical profession persist in chalking women's experiences up to psychological stress. One of the great challenges of a chronic disease such as endo is that one goes through all the painful psychological stages of denial, anger, bargaining, grief, and acceptance over and over. What a test of a human being this chronic illness is!

Third, this sourcebook supplies a basis for *future writing, study,* and *evaluation* of this frustrating disease. It is not the end point in the endometriosis journey. While we have learned an amazing amount about the disease since the association was formed in 1980—when no brochures or lay books were available and very little research had been done—we still do not have the answers we all want: what causes the disease, how to cure it, how to prevent it.

Fourth, this sourcebook presents *original* writing. All the material in this book is new since the last book (with the exception of the article "The Enigma Called Endometriosis," a repeat of the first chapter from *Overcoming Endometriosis*). This book is not a revision of *Overcoming Endometriosis* but additional, original material. We see the two books as companions and expect that most women with endo will want both; in addition, informed women with endometriosis will want to keep up with current and late breaking information by following the association's newsletter. (See the back of this book for information on getting in touch with us.)

The material is original in another way, too. Rather than just reporting information, we attempt to sift and winnow through the conflicting, confusing morass of data, opinions, politics, and marketing efforts in the field of endometriosis. An example is our chapter on surgery, an area of rapid change, indeed a virtual revolution (in which the association has been a key player) in the last decade. Solid *data* is sparse for a number of reasons. Often, because limited research has been done or because the basic mechanisms underlying endo are not understood, it's hard to know what research findings mean. And what data is available is often misleading—at times both practitioners and patients seem to be grasping at straws in a desire to find answers to tough treatment decisions.

Opinion, however, is abundant, fed by the need to do something about the disease. Academicians often complain about practicing clinicians and patients attempting treatments that are not scientifically proven. However, as Karen Lamb, Ph.D., director of the Endometriosis Association Research Registry for many years, was fond of saying, what are these women supposed to do—roll over and die until medicine and science have answers? When your life has come grinding to a halt due to the disease, you have to do the best you can with the knowledge that is available. You can't wait for science to catch up. (However, you can, as the association has done, push it.)

Politics, too, is a player. Politics in the field of medicine? Laypeople are often surprised to learn this. Little have most suspected that, as in every other field, people in medicine and science are building a career, trying to make a name for themselves, knocking the competition, trying to make money. The changes in the medical field (to managed care in the United States and efforts worldwide to control costs and the dangerous crunch on research dollars) have intensified the problem.

In clinical practice, for example, surgeons who really enjoy doing the complicated surgery often required for endo can see enough patients to gain the necessary experience to become specialists, the kind of surgeons that patients will scrimp and save to go to in spite of lack of coverage by insurance or governments, only by building a name. And in research, if scientists' only chance of obtaining some of the very scarce research funds is to produce results, they may become unwilling to share important information with other researchers—their competitors for funding—even though such sharing might help push the whole field forward. (The association has been a key player in helping to obtain funding for research and in helping to promote active sharing of information and resources in the research community.) It is sad and ironic that research funds made available in 1983 for endo went unused because no proposals were submitted for the funds (there was so little interest in endo at that time!). But in 1991, when funds were appropriated by Congress due to the efforts of the association, so many excellent proposals were submitted that most went unfunded. (Indeed it is primarily because of the association that the great surge of interest in and research on the disease has occurred in the last decade. Women with endometriosis and their families will need to continue to fund research and to keep people aware of the disease if we expect ongoing progress.)

Finally, *marketing* is a factor. As association advisor David Olive, M.D., writes in the medical textbook *Infertility and Reproductive Medicine Clinics of North America: Endometriosis*, "a number of prima donna physicians who claim to specialize in the diagnosis and treatment of endometriosis bring their singular bias to bear on large numbers of patients, often without scientific data to support their views. Often these physicians fail to report their results, and publicize wildly successful claims. . . . It is imperative that women suffering from the disease understand what is known (and not known) about endometriosis. This requires thoughtful dissection of all existing information with a critical eye, rather than blind acceptance of promotional efforts by selected clinicians."

This thoughtful dissection is not easy, as the difficulties we faced preparing our GnRH chapter illustrate. The newness of these drugs meant not only that there was limited data on them but also that we constantly had to be aware of the marketing of the drugs as a factor and sort it out from reality. Because of the huge cost—now estimated at about $100 million—involved in bringing a new drug to market, companies must aggressively market drugs to recoup their investment. So women with endometriosis must remember that they're hearing about a new drug not because it is necessarily better than older options but rather because of an intensive marketing campaign. Older drugs are marketed little or not at all because the drugs are often off-patent and thus no one company stands to make money from advertising the drug. Keep in mind that these older options also are often much less expensive, since the companies making them recouped their development costs long ago. (See Chapter 3, "Medical Treatment for Endometriosis: Overview and Alternative Options," for more information on these older alternatives.)

Sorting through the research studies is a critical part of "thoughtful dissection." Was the study in question truly a good one? Was it applicable to women with endometriosis? Did it make a difference, for instance, whether a GnRH study of side effects involved women with fibroids rather than women with endo? Or, as in the case of another study on short-term memory loss in women taking GnRH agonists, did the fact that the study had only been reported at a meeting and had not been published in a good research journal mean that the information should not be included? (Publication in a good research journal generally means the data has been subjected to a process called *peer review* by other researchers. Peer-reviewed journals and the papers in them are more highly regarded as solid research in the medical community.) Ultimately we opted not to include the first study, on fibroids. One of our reviewers argued persuasively that the women in the study were somewhat older than most women with endometriosis typically taking GnRH agonists. This meant that many of the menopausal complaints in the fibroid group may have been in part exacerbated by their already lower levels of estrogen. (Other studies specifically on women with endo and their side effects on the drugs *were* used, of course.) In contrast, we opted to include the second study, on short-term memory loss. Reports to the association indicated this was a side effect some women with endo were experiencing, and that they were concerned about it. Also, research in other areas of women's health has provided some support for an estrogen/memory relationship. Again, however, we had to wade through unhelpful opinion. In talking with a physician on the side effects of GnRH, he cautioned us not to carry all the information because it would "scare" women. The association has always believed women have the right to important information that might impact their health and that they can handle it.

Struggling through this process, I was reminded again of the tremendous value of an organization like the association. We are proud of the fact that the solid, useful information we are able to produce on GnRH drugs and on other topics throughout the book, despite the obstacles, is widely regarded as the most balanced available for the layperson. (I am reminded of the journalist who, while researching a story on endometriosis, was thoroughly amazed by the conflicting, confusing opinions she got from interviews with 15 different doctors. Only in the association, she said, did she find balance and clarity.) Because we act as a clearinghouse and can pool the experiences of hundreds and sometimes thousands of women and because we represent women, not a product or a service or a practice, we are not completely dependent on the willingness of physicians, researchers, and drug companies to study well and share completely this kind of information. (Not to mention that a clearinghouse is needed because, with so much new information coming forth, no one person could possibly keep up with the whole field.) With 15 years of background and growing sophistication we are indeed able to struggle through that process.

The *entire* endo field, in fact, is growing in sophistication—more and more members of the medical community are insisting on well-designed research and clinical studies and questioning old ideas about the disease, a wonderful development that the association has been very much behind. It was reassuring to discover, for instance, that the chart on the side effects of danazol originally prepared by our Research Department in 1983, when there was little data, is no longer the only available compilation of such data.

Struggling through the type of process I've just described is not something newcomers or the typical girl or woman with endometriosis could possibly do. As Dr. Olive wrote in his textbook on endo, "Local and national associations serve a critical purpose as educators in the community. Newly diagnosed women, as well as those merely suspected of having the disease, are bombarded with an array of often conflicting information. Consumer organizations can provide an unbiased source of information and guidance for these women. Educating the patient population is guaranteed to provide the greatest impact in promoting quality care for those suffering from endometriosis."

The association's role in producing original materials, besides providing vital information needed by women with endometriosis, also helps bring to the forefront issues that need to be addressed. For instance, in 1988, when we pulled together all the information and experiences we could to do our pioneering article on endometriosis and the intestines, it was a neglected area of endometriosis (even though 79 percent of women with endometriosis report bowel symptoms of one kind or another, according to reports to the association's Research Registry). Our article helped push the field to new recognition of these symptoms and to develop methods of addressing these problems, rather than ignoring them as had been the case in the past. Another example is our recent article on somatization disorder, the scandalous tendency to label people with confusing physical symptoms as having mental disorders (see Chapter 9, "It's All in Your Head"). This article, now also being published in an ob-gyn journal and publicized through my speeches at the Fourth World Congress on Endometriosis in Brazil in 1994 and the NIH Endometriosis 2000 conference in the spring of 1995, is opening discussion on this tough subject.

Thus is progress made. And, despite our many remaining questions, *much* progress has been made. In the eight years since our first book was published there has been an explosion of information and new treatment options—new ways of coping with chronic pain, the surgical revolution already mentioned, new medical treatments, new understanding of how to cope with the disease and how those of us who have it can support each other.

Awareness of the disease has increased tremendously also—another very hopeful sign. In a survey conducted in 1994 by a U.S. professional polling company, 69 percent of the women surveyed claimed to have at least heard of endometriosis, and 66 percent were able to select the correct definition of the disease from a list. This is a remarkable increase in awareness—given that in the early eighties most people had not heard of the disease—and a testament to the unending outreach and education on the disease that women with endometriosis have carried out.

Research breakthroughs are also occurring. Most important of these is the association's work linking the environmental pollutant dioxin to endometriosis. (See Part IV, "New Research Directions," for more information.) For the first time we know specific agents that can cause spontaneous development of the disease in animals. We also may have important clues about why there are now millions of women with endometriosis all over the world whereas in the past the disease was considered rare (although, given the lack of study in the past, we may never know how many it actually affected).

Finally, most hopeful of all, the message that endometriosis is an important disease affecting many millions of women has spread worldwide since the publication of our last book. And therein lies great hope. As I have met courageous women with the disease from other countries, I have time and again been impressed by the realization that we can, working together around the world, conquer this disease. I think of our contact person in Algeria, who can't even have a pelvic exam despite severe pain because she's not married and a pelvic might affect her hymen, which would make potential marriage partners consider her "damaged goods"! Imagine the courage it takes to work to increase awareness of endometriosis in a social climate like that. I think of our organizers in Brazil, who, despite the obstacles imposed by terrible poverty, have started groups for women with endo and outreach campaigns. I marvel at the courage and determination of people like Sumie Uno, Yasuko Ako, and their companions, who founded the first women's health center in Japan, a country where consumer activism, particularly in women's health, is unheard of. As I talk to the 150 or so women attending the first-ever public meeting for women with endometriosis in Japan and hear some say that the association has inspired a desire to offer the same programs in their country, I brim over with pride and inspiration.

How lucky we are, endo or not, that we can bond so deeply as women around this disease, beyond cultural and language barriers. As I have had the opportunity to meet our leaders and members around the world, I've often thought that there is nothing these women cannot do, strengthened by the struggles of the disease, determined, and united. Together we will cure endometriosis!

EDITOR'S NOTE: Just as *multiple sclerosis* was shortened to MS decades ago, we made the decision to shorten *endometriosis* to *endo* for lay use. Educating about the disease and making it a little more manageable and a little less formidable starts with the public's being able to pronounce its name.

■ *Mary Lou Ballweg is president and executive director of the Endometriosis Association, an organization she cofounded in 1980. Besides founding and leading the association for the last 15 years, she has overseen publication of the association's two books, its educational videotapes, an extensive body of literature on the disease, development and execution of a $1.3 million educational awareness campaign, two public service announcement campaigns, and numerous other outreach efforts. Together with Dr. Karen Lamb, she established the world's first research registry for endometriosis. She was responsible for a major breakthrough in endometriosis research linking dioxin and the disease that has received attention in leading scientific journals and prompted numerous additional research studies. She was instrumental in establishing an association research program for endometriosis at Dartmouth Medical School.*

Prior to founding the Endometriosis Association, Ms. Ballweg was a communications consultant with her own national business, scriptwriter-director at a film and public relations company, and managing editor of a monthly magazine. She was also one of the founders of a women's community health clinic and has been recognized in numerous Who's Who listings.

The Enigma Called Endometriosis

By Mary Lou Ballweg

Endometriosis is a puzzling disease affecting women in their reproductive years. The name comes from the word *endometrium,* which is the tissue that lines the inside of the uterus and builds up and sheds each month in the menstrual cycle. In endometriosis, tissue like the endometrium is found outside the uterus, in other areas of the body. In these locations outside the uterus, the endometrial tissue develops into what are called *nodules, tumors, lesions, implants,* or *growths* (see Glossary for definitions of these terms). These growths can cause pain, infertility, and other problems.

The most common locations of endometrial growths are in the abdomen—involving the ovaries, the fallopian tubes, the ligaments supporting the uterus, the area between the vagina and the rectum, the outer surface of the uterus, and the lining of the pelvic cavity. Sometimes the growths are also found in abdominal surgery scars, on the intestines or in the rectum, and on the bladder, vagina, cervix, and vulva (external genitals). Endometrial growths have also been found outside the abdomen, in the lung, arm, thigh, and other locations, but these are uncommon.

Endometrial growths are generally not malignant or cancerous—they are a normal type of tissue outside the normal location. (However, in recent decades malignancy has occurred or been recognized in conjunction with endometriosis with increasing frequency.) Like the lining of the uterus, endometrial growths usually respond to the hormones of the menstrual cycle. They build up tissue each month, break down, and cause bleeding.

However, unlike the lining of the uterus, endometrial tissue outside the uterus has no way of leaving the body. The result is internal bleeding, degeneration of the blood and tissue shed from the growths, inflammation of the surrounding areas, and formation of scar tissue. Other complications, depending on the location of the growths, can be rupture of growths (which can spread endometriosis to new areas), the formation of adhesions, intestinal bleeding or obstruction (if the growths are in or near the intestines), interference with bladder function (if the growths are on or in the bladder), and other problems. Symptoms seem to worsen with time, though cycles of remission and recurrence are the pattern in some cases.

Symptoms

The most common symptoms of endometriosis are pain before and during periods (usually worse than "normal" menstrual cramps), pain during or after sexual activity, infertility, and heavy or irregular bleeding. Other symptoms may include fatigue, painful bowel movements with periods, lower back pain with periods, and diarrhea and/or constipation and other intestinal upset with periods. Some women with endometriosis have no symptoms. Infertility affects about 30 to 40 percent of women with endometriosis and is a common result with progression of the disease.

The amount of pain is not necessarily related to the extent or size of growths. Tiny growths (called *petechial growths*) have been found to be more active in producing prostaglandins, which may explain the significant symptoms that often seem to occur with small implants. Prostaglandins are substances produced throughout the body, involved in numerous functions, and thought to cause many of the symptoms of endometriosis.

Theories About the Cause of Endometriosis

The cause of endometriosis is not known. A number of theories have been advanced, but no one of them seems to account for all cases. One theory is the retrograde menstruation or transtubal migration theory—that during menstruation some of the menstrual tissue backs up through the fallopian tubes, implants in the abdomen, and grows. Some experts on endometriosis believe all women experience some menstrual tissue backup and that an immune system problem and/or hormonal problem allows this tissue to take root and grow in women who develop endometriosis. Another theory suggests that the endometrial tissue is distributed from the uterus to other parts of the body through the lymph system or the blood system. A genetic theory suggests that it may be carried in the genes of certain families or that certain families may have factors predisposing them to endometriosis.

Another theory suggests that remnants of tissue from when the woman was an embryo may later develop into endometriosis or that some adult tissues retain the ability they had in the embryo stage to transform into reproductive tissue under certain circumstances. Surgical transplantation has also been cited as a cause in cases where endometriosis is found in abdominal surgery scars, although it has also been found in such scars when direct accidental implantation seems unlikely. Other theories are being developed by the association and others researching endometriosis.

Diagnosis

Diagnosis of endometriosis is generally considered uncertain until proven by laparoscopy. Laparoscopy is a minor surgical procedure done under anesthesia in which the patient's abdomen is distended with carbon dioxide gas to make the organs easier to see and a laparoscope (a tube with a light in it) is inserted into a tiny incision in the abdomen. By moving the laparoscope around the abdomen, the surgeon can check the condition of the abdominal organs and see the endometrial implants if care and thoroughness are used.

A doctor can often feel the endometrial implants upon palpation (pelvic examination by the doctor's hands), and symptoms will often indicate endometriosis, but medical textbooks indicate it is not good practice to treat this disease without confirmation of the diagnosis. (Ovarian cancer, for instance, sometimes has the same symptoms as endometriosis.) A laparoscopy also indicates the locations, extent, and size of the growths and may help the doctor and patient make better-informed, long-range decisions about treatment and pregnancy.

Treatment

Treatment for endometriosis has varied over the years, but no sure cure has yet been found. Hysterectomy and removal of the ovaries has been considered a "definitive" cure, but association research has found such a high rate of continuation/recurrence that women need to be aware of steps they can take to protect themselves. (See Chapter 2.) Painkillers are usually prescribed for the pain of endometriosis. Treatment with hormones aims to stop ovulation for as long as possible and can sometimes force endometriosis into remission during the time of treatment and sometimes for months or years afterward. Hormonal treatments include oral contraceptives, progesterone drugs, a testosterone derivative (danazol), and GnRH agonists (gonadotropin-releasing hormone drugs). Side effects are a problem with all hormonal treatments for some women.

Because pregnancy often causes a temporary remission of symptoms and because it is believed that infertility is more likely the longer the disease is present, women with endometriosis are often advised not to postpone pregnancy. However, there are numerous problems with the "prescription" of pregnancy to treat endometriosis. The woman might not yet have made a decision about childbearing, certainly one of the most important decisions in life. She might not have critical elements in place to allow for childbearing and child rearing (partner, financial means, etc.). She may already be infertile.

Other factors may also make the pregnancy decision and experience harder. Women with endometriosis may have higher rates of ectopic pregnancy and miscarriage, and one study has found they have more difficult pregnancies and labors. Research also shows there are family links in endometriosis, increasing the risk of endometriosis and related health problems in the children of women with the disease.

Conservative surgery, either major or through the laparoscope, involving removal or destruction of the growths, is also done and can relieve symptoms and allow pregnancy to occur in some cases. As with other treatments, however, recurrences are common. Surgery through the laparoscope (called *operative laparoscopy*) is rapidly replacing major open abdominal surgery. In operative laparoscopy, surgery is carried out through the laparoscope using laser, electrosurgical equipment, or small surgical instruments. Radical surgery, involving hysterectomy and removal of all growths and the ovaries (to prevent further hormonal stimulation), becomes necessary in cases of long-standing, troublesome endometriosis.

Menopause also is believed to end the activity of mild or moderate endometriosis, although little research has been done in postmenopausal women. Even after radical surgery or menopause, however, a severe case of endometriosis can be reactivated by estrogen replacement therapy or continued hormone production after menopause. Some authorities suggest no replacement hormone be given for a short time after hysterectomy and removal of the ovaries for endometriosis.

A wide range of alternative treatments including nutritional approaches, traditional Chinese medicine, allergy management techniques, and others are being used by some women with endometriosis with varying degrees of success.

Learning About Endometriosis

Endometriosis is without question one of the most puzzling conditions that affect women. More is being learned about it as time goes on, and this knowledge is dispelling some of the assumptions of the past that now have been disproven or are suspect. One of these past assumptions was that nonwhite women did not generally get endometriosis. This has now been shown to be untrue—often nonwhite women in the past were not getting the kind of medical care to have endometriosis diagnosed.

Another myth about endometriosis was that very young women did not get it—an idea that probably arose because formerly teenagers and younger women endured menstrual pain (often one of the early symptoms) in silence and did not get pelvic exams until the disease progressed to unbearable proportions. It was also believed in the past that endometriosis more often affected well-educated women. Now we know that this notion developed because well-educated women were those getting the best medical care and were more often persistent enough to obtain explanations for their symptoms.

Another assumption that has at times been made about endometriosis is that it is not a serious disease because it is not a killer like cancer, for instance. However, anyone who has talked with many women with endometriosis about their actual experiences with the condition soon learns that while some women's lives are relatively unaffected by it, too many others have suffered severe pain and emotional stress, have been unable to work or carry on normal activities at times, and have experienced financial and relationship problems because of the disease. Perhaps someday soon we will understand this perplexing disease and be able to end all the myths, pain, and frustrations that sometimes go with it!

How the Endometriosis Association Can Help

The Endometriosis Association is a self-help organization of women with endometriosis and others interested in exchanging information about endometriosis, offering mutual support and help to those affected by endometriosis, educating the public and medical community about the disease, and promoting research related to endometriosis. Ending the feeling of being alone, sharing with others who understand what one is going through, counteracting the lack of information and misinformation about endometriosis, and learning from each other are ways those affected by the disease help each other.

The association is an international organization with headquarters in Milwaukee, Wisconsin (USA), members in numerous countries, and chapters and activities growing worldwide. Elected officers guide the association, with help and suggestions from an advisory board of medical professionals and others. The association was founded in Milwaukee in 1980 by Mary Lou Ballweg and Carolyn Keith and was the first group in the world dedicated to helping women with endometriosis.

The Support Program provides a wide range of services to help women and their families. These include support groups, formal and informal counseling/crisis call assistance, networking, and other help to aid the woman with endometriosis to best cope with her disease. At the local group level, meetings and activities are planned according to groups' wishes. Usually some meetings are planned to allow informal information sharing about endometriosis and support and help for problems arising from it. Other meetings offer speakers and presentations on the disease, self-help care, infertility, medical research, and so on. Group activities also may include fund-raising and outreach into the community to teach about endometriosis.

The Education Program provides a wide range of literature, books, videotapes, audiotapes, and other educational items to help individuals, the public, and the medical community learn about the disease. Members of the association receive a popular newsletter covering the latest treatment and research news as well as activities of the association. The association also provides ongoing help to the media and medical community to aid in the dissemination of accurate information about endometriosis.

As part of its Research Program, the association also conducts research on endometriosis, including a special program at Dartmouth Medical School and continuing work on the relationship between dioxin and endometriosis. The association also serves as a clearinghouse for information on endometriosis. Researchers interested in working with the association should write to the Research Review Panel, Endometriosis Association, at the headquarters office. Donations to help continue the work of the Endometriosis Association are very much needed and appreciated.

How You Can Get More Information

Join the association. A wide variety of informative, accurate, and highly acclaimed literature on endometriosis and related health problems, developed by the association, is available to members. Our popular book entitled *Overcoming Endometriosis* has been reprinted five times. It can be ordered from the association for $10.95 U.S./$13.65 Canada plus shipping and handling ($1.75 U.S./$2.50 Canada) or from your local bookstore. The association also has available educational videotapes, cassette tapes of speeches by leading experts on the disease, booklets, kits, and newsletters. For a free information packet including our *Materials to Help You* catalog, call or write to us.

If you are not diagnosed with endometriosis but wonder if you might have it, the *How Can I Tell If I Have Endometriosis?* kit is available. Contact the association for the kit.

To become a member, fill out the membership form at the back of the book and mail it with your dues to:

International Headquarters
Endometriosis Association
8585 N. 76th Place
Milwaukee, Wisconsin 53223-2600
1-800-992-3636 (North America)
Join Us Today! You'll Be Glad You Did.

This information is available as a brochure in quantity to gynecologists, hospitals, pharmacies, and women's clinics. Please specify whether you want the brochure in English, Spanish, French, Dutch, Chinese or Taiwanese, Japanese, German, Korean, Polish, Italian, Portuguese, Russian, or Arabic.

Joe with Endo

By Mary Lou Ballweg
Illustrated by Meri Lau

One of the most popular parts of our first book, *Overcoming Endometriosis*, was the cartoon series "Joe with Endo." Joe, a young man with endometriosis, seems to have helped thousands of people understand that endometriosis should be taken seriously. He helps show, with humor, that if a disease like endometriosis were affecting millions of young men rather than millions of young women, society would think of it differently. After all, if there were millions of Joes out there, young men whose dreams were in danger of being destroyed by a disease, whose ability to function sexually was at risk, whose fertility was at risk, whose ability to build a satisfying work life and carry out the normal activities of living was at risk, and who even would face the threat of castration, no one would dare say it was unimportant.

Joe seems to help men relate to the disease. Once, after a speech in Portland, Oregon, when I had shown the "Joe with Endo" series (in colored slide form and live voice-overs of the dialogue), a male physician came up to me to say how effective the cartoon series was. He said he'd always thought he was empathetic with his female patients but not until he saw

In Overcoming Endometriosis, *we met Joe, a young man whose dreams were shattered by a mysterious disease called endometriosis. Joe went through a lot of frustrating experiences not unlike that of millions of women with endometriosis.*

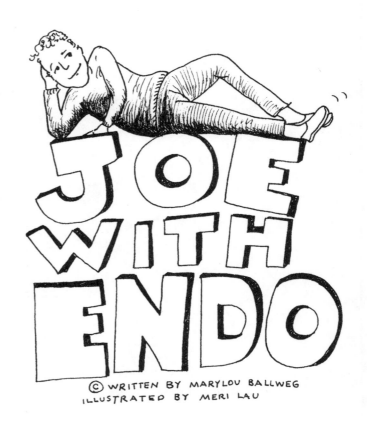

© WRITTEN BY MARYLOU BALLWEG
ILLUSTRATED BY MERI LAU

"Joe with Endo" had he found himself squirming in his seat, really identifying with those with the disease for the first time.

Joe also helps with his black humor. He helps me leave audiences laughing at the end of what can sometimes be discouraging meetings (because we don't yet have the answers we need for this disease). Joe is particularly funny when I share the podium with a doctor who is willing to take the part of Joe. (Camran Nezhat, M.D., had the audience rolling in the aisles when he did the part for a San Francisco association chapter audience.)

Joe has also brought his important message to other parts of the world. In the summer of 1994, at the first public meeting of the Japan Endometriosis Association in Osaka, I was pleased to find that Joe was able to transcend language and cultural differences with his message (with the skillful translation help of Sumie Uno). The Japan Endometriosis Association also printed "Joe with Endo" in its newsletter—what a treat to see Joe speaking Japanese!

We're thrilled that the very talented artist and teacher Meri Lau has again drawn Joe as only she can. We especially appreciate her efforts this time, since she'd just given birth to her son, Sam, at deadline time. Thank you, Meri!

We hope you enjoy Joe while recognizing the real tragedy behind him. That is that everything that happens to Joe is based on the actual experiences of thousands of women with endometriosis. Let's change that!

■ *Meri Lau is an art teacher for the Madison, Wisconsin, Metropolitan School District at the elementary level, taught art in the Milwaukee Public Schools for seven years, earned a master's of science in art education at the University of Wisconsin–Milwaukee, and continues to advocate for the inclusion of children with severe disabilities in art. She and her husband recently celebrated the birth of their son.*

Joe is a typical young man in his twenties. He has all the realistic dreams of a young man— the perfect life, perfect wife, perfect job, perfect house, perfect family, perfect body. There's just one problem. . . .

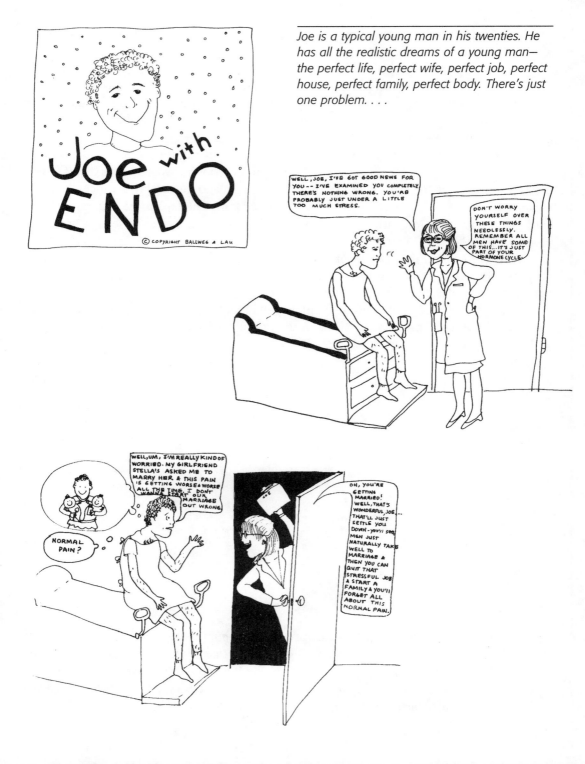

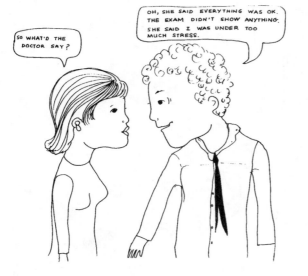

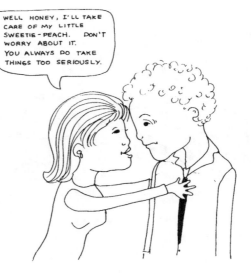

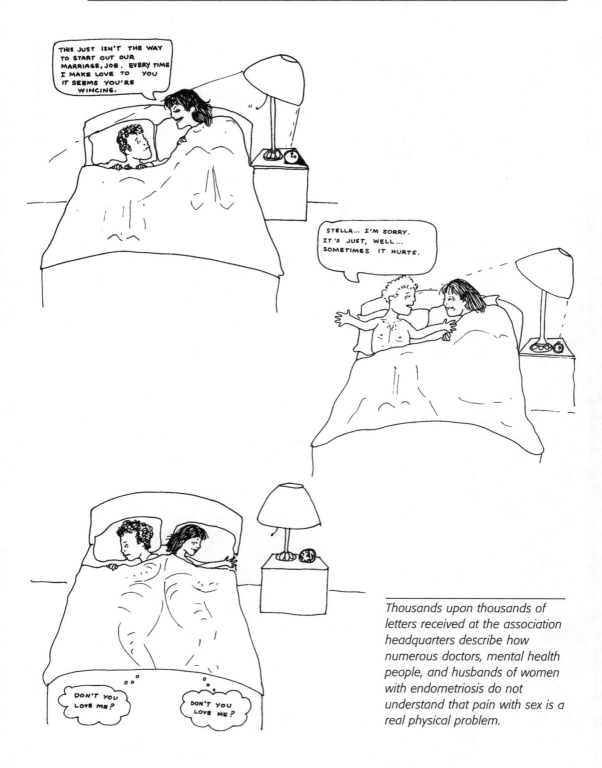

Thousands upon thousands of letters received at the association headquarters describe how numerous doctors, mental health people, and husbands of women with endometriosis do not understand that pain with sex is a real physical problem.

Note: When we conducted our first analysis of 365 case histories of women with endometriosis, we were horrified to find a percentage of the women had been given tranquilizers for symptoms and told it would take care of their problems!

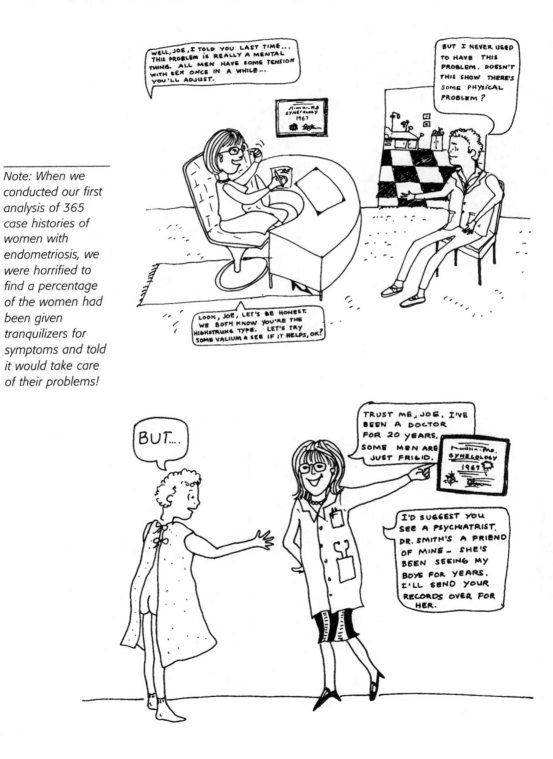

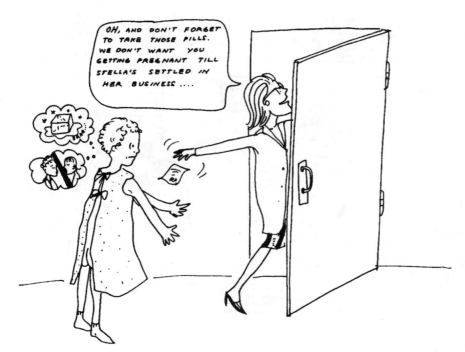

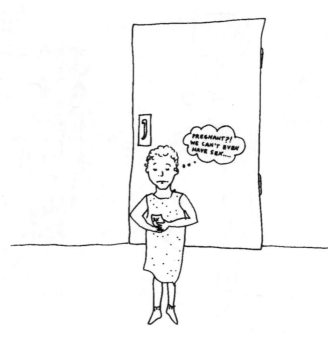

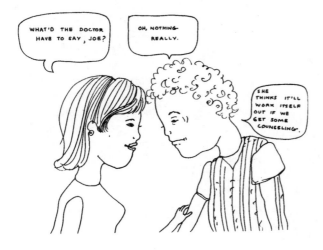

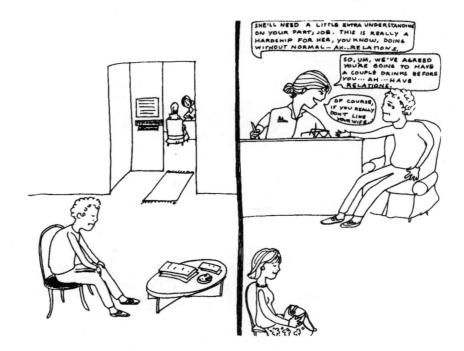

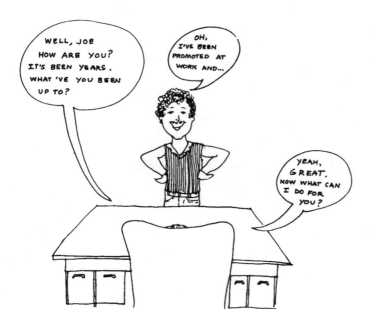

A couple of years later. Joe's health, on the birth control pills, has improved tremendously. He's been promoted at work and his former pain with sex and the problems between Stella and him because of it have been alleviated.

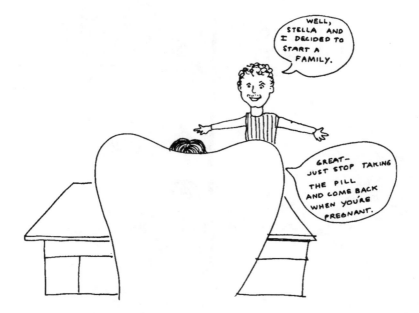

A year later . . .

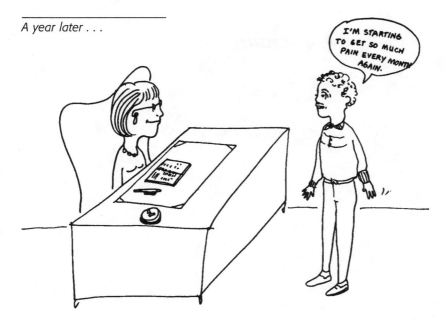

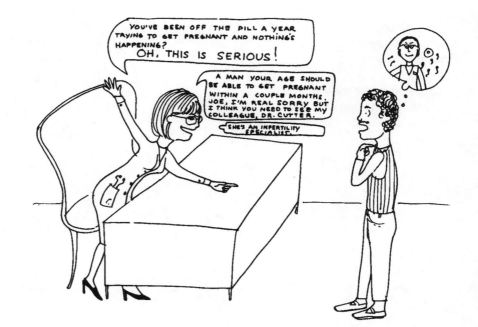

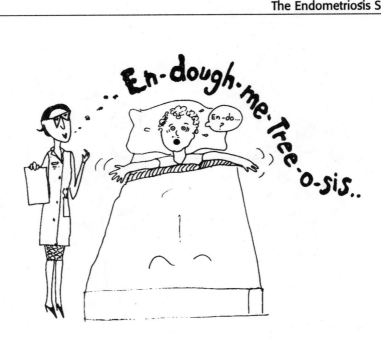

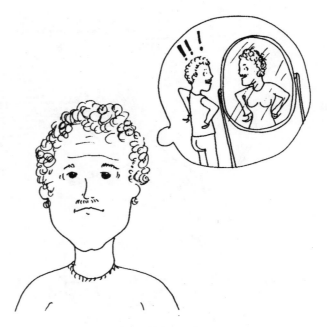

Joe is put on a female hormone to treat the disease. He is told "the side effects are well tolerated by most patients." But privately, he agonizes over his development of breasts.

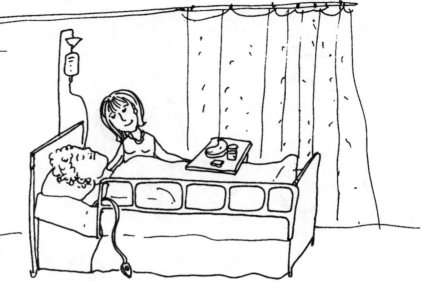

Fortunately, the breasts Joe developed as a side effect of the female hormone go away after the drug is stopped. But by then the disease is back. Major abdominal surgery is the next step.

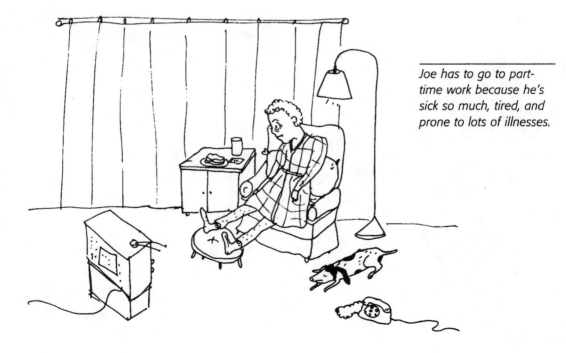

Joe has to go to part-time work because he's sick so much, tired, and prone to lots of illnesses.

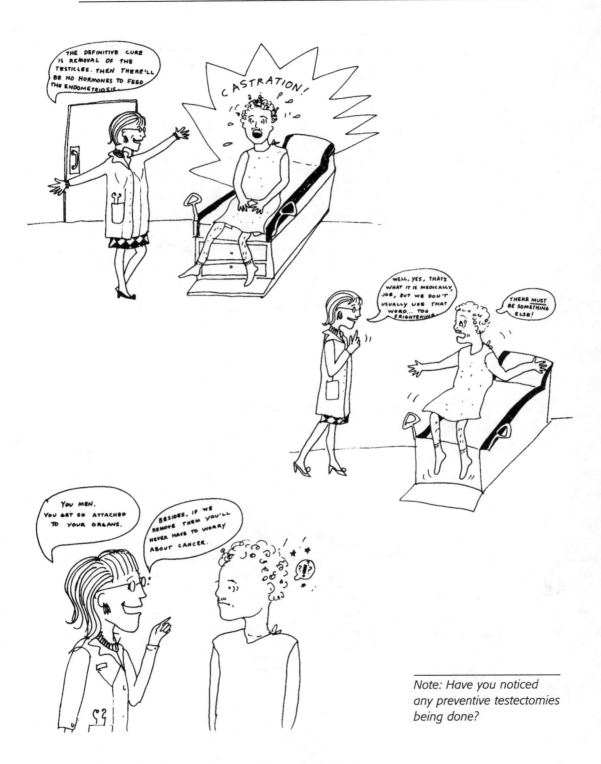

Note: Have you noticed any preventive testectomies being done?

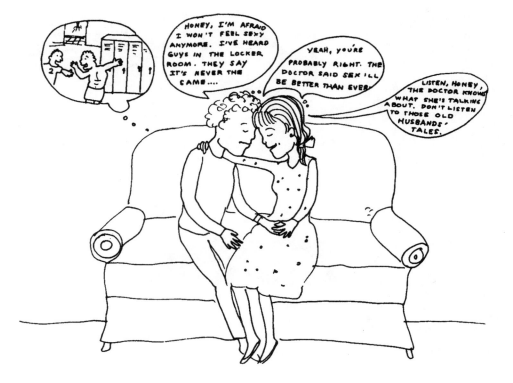

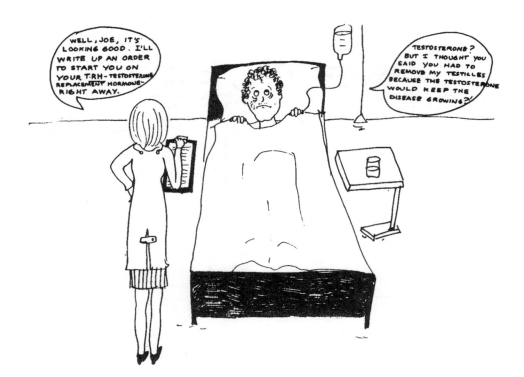

Note: The most tragic stories heard by the association are those of women who've gone all the way to the end of the road to hysterectomy and removal of the ovaries but still have endometriosis! It defies reason to remove the ovaries one day in order to remove the hormonal stimulation of stray endometrial tissue and then give the woman hormones the next day. A better approach is waiting three to nine months to give stray endometrial tissue a chance to die out and then go on hormone replacement.

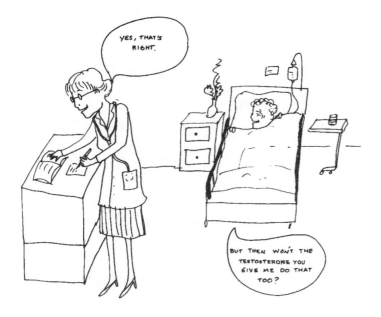

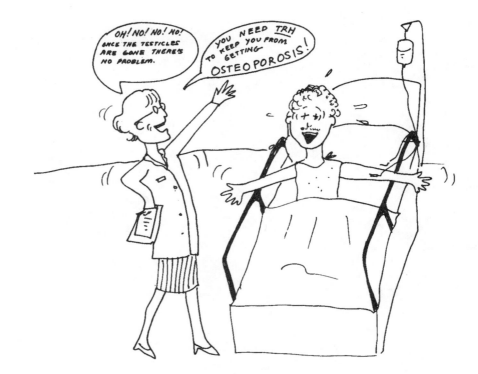

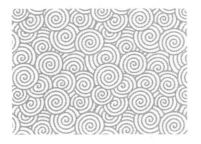

PART II

∞

Treatments for a Puzzling Disease

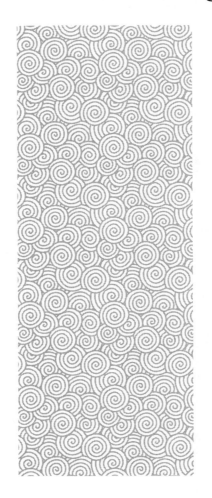

1

❧❧

Endometriosis and Pain

By Barbara Mains

"*Like menstrual cramps but much worse. Very intense pain.*"

"*A burning sensation, just below the pubic hairline, on the right side. Hot, prickling—as if my ovary was sitting in a bed of thistles. It was there all month long but worse around ovulation. During ovulation I sometimes thought I would go out of my mind.*"

"*. . . In several different places, but the worst was my low back, which became extremely sensitive to pressure of any kind. I couldn't find a comfortable position to sit down for more than a few minutes at a time, which made driving to work a real challenge! I couldn't sleep lying on my back. . . . It got so that we stopped making love because the back pain would last for days afterward. They told us to try different positions, and we did, but it didn't make much difference. When you're still on painkillers three days later, you have to ask yourself whether it's worth it.*"

"*Knifelike pain, right through the rectum, without warning. One moment I'd be standing in line for a movie, talking with a friend, and then I'd be doubled over, trying not to black out. . . . The worst was telling people where the pain was. No one wants to hear about this symptom—believe me—and then they don't want to accept that it's related in some way to bad periods. I don't think there's anything harder than having to live with a symptom nobody is even willing to hear about.*"

"*Indescribable. . . . It affected every decision I made all day, every day. It affected my ability to love other people and eventually to love myself. . . . When you're in pain for a long time, your imagination shrivels up, and it gets harder and harder even to imagine your life without the pain.*"

"My doctors wanted me to attend a three-week chronic pain clinic. I had the assumption they would give me a physical and then proceed to find a way to help my condition. Boy, was I wrong. I was never looked at. It dealt strictly with your mind. You had to try to pretend you didn't have any pain."

Introduction

Pain may be the most common symptom of endometriosis, but its significance as a symptom has not always been recognized; nor is pain the symptom that leads most readily to diagnosis. For many women with endometriosis the struggle to be heard and to have their pain accepted as real has been almost as damaging as the disease itself. Despite hard-won advances in our understanding of this disease, myths about endometriosis and pain persist today and continue to delay diagnosis and obstruct management of the disease. The association's daily mail tells the story: many women with endometriosis-associated pain are still fighting an uphill battle to be believed, to get diagnosed promptly, and to find effective help. "I'm not a lawyer," one member wrote, "but sometimes when I'm preparing for a consultation with my doctor I feel as if I were presenting a case in court."

Perhaps we can take heart from recent victories in related fields. Research into the cause of menstrual cramps, for instance, has already brought about significant changes in attitude toward painful menstruation. For centuries women as well as doctors mistakenly believed that painful menstruation, like painful childbirth, was the price some women paid for being female—an unhappy fact of life, inevitable, and too routine to justify serious investigation. Recognition of menstrual pain was further delayed by the taboos commonly attached to menstruation itself, in some cultures an inherently shameful event. At their worst these attitudes taught women to blame themselves for menstrual pain. But when research uncovered the biochemical basis for that pain—and the role of prostaglandins (see Glossary) in uterine contractions was established—many physicians changed their tune. Menstrual cramps were real, because science had produced an explanation. Moreover, menstrual cramps could be treated. New medications came onto the market (the prostaglandin synthetase inhibitors, also called the NSAIDs—nonsteroidal anti-inflammatory drugs), and life was changed for millions of women.

The moral: symptoms are real once they've been explained. Attitudes change when the basic research gets done.

Endometriosis-associated pain frequently includes menstrual cramps, as well as pelvic pain or low-back pain that worsens with menstruation, among a long list of pain symptoms that may also occur at other times of the month and in a range of locations. Because the basic research on endometriosis hasn't been done yet, mechanisms to explain the different kinds of pain are sketchy at best. As the fog clears and a more detailed picture of the disease emerges, social and medical attitudes toward the pain associated with endometriosis are destined to improve.

In the meantime, the following definition of pain is worth remembering:

"Pain . . . is present when the person who is experiencing it says it is."[1]

Research Recap: Endometriosis and Pain

When researchers describe endometriosis as "puzzling," they're often referring to the paradox of pain. Pain may be the hardest part of the puzzle to solve: the lack of a consistent fit between the symptoms and the amount of disease (as defined by current classification systems). Several studies have now established what women and doctors have long observed: the pain associated with endometriosis does not always correlate with the quantity or stage of disease.

In 1990 an Italian research team led by Luigi Fedele[2] found no relation between pain symptoms and the revised American Fertility Society stage of disease. The Milan-based group was among several groups of investigators unable to find a relationship between pain symptoms and stage or location of disease. But in 1992 Fedele's group published contradictory findings from a new study[3] of infertile women with endometriosis: in this sample the severity of pelvic pain and painful periods did correlate with the extent of disease. Further research—and development of a new classification system—will be necessary to resolve this contradiction.

Paolo Vercellini and colleagues looked closely at different types of lesions, separating women who had only typical (black) lesions from women who had only atypical lesions (any other color); women who had both typical and atypical lesions were put in a third group. In this study,[4] the women who had only typical lesions were more likely to suffer dyspareunia (painful sex), but no relationship was found between type of lesion and any other pain symptom, including painful periods and chronic pelvic pain. In an effort to explain the different kinds of pain associated with endometriosis, the authors wondered aloud whether "fresh, papillar atypical lesions exposed to peritoneal fluid" might provoke different kinds of pain than "old, black nodules immersed in infiltrating scars." (Although important in pain theory, this distinction may not apply to individual women, in whom both kinds of lesions might be found at one time.)

A paper published in the same year by association advisor Dan Martin and B. Ripps[5] reported that the appearance of the lesion did not correlate with focal tenderness (discomfort or pain felt at a specific site) when pressure is applied to that site. Interestingly, the same team found that depth of infiltration (how deeply the lesion invades the tissues of the pelvis) did correlate with focal tenderness.

Several other researchers have found depth of disease to be important. Belgian researcher Freddy Cornillie and co-workers found deeply infiltrating endometriosis (penetrating more than five millimeters) to be strongly related to pelvic pain.[6] In a related prospective study,[7] Philippe Koninckx found depth of infiltration to be the single most important factor in pelvic pain.

Association advisor David Olive summarizes these findings: "It seems that the anatomic location and the depth of penetration of endometriosis lesions are the critical factors in determining pain—that is, very superficial lesions tend not to produce much pain unless they are in a crucial anatomic location. Deep, penetrating lesions seem to produce a lot of pain almost no matter where they are located, but if they are at a crucial location, the result can be excruciating pain."[8]

As readers will appreciate, these are important findings for surgeons—and for women with endometriosis who choose surgery to relieve pain. Dr. Olive continues: "Running a laser beam or electrical current over the top of the lesions isn't the way to go, as far as we know, because the depth of the lesions does seem to be a factor in causing pain. Surgical treatment requires excision or destruction of the lesion to its full depth."

Deeply infiltrating disease seems to be found more often in certain parts of the pelvis, particularly the cul-de-sac, the uterosacral ligaments, and the uterovesical fold (between the uterus and the bladder). Some forms of deeply infiltrating disease may be more palpable (felt by touch) than visible, and these may be missed easily at laparoscopy. Endometrial lesions in the rectovaginal septum (the membrane separating the vagina and the rectum) may be very difficult to locate through the laparoscope and can perhaps be palpated only during menstruation.

(It's worth noting that depth of disease is not a major factor in any of the current classification systems, which stage endometriosis by adding up the total number of lesions and adhesions. The classification system in common use—the revised American Society for Reproductive Medicine system—was an attempt to predict pregnancy rather than pain relief or recurrence and remains weighted toward ovarian disease. The society, formerly called the American Fertility Society, has put together an international committee to design a new classification system. One recent paper[9] out of Brussels proposes that depth of disease, color, and metabolic status of the lesions and pain should all be taken into account. As a first step the society is now testing evaluation forms[10] that will match up pain symptom information with operative descriptions of the disease.)

How does endometriosis cause pain? Probably by both chemical and mechanical interference with pain receptors (nerve endings) in the pelvis:

1. The disease may compress or stretch pain receptors (especially during periods when the tissues expand rapidly, such as menstruation or pelvic congestion).
2. Endometrial cells have been shown to release inflammatory chemicals, including prostaglandins and histamine (substances that irritate pain receptors). When it ruptures, an endometrial cyst also releases these irritating substances.

3. Endometriosis may act on pain receptors to make them more sensitive in two ways:
   - The prostaglandins (and other inflammatory substances) appear to lower the receptor threshold, making the receptors more sensitive to repeated stimulation.
   - Fibrosis (scarring) can block or restrict access to blood vessels and deprive receptors of oxygen. The same scar tissue also traps aggravating metabolic waste products nearby.
4. Endometriosis may cause pain when it invades tissues or organs, including the urinary or gastrointestinal tracts.

Endometrial lesions obviously play an important role in endometriosis-associated pain. Could there be other causes? This provocative question pushes at the very limits of our knowledge about the disease process. Lesions are visible disease, but what we now call the absence of endometriosis may turn out to be the presence of microscopic disease.

Could microscopic endometriosis cause pain? It's important to remember that other kinds of pain can exist without cellular evidence. One cannot say that just because a brain tumor can be shown on a brain scan and a tension headache cannot, the person with the brain tumor has pain and the person with the tension headache does not have pain. Pain reaches the brain via multiple pathways, some of which have been charted only recently. Are there others? Could a high level of inflammatory activity in the pelvis send pain signals along these pathways, even before visible lesions have been documented?

Unanswered questions about the cause(s) of endometriosis lie underneath the many questions about pain. Perhaps the investigations of immune and toxic mechanisms, now under way, will point to new answers.

Notes

1. *Miller-Keane Encyclopedia & Dictionary of Medicine, Nursing & Allied Health*, 5th ed. (Philadelphia: W. B. Saunders Company, 1992).
2. L. Fedele et al., "Stage and Localization of Pelvic Endometriosis and Pain," *Fertility and Sterility* 53 (1990): 155.
3. L. Fedele et al., "Pain Symptoms Associated with Endometriosis," *Obstetrics and Gynecology* 79 (1992): 767–69.
4. P. Vercellini et al., "Peritoneal Endometriosis. Morphologic Appearance in Women with Chronic Pelvic Pain," *Journal of Reproductive Medicine* 36 (1991): 533–36.
5. B. A. Ripps and D. C. Martin, "Focal Pelvic Tenderness, Pelvic Pain, and Dysmenorrhea in Endometriosis," *Journal of Reproductive Medicine* 36 (1991): 470–72.
6. F. Cornillie et al., "Deeply Infiltrating Endometriosis: Histology and Clinical Significance," *Fertility and Sterility* 53 (1990): 978–83.
7. P. R. Koninckx et al., "Suggestive Evidence That Pelvic Endometriosis Is a Progressive Disease, Whereas Deeply Infiltrating Endometriosis Is Associated with Pelvic Pain," *Fertility and Sterility* 55 (1991): 759–65.

8. J. M. Still, "Endometriosis—Etiology and Treatment: State of the Art, Status of the Research," *Today's Woman* (February 1993):10–14.

9. I. Brosens et al., "Improving the Classification of Endometriosis," *Human Reproduction* 8, no. 11 (1993): 1972–75.

10. The American Fertility Society, "Management of Endometriosis in the Presence of Pelvic Pain," *Fertility and Sterility* 60 (1993): 952–55.

■ *Barbara Mains, Toronto, Ontario, former director of Canadian projects, has worked for the association for several years on Canadian and education program projects. Previously she served as recording secretary on the association's board and as one of the organizers of an association support group in Toronto.*

Barbara recently chaired the pain subcommittee of the Society of Obstetricians and Gynaecologists of Canada (SOGC) consensus conference on endometriosis. This working group of 17 formed in 1992 when the SOGC put together a national committee of physicians (plus Barbara) to develop guidelines for managing endometriosis. This article is the result of our request that Barbara share pertinent new information on endometriosis and pain with our readers, based on the in-depth review carried out by her pain subcommittee.

Common Questions About Endometriosis and Pain

By Barbara Mains

Pain presents researchers with a great number of questions, for which current knowledge can suggest only tentative answers. The questions that follow are among those the association is asked frequently:

Q: Why do some women with tiny amounts of disease have severe pain, while other women with extensive disease report no pain at all?
A: Nobody knows. (To complicate the issue, some women with extensive lesions do suffer severe pain.) Some ideas? The absence of pain in some women with extensive disease may indicate that most of their lesions are biochemically inactive, less likely to release the inflammatory substances that can cause pain. The classic black powder-burn lesions traditionally associated with endometriosis and often described as old or burned-out disease have been shown to secrete less prostaglandin than lesions of other colors. The most active lesions are thought to be the petechial (tiny reddish) lesions, which some researchers are calling early disease. But lesions of several different colors have been found at the same time in some women.

The problem could well be our definition of the disease as lesions of endometrial tissue and our assumption that symptoms are necessarily dictated by these lesions. It's important to remember that we don't yet know the natural history of endometriosis and whether the disease follows different time lines in different women.

Q: Why do some women still have pain after "all disease has been removed"?
A: Implants may not be the only cause of pain. This means that the answer to this question will have to be multiple choice—one or more of the following may be true in some women:
1. All disease was not removed.
2. All visible disease was removed, but microscopic disease remains.
3. All visible disease was removed, but retroperitoneal disease remains (underneath the surface), very difficult to see and sometimes difficult for the surgeon to palpate.
4. All visible disease was removed, but adhesions remain. Adhesions may also have formed after the surgery. (See "Adhesions and Endometriosis: The Puzzle Continues" at the end of Chapter 2.)
5. Even after all visible disease and adhesions have been removed, endometriosis may cause pain in other ways, by mechanisms that have yet to be established. Dysregulation of the immune system may make pain receptors more sensitive or interfere with the coding of pain signals.

Q: Why does the pain sometimes spontaneously go away?

A: This is another of the mysteries that surround endometriosis-associated pain and remind us how little we know about the disease process. Several members have written to report improvement in their pain symptoms not associated with surgical or medical or alternative treatment: "I just got better, without doing anything." Perhaps the lesions are still present in these women but for some reason are now less metabolically active. Perhaps the human body can in some cases regulate an underlying dysfunction so that the disease process slips into low gear. Although some women enjoy lasting health, many report that symptoms associated with endometriosis eventually return.

Q: Why does hysterectomy sometimes cure the pain, sometimes not?

A: Pain relief after hysterectomy may depend on the location of the disease as well as the nature of the pain. When the pain is limited to menstruation, hysterectomy will often—but not always—be effective. (Although they no longer menstruate, some women whose uterus has been removed—but who still have their ovaries—report that low-back pain and other kinds of pelvic pain return during what would have been the menstrual phase of their cycles.)

Those women in whom the uterus was removed while disease was still present in the pelvis seem more likely to suffer persistent pain. A nodule in the cul-de-sac, for instance, will probably continue to cause pain with sexual activity or bowel movements, whether or not the uterus is removed.

In some cases relief from pain may be due to other factors, not absence of the uterus. During hysterectomy several dense nerve bundles in the pelvis may be severed or damaged as the uterus is removed. Transmission of pain signals may be interrupted or weakened, providing substantial relief to some women.

The coding of pain signals is often disturbed after trauma, especially amputation. Phantom-limb pain (the perception among amputees that the amputated limb is still attached) probably occurs when the brain interprets these distorted signals as evidence of the limb's continuing presence. In some women with extensive or long-standing disease—especially disease embedded within scar tissue—these well-established pain signals may continue to travel to the brain after the uterus and/or the ovaries have been removed.

Complex issues are involved in making a decision for or against hysterectomy for endometriosis. For a full discussion of these issues, the problem of recurrence after hysterectomy, and the role of the ovaries and estrogen replacement therapy, see the articles on hysterectomy in Chapter 2.

Q: How can I get the doctor to believe I'm in extreme pain?

A: "Let a sufferer even try to describe pain . . . to a doctor," wrote British author Samuel Johnson, "and the language runs dry." Words often seem inadequate to describe the pain of endometriosis, but try to be as precise as possible. The doctor will want to know

  1. the character of the pain (sharp, dull, burning, aching)

2. the location
3. when it began and how long it lasts
4. what makes it better and what makes it worse
5. accompanying symptoms, including headaches, dizziness, nausea or vomiting, heavy blood flow, diarrhea, or constipation

It's important to see the doctor while your symptoms are happening rather than 10 days later. You may find it worthwhile to keep a diary of your symptoms, since many women with endometriosis find that a pattern emerges or that an established pattern has begun to change. If you're using painkillers, be sure to record the quantity used as well as the effects of the pain on your life (time lost from school, work, family life, or social activities). The pelvic pain map designed by association advisor Arnold Kresch, M.D. (and included in Chapter 2), makes it easier to document the location of pain symptoms.

As a last resort, change doctors. If the doctor dismisses your symptoms or isn't willing to work with you to reduce the level of pain, you've got the wrong doctor. Remember, you are entitled to competent, compassionate care, whatever the cause of your symptoms. (If there's a support group that meets in your area, ask women about their experiences with their physicians. You may also want to ask the association for a contact list for your area: you'll be sent the names of members who live near you and who have indicated willingness to share their experiences with other women. Also see Chapter 11, "Building the Doctor-Patient Relationship.")

Q: What do I do when doctors won't give me painkillers?
A: Schedule an appointment with the doctor to discuss pain control. In some cases it may help to take a supportive partner or friend with you for moral support (and to bolster your statements with a few of his or her own about the impact of the pain on your life). Explain that the pain relief is not adequate and briefly outline the effects of the pain on your work life and personal relationships. Be honest and straightforward about your use of painkillers; you and your doctor need to work together for effective pain control while minimizing the risks to you.

No progress after this discussion? It may be time to make a change (see previous answer). You may also want to consult a pain management specialist.

Q: What do I do when I'm in terrible pain? Should I go to the emergency room?
A: The emergency room is probably not your best option for pain management, except in rare circumstances. Emergency staff do not usually have sufficient training to manage endometriosis, and they will nearly always refer you back to your own doctor or to the nearest gynecology clinic. You'll probably be put through a long battery of tests to rule out other conditions, and you may not always be handled sensitively.

Remember that unless you show up with a life-threatening symptom, emergency surgery is usually not in your best interest. Endometriosis surgery requires a skilled gynecologic surgeon, trained to recognize the many appearances of endometriosis and experienced in removing disease in the least invasive manner. Such a surgeon is unlikely to be on duty the night you show up in emergency, and operating conditions are usually not ideal in this environment.

If you show up with severe pain, the emergency room may or may not be willing to provide you with narcotics (morphine, meperidine, etc.). Individual doctors tend to interpret the guidelines for administering narcotics differently, and emergency room physicians tend to be on "high alert" for narcotics abuse. This is why your best route to emergency pain relief is through your own physician, who knows you and knows your history.

If you absolutely have to go to the emergency room, try to reach your doctor first: your gynecologist or your family doctor, whoever is helping you with pain management. (If you can't get through, leave a message with the paging service.) Ask your doctor to phone the emergency room and give the attending physician some background on your case. ("Louise is one of my patients. I diagnosed her with stage III endometriosis a year ago, when she had a lot of problems with rupturing endometrial cysts. She's scheduled for surgery again next month, but she's coming into emergency tonight because she's in acute pain.") That phone call will make all the difference to your reception—and save time for both you and the emergency team.

EXCEPTIONS: In rare circumstances endometriosis can be life-threatening. Intestinal and ureteral obstruction (blockage of the colon or ureters) and peritonitis following the rupture of ovarian cysts are serious events. Any of the following symptoms call for prompt medical assessment: dizziness, fainting, or loss of consciousness; hemorrhagic (very heavy) bleeding; sustained fever; inability to pass urine; protracted vomiting.

Acute pelvic pain may also be a symptom of pelvic inflammatory disease, appendicitis, ectopic pregnancy, colitis, or enteritis, among other conditions. It's perfectly possible—though not common—to have one of these conditions and endometriosis at the same time. When in doubt, call your doctor's office first.

Q: I'm in terrible pain, but my doctor says there's nothing left to try. Where do I go next?

A: Would you consider consulting a pain management specialist? Some members who have exhausted the treatment options for endometriosis obtain pain relief by working closely with these specialists. Testing might include thermography (mapping the body's surface temperature), spinogram (measures the involvement of spinal pathways), selected blind nerve blocks (injections to identify the nerves or nerve bundles involved in pain), provocation tests, and neurological assessments. These tests may give you more information about the causes of your pain and the pathways involved—information that may help you make decisions about surgery and medication.

A physician who specializes in pain management will be able to fine-tune your pain medication to give you better relief at lower doses or with fewer side effects. Many pain specialists are involved in research, which may give you the opportunity to try out new treatment modalities as they're being developed.

Pain management specialists tend to work at teaching hospitals, and most have long waiting lists. Referral from a doctor is usually necessary.

Q: How do I find a pain clinic?

A: Your doctor, your doctor's office, and the hospitals in your area are primary information sources; local medical societies may also provide this information. In some cities pain clinics are listed in the yellow pages. The National Chronic Pain Outreach Association (see "Additional Resources") maintains listings for pain clinics in both Canada and the United States.

Pain clinics are often, but not always, affiliated with hospitals or medical schools, and most will insist on doctor referral. It's important to know the clinic's mandate: diagnostic pain clinics will put you through an intensive work-up to identify the cause(s) of your pain; therapeutic pain clinics use a combination of medication, adjunctive treatments (biofeedback, physiotherapy, etc.), exercise programs, and group counseling to relieve pain, improve general health, and build coping skills. Most patients go to therapeutic pain clinics as a last resort, having exhausted the standard medical and surgical avenues.

Pain clinics treat many different kinds of chronic pain, including migraine and cluster headaches, sciatica, neuralgia, arthritis, and pain related to injuries. Clinic staff (neurologists, anesthesiologists, internists, physical therapists, dentists, surgeons, and psychologists, among others) may or may not be up to date on the many complexities of endometriosis-associated pain.

Certainly reports from members who have tried pain clinics are more negative than positive. The multidisciplinary approach advertised by one reputable pain clinic "rapidly dwindled to a single option," wrote a member who consulted the clinic for disabling low-back and pelvic pain that worsened with menstruation. That treatment option turned out to be psychotherapy, which this member didn't find useful. It may be that without special training the cyclicity of the pain makes endometriosis-associated pain more challenging to treat. Nonetheless, some women may find pain clinics helpful.

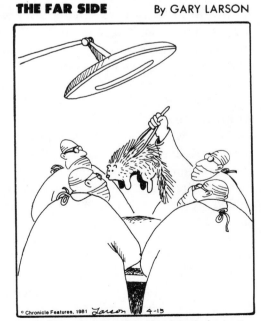

THE FAR SIDE   By GARY LARSON

"Well, I guess that explains the abdominal pains."

Pain Management

By Barbara Mains

Update on Pain Medications

Women with endometriosis often turn to pain medications for relief. For discussion of the advantages of, disadvantages of, and contraindications for the most commonly used painkillers—as well as side effects and important warnings—see Chapter 2, "Pain Medications for Endometriosis," in the association's first book, *Overcoming Endometriosis*. This update expands on the information in that chapter and covers medications/formulations that have entered the market since it was published.

Nonsteroidal Anti-Inflammatory Drugs (NSAIDs)

The nonsteroidal anti-inflammatories are used widely to relieve painful menstruation as well as the pain associated with endometriosis. Some drugs in this class can now be obtained over the counter: naproxen sodium (prescription names: Anaprox, Naprosyn; over the counter: Aleve) in the United States, and ibuprofen (available in many brands) in both the United States and Canada. The new kid on the NSAID block is ketorolac tromethamine (brand name: Toradol), available in both countries on a prescription basis.

As the NSAID family expands, more information emerges about its different members. NSAIDs don't all act in exactly the same way, and they aren't necessarily interchangeable. Some formulations (Ponstan/Ponstel, Toradol, Idorac) provide a high level of analgesia (pain relief) with relatively low anti-inflammatory activity. At the other end of the spectrum are NSAIDs like indomethacin, which provides a high level of anti-inflammatory activity with a lower level of analgesia. Ibuprofen, used by many women with endometriosis, falls somewhere in the middle of the range. The more anti-inflammatory activity, the greater the risk of gastrointestinal damage (ulcers, internal bleeding).

Not all women with endometriosis are able to tolerate the anti-inflammatories (stomach distress and dizziness are the side effects most commonly reported by members). But many women who can tolerate this family of medications obtain a high degree of pain relief. "A lifesaver," one member wrote to us of Ponstel. "This drug has totally turned around my ability to cope." Another member told us that she had reversed her decision to undergo a hysterectomy after taking Toradol.

Remember that NSAIDs work best if taken before pain is severe. If you're buying them over the counter, be sure to let your doctor(s) know you're using them, and to report any side effects. (If you're taking them frequently, you may want to run tests every six months for signs of blood in the gastrointestinal tract.)

Narcotics

Anti-inflammatories provide pain relief by interfering with the signals that run along the body's peripheral pathways. Opiates, such as morphine and codeine, and opioids, such as Demerol, act on the central nervous system (CNS) to slow down the pain traffic altogether. Although often effective in relieving severe pain, these drugs are frequently associated with CNS side effects such as drowsiness, as well as constipation. In high doses opiates may produce problematic side effects such as respiratory depression.

A current trend in the management of chronic pain is toward lower doses of opiate, boosted with a small dose of NSAID. Some combinations have a synergistic effect, so the patient gets better pain relief with less sedation. "Piggybacking" works only for certain combinations of drugs, however: put two NSAIDs together, and all you're adding is side effects. Because the choice of medications and their precise ratios are critical, it's important to work with an experienced physician to find the combination that works best for you while minimizing the risks. Experimentation, without the advice of a knowledgeable professional, is a recipe for disaster.

The combination of opiate with first-line analgesics isn't a new idea. Some association members will remember when "222s" were the painkiller of choice: a popular blend of aspirin, the first anti-inflammatory medication, with codeine. As more NSAID formulations have come onto the market, pain management specialists have broadened the mix to take advantage of these additional pathways to the brain. Some pain specialists are now prescribing low-dose narcotics with accompanying anti-inflammatories, with antihistamines, and in some cases with muscle relaxants. This approach is gaining popularity with pain specialists but has not yet been adopted by most primary care practitioners.

Among the newer opioid formulations is a nasal spray. Butorphanol (trade name: Stadol), a synthetically derived opioid, is now available in the United States by prescription. The drug is marketed for managing outpatient pain after surgical procedures and for migraines but might prove helpful for women with endometriosis-associated pain who cannot take other pain medications.

Topical Medications

Several members report success in controlling pain with over-the-counter topical liniments (creams or gels massaged into the skin). A traditional remedy for congestion, capsicum ointment, made from the pulverized seeds of hot peppers, is used by some practitioners to improve circulation and relieve pain. Applied directly to the pain site or to the trigger points used in acupuncture, capsicum and similar ointments (trade names: Zostrix, Capsagel) are believed to increase production of endorphins and enkephalins in local tissues. Some women with endometriosis get pain relief by applying the gel to trigger points on the inside ankle. Topical lidocaine (trade name: Emla) blocks pain signals by freezing the adjacent tissues: this dermal analgesic has been available without prescription since 1991.

How Women with Endometriosis Are Coping with Pain

Relief of pain is a compelling goal for many women with endometriosis—but it is not their only goal. Pain relief does not change the course of the disease. Until the natural history of the disease and its causes are known, women with endometriosis will continue to undergo hit-and-miss treatments that may or may not bring pain relief, which may or may not be lasting.

Perhaps the biggest challenge in educating the general public and the medical community about endometriosis has been the challenge of overcoming the myths about pelvic pain and teaching them to look at it for what it is. Pain is a symptom. Pain is a symptom of endometriosis, as pallor (paleness of the skin) is a symptom of anemia (a condition of reduced oxygen delivery to the blood or tissues of the body). In other words, the pain of endometriosis is not a penalty some women must pay for being female and having periods. The pain of endometriosis is not a punishment for delayed childbearing, for abortion, for using oral contraceptives, or for not using oral contraceptives. The pain of endometriosis is not some kind of test or trial through which we must pass to become better people. Pain is, pure and simple, a symptom of endometriosis.

Punitive attitudes toward pain aren't just floating around in society at large. They're inside all of us, internalized by the attitudes toward women's bodies that we absorbed as we grew up and that tend to emerge at times of crisis. If you notice that you're blaming yourself for pain, get support. Talk to other women in your support group or to members who live in your area. Talk to one of the association's crisis callers. Read the coping section of this book (Part III). Reread key materials that have helped you in the past (try the sections on dealing with the emotions in *Overcoming Endometriosis*).

Pain researchers now recognize that the experience of pain includes an emotional response, which might range from anxiety (usually accompanies acute pain) to reactive depression (common with chronic pain). Pain involves the limbic system of the brain, memorably described by poet Diane Ackerman as that "mysterious, ancient, and intensely emotional section of our brain in which we feel, lust, and invent." It is actually impossible to experience pain without having an emotional response to the pain, and everyone in pain has an emotional response. Our emotional response to pain may be one mechanism by which the human body ensures that we take it seriously, rather than ignoring it or accepting it as inevitable.

Chronic pain imposes heavy restrictions on us. "Pain is greedy, boorish, meanly debilitating," wrote Virginia Woolf. Remember to give yourself the same support you'd give to any other woman with endometriosis.

Be easy on yourself: you're coping as best you can.

He Suffers from Excruciating Discomfort

By Kevin Cowherd

EDITOR'S NOTE: Coping with pain is a challenge. Sometimes humor helps. For that reason we offer this humorous article about pain and the way some medical people talk about it.

A lesser man probably would be in the hospital now, instead of gritting his teeth and plugging away at the word processor and fighting off the pain.

I'm sorry . . . did I say pain? I meant discomfort. This is what my doctor says I'm experiencing now: discomfort.

Being unschooled in modern medical terminology, I originally had labeled the sore, throbbing, think-I'm-gonna-scream feeling as pain. But the good doctor who examined me referred to it repeatedly as discomfort, so discomfort it must be.

The discomfort began the other day, when a chunk of firewood the size of a filing cabinet dropped on my foot.

There was so much initial discomfort, in fact, that I began jumping up and down very rapidly, in the manner of a piston thrusting in an engine.

The discomfort also caused me to scream all manner of nasty things that cannot be repeated here and that made the children run from the room.

In the interest of perhaps easing this discomfort, I called the doctor's office.

The phone was answered by an earnest young woman, who listened carefully as I explained (between wracking sobs) that a chunk of firewood the size of a toolshed had just dropped on my foot.

"Are you in any discomfort?" she asked.

"Now that you mention it," I said, "I am experiencing some discomfort. The room is starting to spin . . . feel a strange sense of warmth and . . ."

The earnest young woman urged me to make my way to the doctor's office as soon as possible.

After the obligatory 40 minutes spent in the waiting room—try thumbing through *People* magazine and concentrating on this Milli Vanilli lip-sync business while your foot balloons to the size of a pumpkin—I was ushered into an examining room.

"Understand you're experiencing some discomfort," the doctor said.

"Why, yes," I said, collapsing into a heap and startling one of the nurses. "There seems to be some discomfort in the general area of these two toes, the ones that have turned black."

"Yes, that would cause some discomfort," he said.

I said: "Well, it certainly . . . uh-oh, room starting to spin again . . . eerie twilight . . . can't wait for *Godfather III* to open . . . understand Pacino turns in a performance that . . ."

It's funny, but as I lay there babbling and drifting in and out of consciousness, I thought of the word *discomfort* and how it has evolved in the lexicon.

I used to think discomfort was, oh, a small pebble in your shoe. Or perhaps a mild itch to one side of your shoulder blade that you couldn't quite reach.

But now I see that the term *discomfort* is more accurately applied to the feeling one experiences when a piece of wood the size of a baby sequoia drops on one's foot and causes one to run about the room in the highly agitated manner of someone who has just stepped into a bear trap.

By expanding the parameters of the term *discomfort*, we may also note that women in the throes of childbirth can be said to be experiencing "discomfort."

Oh, I know what you're thinking. You're thinking: "My God, look at that poor woman in labor over there, gripping the bed rails and thrashing about violently and screaming for someone to pull out a .45 and put her out of her misery."

"Mister, that ain't discomfort. That's 100 percent pure, unadulterated, industrial-strength pain."

Sorry, no. Not according to the medical profession. As I understand it, only if the woman were delivering a baby and simultaneously having her arm hacked off with a dull axe would she be experiencing "pain" in the modern-day sense.

Otherwise a woman in labor is simply feeling the typical discomfort that comes when an eight-pound, five-ounce baby makes its way down a narrow birth canal more suited for the transportation of a marble. In any event, there will be no more talk here of childbirth and those whiners who consider it discomforting, as I am now occupied with my own discomfort.

The sore foot is now wrapped in a light bandage, which seems to be doing absolutely no good. However, these tiny pills prescribed by the doctor are working fabulously and have me in a positively chipper mood. In fact, I thought I just saw Humphrey Bogart over by the window. Or maybe it was Napoleon.

As I left his office, the good doctor asked me to return in a couple of days to undergo a testing procedure that he didn't have time to fully explain.

"It might sting a little" is all he said.

Hmmm. Wonder what he meant by that?

■ *Article by **Kevin Cowherd**, reprinted with courtesy of* The Baltimore Sun. *Cowherd's article appeared in* The Baltimore Sun *in November 1991.*

The Stigma of Chronic Pain

By Catherine Avery

A church organist is asked to stay at her bench during the entire service despite chronic arthritis pain. The same church provides an interpreter for the deaf and wheelchair ramps for the disabled. It also allows a pregnant organist to move about the church freely to ease her back.

A woman with chronic back, hip, and leg pain is publicly upbraided by a stranger for parking in a handicapped spot even though she has handicapped plates on her car.

A male moviegoer, standing in the back of the theater to ease his aching back, is asked insistently to take his seat by the usher.

A pain patient's parents tell her to quit acting like a baby. "Where's the blood running out?" her mother asks her.

An anesthesiologist is suspected of angling for a disability when colleagues hear he is suffering from chronic neck pain due to a whiplash injury.

What do these scenarios have in common? They are all vivid, real-life examples of the stigma of chronic pain.

Stigma: A Fact of Life for Those with Chronic Pain

"It's easy to be paranoid when you hurt like hell and you're at the mercy of the health care system," says Dr. Bernard Filner, a Rockville, Maryland, pain management physician and chronic pain sufferer. He sustained a whiplash injury in a car accident 10 years ago and still experiences neck pain and headaches.

Stigma, defined by the *Random House Dictionary* as "a blemish on one's record or reputation," is a pervasive fact of life for people with chronic pain.

The most widespread misconception about chronic pain is that it results from a psychological disturbance. Other common misconceptions are that those with chronic pain should be able to tolerate pain better as time goes on, that they are using pain to obtain narcotics, and that they exaggerate their pain for secondary gains—that is, for sympathy or financial gain.

The impact of stigma on chronic pain sufferers is devastating. "Stigma is a magnifier of pain," says Roberto Anson, 41, of Silver Spring, Maryland. "It boils down to one word—discrimination."

Chronic pain often presents sufferers with a real catch-22 dilemma. If they talk about their pain, they risk being perceived and labeled as hypochondriacs or even worse—fakers or malingerers. On the other hand, if they hide their pain, others don't believe the pain is significant. It is enough to tax the patience of the most stoic person.

Health care professionals who see pain patients every day agree emphatically that stigma makes an already bad situation worse. Dr. Paul Buongiorno, a Fairfax, Virginia, psychiatrist who serves as medical director for northern Virginia's Fair Oaks Hospital's Pain Management Program, sees patients daily who suffer from guilt, demoralization, and depression due to the negative perceptions of others. "Others feel you should pull yourself up by your bootstraps," Buongiorno says. "I don't believe that, though. You can't just talk yourself out of it."

Dr. Richard Baither, a Fairfax, Virginia, psychologist who treats chronic pain patients, refers to the Job syndrome. "People remember Job's patience," Baither says. "They feel they must have sinned. They ask themselves, 'What did I do wrong for these bad things to happen?'"

Noreen Freedman, a nurse and the coordinator of the Pain Resource Center at Washington Adventist Hospital, in Takoma Park, Maryland, says that her patients report a real sense of frustration about the public's perception of chronic pain. "You look fine; you must feel wonderful," others say, according to Freedman. "Pain is something you wear on the inside, not on the outside," she notes. Freedman observes that men tend to emphasize the way chronic pain affects their work, while women tend to focus on the way it affects their relationships.

Stigma can be manifested in various ways—by raised eyebrows at work, by friends asking "Shouldn't you be feeling better by now?" and even by family members looking the other way or minimizing the problem.

Social biases are also apparent—theaters, restaurants, and the workplace are all designed for pain-free people, despite the staggering statistics that as many as one in three suffers from chronic pain.

In addition, very recent articles in the pain management literature demonstrate that negative stereotypes are alive and well even among professionals. Consider the following:

• A researcher who studied chronic back pain patients says his results support the theories of psychiatrist Thomas Szasz that chronic pain may become the "career" of patients who are "deeply committed" to the "sick role." The researcher concludes that medical treatment for such patients is ineffective since it "reinforces the pain patient role."[1]

• Another researcher concludes that receiving disability payments for work-related injuries sets in motion a "stimulus-response-reward cycle" that is hard to break. Receiving workers' compensation payments, he believes, is likely to mean that the patient will always have chronic pain. The same researcher warns that "pathologic dependency," whether on one's family, physicians, or drugs, is a "major obstacle to treatment" of chronic pain. He states that doctors who fail to recognize this "are destined to become entwined in the patient's dependency and become themselves an 'enabler' of the patient's problem."[2]

• Still another article reported on a survey of physicians' attitudes toward chronic pain patients. While most of the 103 doctors surveyed as a group did not show evidence of negative bias toward chronic pain patients, there were key differences among different medical specialty groups. For example, anesthesiologists tended to believe that malingering is common among pain patients.[3]

• A psychologist who specializes in hypnosis argues that the management of chronic pain is actually the management of anxiety. He refers to the "seductiveness of demanding and receiving help from significant others" and "the mildly pleasant and/or euphoric effects of medication" that render pain "eventually necessary." He also cites examples of patients who use headaches to avoid sex and playing with their children and back pain to avoid mowing the lawn. The same pain management expert describes a helpful technique to unmask those pain patients who are receiving secondary gains from their pain. He asks four simple questions, including, "Do you want to get better?" An angry response to this question indicates a poor prognosis, while a simple, submissive "yes" indicates a good prognosis.[4]

• Even recent medical research provides evidence of the stigma of chronic pain. The news media recently reported the development of a machine that determines whether patients are telling the truth about how much pain they have by recording how patients move and how much force they exert in various directions. Insurance companies are reportedly showing great interest in this new device.[5]

Indeed, people with easily visible proof of pain such as swollen joints, wheelchairs, canes, or neck braces often report this tangible evidence of pain offers them validation in the eyes of others. Pain sufferers emphasize that a major factor behind the stigma is the invisible nature of most chronic pain.

"You don't look like you're in pain," people tell Marty Heinrich, 39, of Damascus, Maryland. She asks them, "What does pain look like?" She has had chronic pain, originating with a broken back, since childhood.

Where Does Stigma Come From?

Stigma arises from external sources such as health care professionals, family and friends, the public at large, government agencies and insurance companies, and even other chronic pain sufferers. Stigma also can arise from within, with pain sufferers often experiencing guilt and blaming themselves for their pain.

Health care professionals often present formidable psychological obstacles to chronic pain patients. They want their treatments to produce results, and when this doesn't happen some blame the patient, believing that the patient hasn't followed instructions properly, is receiving secondary gains from being in pain, or is simply imagining the pain.

Marty Heinrich visited her doctor after her second back surgery, still suffering from chronic back pain. "There's nothing wrong with this fusion," the doctor told her. "It's a beautiful fusion. You need a psychiatrist." She says that health care professionals have asked her, "Why are you hanging on to your pain?" or "What's the payoff you're getting?"

Linda Lockaby, a Fort Meade, Maryland, musician, has suffered from a variety of pain symptoms for the past five years, including rheumatoid arthritis, a nerve disorder in her shoulder, and myofascial pain. She reports that a rheumatologist diagnosed her as depressed, citing her weight loss and frequent bladder infections. He wasn't able to fit her symptoms with his diagnosis of arthritis, so he advised her, "Just relax and see a psychiatrist."

Filner notes that patients tend to be sent from one doctor to another in search of relief. "It puts the burden on the patient," he says. Only once in several years of working with pain patients has Filner treated a true malingerer.

Even when doctors acknowledge that chronic pain is not rooted in psychological disturbances, Filner believes that they may focus too much on helping patients accept their pain and not enough on finding ways to alleviate it. He wishes doctors would spend at least as much time ruling out additional treatment possibilities as they do in telling patients they just have to learn to live with the pain. "Many treatment options are available today," he says, "and more will be available tomorrow. I won't stop looking for causes and new treatment approaches." He terms his practice a "court of last resort."

Most pain patients report that family members, especially spouses, feel a sense of frustration that they can't do more to alleviate the pain. Jill Gendleman, 39, of Bethesda, Maryland, has low back problems originating from scoliosis in her childhood, as well as almost daily headaches. Her husband of one year tries to help but feels frustrated that he can't make the pain go away.

Roberto Anson has an 8-year-old daughter and has learned how difficult it is to be a parent who has chronic pain. "It's a challenge because I can't do some things," he says. Heinrich, who has two sons, ages 9 and 15, faces the same challenges. "I tell the boys I can't play ball but I can play Monopoly," she says.

Heinrich finds that families often go to one extreme or the other—either gushing all over the pain sufferer or acting angry and rejecting. As a child she coped by hiding her pain, fearing that her family would reject her as defective and wouldn't love her if they knew the truth.

Lockaby says her mother refers to her daughter's chronic pain as "the little aches and pains of growing older." Lockaby is 34. Further, it has taken her some time to allow friendships back into her life. "People are afraid of us," Lockaby says, "because we look so normal. They're afraid they could be in the same position. They don't know how to act."

In the sixth grade Gendleman was out of school for six months following back surgery. When she went back to school, her classmates avoided her. "It changed my life," she says now. "I became more of a loner. It was devastating." She attributes her classmates' behavior to their fear of "catching it."

Gendleman says a friend from her old job called her recently and commented, "God, I envy your life," referring to the fact that Gendleman has not—because she cannot—worked full-time for the last two years. "Because many people can't relate to what life is like with chronic pain, my life just seems easier," she explains.

Freedman has seen evidence of job discrimination against workers with chronic pain. "The same problem again?" employers often ask pain patients. She notes that chronic pain cannot be validated objectively like heart disease or cancer, so it can be dismissed more easily by employers.

This can be particularly problematic during job hunts. Freedman's patients report that potential employers tend to zero in on long periods when the person has been out of work, which they interpret as a warning flag. The applicant is then told there is someone "more qualified" for the job.

Anson, who has had chronic low-back pain for the past two years as the result of a fall while rollerskating, is a management analyst for the federal government. "People you work with daily forget about your situation," he says. "Sometimes there are assignments that put your health at risk." Anson has a stand-up desk in his office that helps alleviate his pain.

Anson notes the other side of the coin. "Supervisors often make decisions based on their perceptions of what you can do," he says. They may decide that a person with chronic pain might not be up to a particular assignment without first checking that assumption with the individual.

In addition Anson observes that those with chronic pain can be seen as a distraction to others because they move around to increase comfort. "They think we have ants in our pants," he jokes. He often brings a cushion to meetings and arrives early to better adapt to the environment. In restaurants he looks for a spot near the wall where he can stand up unobtrusively.

Filner was a practicing anesthesiologist 10 years ago when his car was hit from the rear while stopped at a red light. It was particularly ironic to have spent his professional life blocking pain in others and then be unable to stop his own. He discovered that when he wore a neck collar after his accident others acted as if there really was something wrong with him. When the neck collar came off, he found out the hard way that no longer wearing tangible evidence of his pain changed the way he was perceived.

As Gendleman says, ours is a production-oriented society. She observes that people often think, If you can't produce, what good are you?

Nowhere is that attitude more obvious or more potentially damaging than when government and insurance agencies use it against pain patients. Psychologist Baither pointed out that insurance companies have learned tactics for not paying chronic pain patients. For example, when a person is injured at work, the insurance company may question whether the injury is really work-related and request a hearing before the state workers' compensation commission. This hearing often doesn't take place until six or nine months later. In the meantime, a person who is unable to work isn't receiving a paycheck and may be shouldering heavy medical bills.

Insurance companies often want people to *prove* that they've been injured on the job, says Baither. "They take an adversarial position—they're not interested in finding out what really happened. They string you out, and meanwhile you have no income and a bundle of medical bills. On top of that, a lot of times they'll pressure you for a settlement."

The perception among many in the government and insurance companies is Why would people go back to work when they're better off not working? However, patients get paid only a small portion of their salaries when they're disabled, Baither points out.

As Filner says, "You get only 30 to 50 percent of your salary on disability, and you spend all your time in doctors' offices and undergoing painful treatments. It totally affects your life. Why would anyone want to do that? It isn't something people want." In fact, recent studies have shown that secondary gains are not a factor in the behavior of the vast majority of pain patients.

Tips to Combat the Stigma of Chronic Pain: An Even Dozen

1. Look for health care professionals with training and experience in pain management. Remember that not all health care professionals are skilled in this field.
2. Join support groups so you can benefit from being with others who have chronic pain. Anson refers to the several hundred years of combined experience found in members of a typical support group. "Share with others and the burden lightens," he observes.
3. Communicate honestly about your pain with your family and friends. Heinrich advises other pain sufferers to strike a balance between talking too much about pain and being dishonest about it.
4. Educate others about the experience of chronic pain. "Be honest about what living with chronic pain is like," Gendleman says. "But try to get control over your emotions first because people have trouble absorbing information when it's loaded with emotion."
5. Accept whatever other pain sufferers are experiencing. "Practice acceptance of both yourself and others," Heinrich advises.
6. Don't reinforce negative stereotypes others might have. Also, don't make assumptions about what others are thinking and feeling about you. Instead, check them out to be sure your perceptions are correct, Baither suggests.
7. Treat yourself with respect! "You have to love and respect yourself before other people can," Lockaby says.
8. Demand respect from others. Challenge negative stereotypes.
9. Accept responsibility for coping with your pain. "You'll be a prisoner of your pain if you don't take charge of your own life," asserts Filner. You're not responsible for your pain—but you are responsible for what you do about it and how you live your life.
10. Give your doctors permission not to cure you, Heinrich advises. "I ask them just to help me be as comfortable and functional as I can be."
11. Resist the temptation to blame yourself for your pain. The question "Why me?" often doesn't have a good answer.
12. Develop a sense of humor, Heinrich advises. When all else fails, a humorous outlook can be your saving grace.

Filner feels the workers' compensation system and insurance plans seem to care more about saving money than getting people better. Insurance plans also tend to promote surgery, believing it to be a "quick fix." In reality surgery not only exposes the person to the risks of a surgical procedure but often ends up more expensive in the long run for everyone because it often makes pain problems much worse.

EDITOR'S NOTE: The author may be referring to the low success rate of surgery for back pain, as well as certain kinds of joint pain. Surgery for endometriosis, on the other hand, in many cases turns out to be the best route to pain relief.

Psychiatrist Buongiorno believes that the health care system has failed chronic pain patients. "Incentives in the system tend to make people with chronic pain worse, not better," he says. "The system is designed for acute care only and doesn't adequately address the needs of patients with ongoing health problems." This can be seen in insurance plans where surgery is covered but pain management programs are not.

Stigma against those with chronic pain also can lead to canceled life and health insurance policies, not to mention insurance applications that are turned down. Lockaby had her life insurance canceled due to her diagnosis of rheumatoid arthritis.

A recent article in the professional literature described the typical odyssey for an injured chronic pain patient beginning with the trek from doctor to doctor and culminating without relief for the patient and only a meager legal settlement. Somewhere along the way the patient gets labeled as a malingerer, which is underscored by the doctors who work for insurance companies. Finally, lawyers contribute to the problem by urging their clients to settle for small sums.

Filner points out that the "independent" medical exams required by insurance companies are anything but independent. Typically the exams last about 15 minutes and are conducted by doctors hired by the insurance company to evaluate patients. "It may be unethical because of conflict of interest," Filner says.

Filner believes that a truly independent examination would be aimed at arriving at a correct diagnosis and appropriate treatment plan rather than at invalidating the patient's complaint of pain.

An unexpected and especially devastating source of stigma can be fellow pain patients. Some people fall into the trap of competing with others over who has more pain, Heinrich says. People sometimes view others who have reached the state of acceptance of their pain as not being in much pain. On the other hand, those who have reached this stage sometimes look down on those still struggling with anger and grief.

Heinrich describes five stages that pain patients seem to experience: denial, anger, bargaining, grief, and acceptance. Those stages have been well documented as the ways in which people cope with loss and death. "You go through these stages when you lose your health," Heinrich asserts.

Sometimes pain patients themselves inadvertently reinforce negative stereotypes. Anson refers to someone he knows who won't look for employment because she has decided that no one would hire her. Such self-defeating attitudes only underscore the negative perception of others.

Reasons for Stigma

Stigma of any kind arises from a multiplicity of sources, both external and internal. A primary psychological underpinning of stigma is fear. When people perceive a threat, they frequently try to ward off their fear by denying that the threat exists. It is as if people say to themselves, "If it happened to you, maybe it could happen to me; therefore, it hasn't happened to you."

Gendleman notes that years ago people didn't talk much about cancer, referring to the disease as the "big C." "They wouldn't even say the word because of fear," she observes.

Another reason for the stigma of chronic pain stems from people inappropriately comparing the minor or short-lived pain they've experienced in their own lives with chronic pain. They reason, "When I hurt my back, I was back at work a few days later" or "I know what a bad headache is like." Heinrich says people often remind her that half the world has back trouble at some point in their lives—they treat her as if she is lazy or not trying hard enough. "If you were a stronger, better, or more courageous person, you'd get over it," she says, describing others' attitudes.

A third reason for the stigma comes from the faulty reasoning that chronic pain must stem from character weakness or psychiatric illness. Come on, nothing can hurt that bad—it must be in your head, the thinking goes. Gendleman remembers a chiropractor advising her to see a psychiatrist after he observed that she was depressed. "Of course I was depressed. Who wouldn't be depressed sometimes living with daily pain?"

"Doctors have treated me like a nut case," Heinrich agrees. "It's the most destructive thing." She firmly believes that in most cases pain leads to depression, not vice versa.

Filner points out that the accepted definition of chronic pain is pain that lasts for six months or more and is not amenable to medical treatment. This latter part of the definition—not amenable to medical treatment—assumes a psychological disturbance, Filner believes.

The stigma of chronic pain has other, more sociological roots in our culture. The attitudes we're all taught as we grow up—to keep a "stiff upper lip" and not show our emotions no matter how much pain and adversity we're faced with—are counterproductive.

Anson feels a particular stigma directed toward men. "In a mixed group, people turn to the men for muscle. One of the frustrations is that my pain is invisible. I walk in on my own; I look fine. They think, What's the problem?" Further, Anson notes, "Men are supposed to handle everything without showing their feelings. Men are not supposed to cry."

Ironically, recent much-publicized findings that positive imagery and visualization can improve health and reduce pain can inadvertently work against chronic pain sufferers and others with chronic medical problems. Sufferers themselves, as well as those around them, may wonder, erroneously, If imagery is capable of reducing pain, doesn't that mean the pain is all in my head in the first place? The logic behind these doubts is faulty since even terminal cancer pain can be eased by imagery and relaxation despite the fact that the pain is caused by malignancy.

Some Good News

Fortunately, chronic pain has been gaining increasing public attention and media visibility. There is reason to be optimistic that the stigma of chronic pain will decrease as the public learns more about chronic pain and recognizes the vast numbers of sufferers in their midst.

The professional literature, too, is showing signs of change in the right direction. A new nursing textbook on pain, for example, contains a thorough chapter on chronic pain that highlights and dispels common myths and misconceptions about pain patients.[6] And more and more articles in the professional journals are addressing the issue of negative bias and stereotyping of chronic pain patients.[7, 8]

Pain patients are speaking out more publicly and getting more publicity. On the national level they are fueling enormous growth in membership of the National Chronic Pain Outreach Association. On a local level they are banding together in support groups to fortify each other. It is only a matter of time until this expanding vitality impacts the public consciousness to squelch the stigma of chronic pain.

Notes
1. R. L. Gallon, "Perception of Disability in Chronic Back Pain Patients: A Long-Term Follow-Up," _Pain_ 37 (1989): 67–75.
2. R. I. Newman, "The Solo Practitioner and the Compensable Back Pain Patient," _Pain Management_ 1, no. 5 (1988): 199–201.
3. B. H. Tearnan and C. S. Cleeland, "The Attitudes of Physicians Toward Chronic Pain Patients," _Pain Management_ 1, no. 4 (1988): 180–184.
4. F. Evans, "Hypnosis and the Management of Chronic Pain," _Pain Management_ 2, no. 5 (1989): 247–255.
5. "Low Back Pain Is Responsible for One-Quarter of All Lost Work Days . . . ," _The Wall Street Journal_, September 26, 1989, section B, 1.
6. M. McCaffery and A. Beebe, _Pain: Clinical Manual for Nursing Practice_ (St. Louis: C. V. Mosby, 1989).
7. N. Hendler, "Chronic Pain and Litigation," _Pain Management_ 2, no. 2 (1989): 65–66.
8. Tearnan and Cleeland.

■ _Catherine Avery is a freelance writer in Washington, D.C., who specializes in health care issues. This article originally appeared in the_ National Chronic Pain Outreach Association _quarterly newsletter,_ Lifeline. _Reprinted with permission of the National Chronic Pain Outreach Association, Inc._

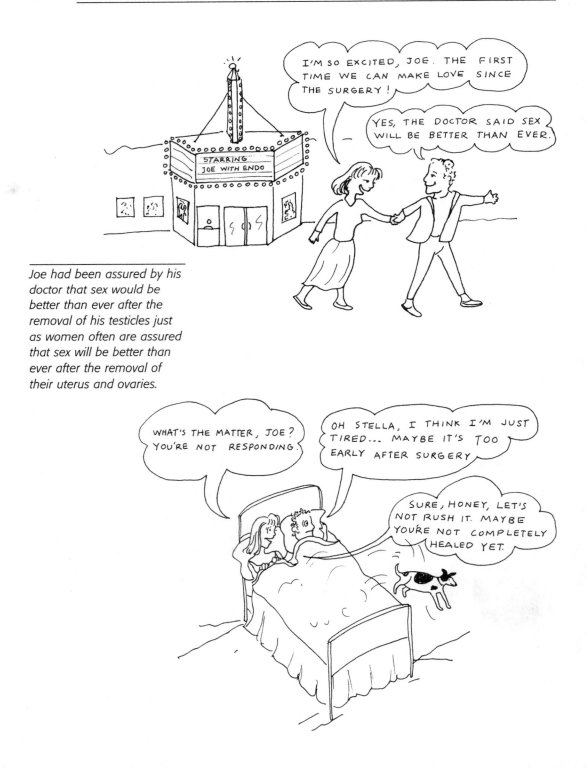

Joe had been assured by his doctor that sex would be better than ever after the removal of his testicles just as women often are assured that sex will be better than ever after the removal of their uterus and ovaries.

2

⊚⊚

Surgical Treatments

Surgery Through the Laparoscope:
The Future Has Arrived

By Charles E. Miller, M.D., and Mary Lou Ballweg

"*I wanted to let you know how much the Endometriosis Association has meant to me in the short time I have been a member. . . . Just when I thought there was no one to turn to concerning my medical problems, I was given the name of Dr. B. by a member of the association. . . . Dr. B. performed laser laparoscopy. . . . Had I not been directed to him, I would have gone through unnecessary major surgery by one of two other doctors I had been seeing, both of whom said there was no way my ovarian cysts could be removed through a laparoscopy!*"

Kay, Pennsylvania

"*I want to thank the members of the association for their many letters describing both symptoms, and treatments and recommendations of doctors. Belonging to the Endometriosis Association has been a major help in my life. I have severe endo, which was diagnosed and removed the first time through major surgery in 1984. Unable to get pregnant after 18 months, I had a diagnostic laparoscopy, which revealed that the endo was back, accompanied by cysts in both ovaries, adhesions and endo on the bowel and bladder. Again I underwent major surgery exactly two years later—this time laser—and 80 percent of the endo was removed. The endo that remained was around my bowel and bladder. And I was placed on danazol for several months. (Two miscarriages followed.)*

"*Throughout major surgery every other year I have managed to keep my career as an assistant professor intact. In order to do this my husband and I no longer take vacations—*

many of you are all too familiar with this. About six months ago I started to have pains on my left side, which my doctors told me to ignore. I knew the endo was back. (Major surgery appears to buy me two years of time.) This time I called association advisor Dr. Camran Nezhat and went to Atlanta, where he performed what I call "miracle surgery"—video-laseroscopy. That is, he was able to remove all the endo, including the endo around my bowels, and I walked out of the hospital the evening of the surgery. I had no pain after the surgery, and besides feeling tired for a couple of days I was fine.

"I feel as if I have been given a gift. Videolaseroscopy is not a cure, but it is a psychological and emotional relief that I didn't have to go through the severe pain that followed major surgery, six weeks' recuperation time, worrying about how the time lost would be viewed by my colleagues and affect my tenure. I have much control back in my life!

"However, I am writing this letter to the association members for a reason. Prior to going to Atlanta I did consult several . . . doctors where I live, [a city] known for its excellent medical care. These doctors (all known specialists) laid out the options that you all know: another laparotomy, and Lupron or danazol were options they told me about. None told me about videolaseroscopy. . . . Why? Because as far as I am aware none of them do this procedure. . . . We have to begin lobbying the medical profession to learn this technique so no more unnecessary major surgeries will be performed! As educated consumers it is time that we demand that this less costly and less physically and emotionally scarring outpatient surgery be available throughout the country. I thank you for making me aware that this surgery exists."

Rosanna, Massachusetts

"I am still paying for the surgery I had three years ago (a laparotomy in which my endometriosis was discovered), as I haven't been able to afford medical insurance. I would love to give you a donation, but I just can't afford to right now—all my financial obligations take up my entire paycheck (and often more) at this time.

"In fact I just spent almost $300 last month on doctor's visits and lab fees related to my endometriosis. . . . The doctor thinks I need more surgery some time within the next two or three months. I was thinking of writing you for advice on this when I got your letter.

"Is there someone from a chapter in my area who might be able to give advice and/or recommended reading about laparoscopy and laser surgery? The doctor said she wants to do this unless she sees something during surgery that necessitates switching to laparotomy. I am scared and want to make an informed decision about what to do next.

"During my first operation I was diagnosed with a severe case of endometriosis, and it is getting much worse with time. I now get my period two times a month and have been taking a lot of painkillers (higher than the recommended doses). . . ."

Mary, California

"The pain from the 'little spot of endo' left on my bowel because the doctor was too scared to remove it during my surgery causes familiar cramping. I still share menstrual-type cramping with my co-workers, although I don't have the heavy bleeding anymore. My lower

abdomen feels at times like it's going to burst. I also have the frequent diarrhea/constipation problems that I experienced prior to my surgery. I feel, at this time, that I will again be in the OR [operating room] at some future time, although I will certainly be much more critical of who does the surgery and more demanding on what is done. . . ."

Susan, Utah

"Because of you, I feel so much better. I read Overcoming Endometriosis *and then traveled to have what I describe as 21st-century surgery. . . . I had not one moment of nervousness or "butterflies" as I was preparing for my outpatient operative laparoscopy.*

"Imagine my surprise the next morning when I got up and, with no pain medication, stood over the sink and washed my hair!

"The total experience was incredible. (In 1984 I had a laparotomy. It took a long time to recover from that six-inch incision.) . . ."

Sylvie, Florida

In the early days of the association it was not at all uncommon to find women with endometriosis who went through major surgery after major surgery. Many of our members had two or three, sometimes even more, major surgeries, each involving a long incision. If there is one development that has removed much disability and some pain from the experience of endo, it is the ability to do major surgery through the laparoscope.

As the preceding letters make very clear, this has been a wonderful development for patients. In an article on laser surgery, *Newsweek* magazine summarized it succinctly in the story of Barbara, a 34-year-old Houston freelance writer who was diagnosed with endometriosis some years ago:

> Barbara underwent major abdominal surgery for removal of the tissue, requiring her to spend a full week in the hospital and six weeks recuperating at home, unable to undertake writing assignments. When her endometriosis recurred—as it very often does—she was luckier. This time her doctor removed the unwanted tissue using a simple laser procedure that required only one day off from work. "I felt completely back to normal within a few days rather than a few weeks," she says.

Barbara and most other patients quickly recognized the dramatic benefits of laparoscopic surgery, but the pioneering physicians on this frontier were accused by their peers of "surgical gymnastics." Supporters of traditional major abdominal surgery routinely stated that until the new techniques could be proven *better* than the old techniques, patients should undergo traditional surgery. Patients, of course, tended to believe that less pain, less cost, less time in the hospital, less recovery time, and less outside scarring gave the edge to the new techniques even if the results only matched but did not surpass those of traditional surgery.

But solid acceptance of laparoscopic surgery for endometriosis and other applications has clearly arrived among endometriosis experts. The major attitudinal shift that has occurred since 1985 was signaled in a lengthy article by Victor Gomel, M.D., in the July 1989 issue of *Fertility and Sterility*. In the article, "Operative Laparoscopy: Time for Acceptance," Dr. Gomel wrote, "It is evident that operative laparoscopy, appropriately employed, offers numerous advantages."

The advantages of operative laparoscopy compared to major abdominal surgery follow.

Operative Laparoscopy	Major Abdominal Surgery
Surgery can be performed immediately, at the same time the disease is diagnosed. If just a diagnostic laparoscopy is performed, the surgeon notes the presence of the disease but does not treat it. Another surgery may have to be performed to treat the disease or lengthy medical treatment with numerous side effects instituted.	*Generally must be preceded by at least a diagnostic laparoscopy*, so at least two surgeries are involved.
Generally performed as a day surgery or on an outpatient basis, rather than requiring a hospital stay.	*In-patient surgery*, which requires a hospital stay of generally 3–5 days.
1–4 small incisions (generally of ¼–½ inch), less outside scar, minimal incision pain.	*Incision of 4–6 inches*, more prominent scar, more pain from incision.
Less blood loss, 2½ times less in one study, in operative laparoscopy compared to major open abdominal surgery.	
Members routinely report far less pain and discomfort following procedure.	*Members routinely report significant pain and discomfort* following procedure.
Hospital costs may be significantly less. An average 49 percent cost reduction was found in one study of operative laparoscopy vs. major abdominal surgery.	
Recovery time generally a few days, but return of energy can require 2–6 weeks, depending on extent of procedures. Most were able to return to work in 5–6 days.	*Recovery time generally 3–6 weeks* with all the resulting lost wages, problems for families, child care, etc. Some women report they're not able to be as active for several months or more after major abdominal surgery.
Results are comparable to or better than major surgery.	

In addition to the known advantages of operative laparoscopy, there are theoretical advantages:

1. Less handling of tissue should lead to fewer adhesions (see Glossary).
2. The tissue remains moist because it is not exposed to air. Again, this decreases adhesions.
3. Low infection rate.
4. Magnification of tissue by the laparoscope (and perhaps by the video system) makes tissue planes and identification of endometriosis easier to note.
5. Laparoscopic surgery allows easier access to the cul-de-sac, where endometriosis can be especially problematic.

Historical Development of Laparoscopy

The laparoscope was first used in North America for diagnosis of endometriosis in 1968. This in itself was a great leap forward from our mothers' generation, for whom diagnosis required major abdominal surgery!

In the 1970s various surgeons experimented with using surgical instruments through the laparoscope. In the eighties, especially since 1985, numerous other surgeons continued refining techniques and equipment used for operative laparoscopy for endometriosis, including simply using traditional surgical tools through the laparoscope. In the nineties, specialized techniques for dealing with endo of the cul-de-sac, intestines, and urinary tract have evolved.

Laparoscopic Treatment Methods

Today a number of methods are used to treat endometriosis through the laparoscope. While they are frequently used in combination, we'll address each separately first for ease of understanding.

Mechanical

Mechanical surgical methods are those using laparoscopic scissors and other traditional surgical tools (graspers, forceps, clamps, etc.) through the laparoscope.

Electrosurgery

Next to mechanical dissection, electrosurgery is the oldest surgical method for the laparoscopic treatment of endometriosis, having been pioneered by European surgeons (Fragenheim and Semm) in the early seventies and in the United States (Eward, Hasson, Sulewski,

Daniell) in the late seventies and early eighties. Electrosurgery involves surgical instruments that use electric current to cut by vaporization, coagulation, or fulguration.

Unipolar and Bipolar

Traditional electrosurgery equipment has included unipolar and bipolar approaches. In unipolar (also called *monopolar*) the electric current travels through the body of the patient. In bipolar the current passes through only the tissue between the jaws of the instrument.

Electrocoagulation raises serious safety concerns, not so much with the experienced physician who understands the limits of the instruments but with the inexperienced surgeon. (Similar concerns, of course, apply to *all* the surgical methods described in this article.) While superficial endometriosis on the uterosacral ligaments and ovaries can easily be electrocoagulated, the use of electrocoagulation for even superficial lesions on the bladder, bowel, and other vital structures, such as the ureter, is potentially very dangerous. Cutting adhesions involving these areas can lead to a similar risk, because the electric current will follow the path of least resistance and can lead to damage.

As a result of these safety concerns, endo on the bladder, bowels, ureters, and other areas of the pelvis often goes untreated when no tool besides electrocoagulation is available. Members routinely report to the association that surgeons have left behind endo on these organs. Some surgeons may not even check these organs for the disease if they lack the ability to remove it. Some use hormonal treatments after surgery to "clean up" what may have been left behind. See Chapter 3 for information about this approach and controversies surrounding it. No medical treatments (or surgical treatments for that matter) have yet been proven to cure endo.

New Electrosurgery Instruments

Within the last few years or so a surprising resurgence of interest in electrosurgery has occurred, apparently because safer instruments have been developed and because these instruments are far less costly than lasers. Elmed Incorporated, one of the manufacturers of electrosurgical equipment, notes in one of its publications: ". . . one must take very seriously the vast cost difference between owning and operating a laser, compared to the proper electrosurgical system, where the same procedures that the $70,000 laser performs can be done with a $3,000 electrosurgical generator!"

Some of the electrosurgical instruments cut with high-frequency current in a manner similar to carbon dioxide (CO_2) lasers: by cellular vaporization. They seal small blood vessels as they go. Dr. Richard Soderstrom, Seattle, an expert on electrosurgery, notes that the tissue effects of electrosurgery are more diverse than those of the CO_2 laser beam. This can be an advantage or a disadvantage, depending on how it is used and the understanding and versatility of the surgeon.

Dr. David Redwine, well-known association advisor who practices in Bend, Oregon, uses electric scissors (three-millimeter monopolar scissors) and is very enthusiastic about it. He notes that the monopolar scissors give him 16 to 40 percent time savings in surgery. The scissors cut with electric current, which creates heat, which vaporizes the cells at the edge of the scissors. In addition to the time savings, the electric scissors are always sharp, he notes, and seal small blood vessels as they cut.

Laser

The use of the laser has become increasingly popular since it was first used in gynecologic abdominal surgery by Dr. Joseph Bellina, New Orleans, in the mid-1970s. Treatment with the CO_2 laser used through the laparoscope evolved in the late seventies and early eighties in France, Israel, and the United States.

The word *laser* is an acronym for light amplification by the stimulated emission of radiation. In the simplest terms a laser is a powerful concentration of energy. Unlike sunlight or light from a bulb, laser light is focused in one direction and wavelength. This results in a tightly concentrated, intense energy beam that can be aimed and controlled precisely.

A number of different surgical lasers are used, each with different properties. The laser that has been used the longest in laparoscopic surgery for endometriosis is the CO_2 laser (first reported in 1979 by Dr. Maurice Bruhat). Others include the argon laser (first reported by Dr. William Keye in 1983), the YAG laser (first reported by Dr. J. Lomano in 1983), and the KTP laser (first reported by Dr. James Daniell in 1986).

Lasers are cutting instruments, vaporizing instruments, and coagulating instruments all in one. This versatility has contributed to the great interest in lasers by surgeons.

Finally, since the laser coagulates as it goes, there is less blood in the operating field, which can make a major difference in visibility. This can help not only in recognition of endometriosis but also in difficult dissections.

CO_2 Laser

The most widely used laser for endometriosis is the CO_2 laser, which can cut and vaporize tissue but, because of its low penetration, is a poor instrument for coagulation. The fact that the depth of penetration can be as little as 0.1 to 0.2 millimeters, however, means it can be used to destroy endometriosis over the bladder, ureter, and bowel. The CO_2 laser also has the smallest zone of heat damage to surrounding tissue, a factor believed to decrease the formation of adhesions.

Being a concentrated beam of energy rather than a physical piece of equipment, the CO_2 laser can reach areas that can be difficult to reach with the scalpel, cautery, or other surgical tools. It also offers precision that is difficult to obtain with other surgical tools— the cut, area impacted, and depth of penetration can be determined exactly.

The CO_2 laser does have limitations. The laser beam is transmitted through a heavy arm via a lens and mirror system. Not only is this arm somewhat awkward, but also if any of the lenses or mirrors are out of alignment, the laser is useless. Further, the smoke generated as the laser cuts and vaporizes can obscure tissue visualization unless properly suctioned. Finally, the CO_2 laser is absorbed in fluid, thus losing its power when a lot of irrigating fluid is used or in a somewhat bloody field.

Laser Comparisons

During the 1980s, other laser wavelengths were developed to try to overcome some of these shortcomings—argon, YAG, and KTP. (The argon is rarely used for endometriosis today, so we will only mention it.) In addition, fibers have been added—the laser beam is directed through the fiber close to or in direct contact with the tissue to be surgically treated. Some surgeons prefer fiber lasers because they allow the surgeon to have a sense of touch between the fiber and the tissue. All three of the fiber-transmitted lasers have greater depth of penetration than the CO_2 laser, although techniques such as shortening the duration of the laser energy and using decreased wattage at the tissue sites lead to less penetration.

Writes association advisor Dr. Dan Martin in "Operative Laparoscopy: Comparison of Lasers with Other Techniques": "Using a laser other than the CO_2 laser increases the potential for damage to the sites other than the pathology being treated. This is particularly an issue when treating lesions on or near the bowel, bladder, ureters, or blood vessels. While some of these lasers have been used at these sites, they nevertheless have greater potential for unnoticed injury than the CO_2 laser."

YAG Laser. When used as a bare fiber (without attaching sapphire tips), the YAG laser has the greatest depth of penetration of the lasers. So it was initially used where greater tissue destruction and coagulation were needed. When sapphire tips are attached to the YAG fiber, the depth of penetration is similar to that with the CO_2 laser, but the coagulation effect is superior because the YAG can penetrate a layer of blood. So, depending on what tip shape is used, the surgeon can easily cut, coagulate, or vaporize tissue.

KTP Laser. The KTP has a depth of penetration greater than the CO_2 but less than the YAG fiber. Because it can penetrate fluids, it can be used to coagulate. It can also vaporize tissue at high power.

KTP/YAG Combination Laser. Another laser being used for endo combines the KTP and YAG lasers, making deep penetration available when desired. The combination laser allows for all the cutting, vaporization, and coagulation normally required in endo surgery.

Ultrasonic Treatment Methods

In addition to the three main laparoscopic treatment methods just described, a new method using ultrasound as an energy source—that is, sound waves at a very high frequency—is being adapted from other types of surgery. Two devices are currently being tested. One is the ultrasonic scalpel (brand name: Harmonic Scalpel), which converts electrical energy and moves across tissue at 55,000 vibrations per second. Proponents say that, unlike electrosurgery or laser, the ultrasonic scalpel generates little heat and less tissue damage than other energy sources. While critics say the ultrasonic scalpel generates more tissue damage, the first author has used the Harmonic Scalpel effectively to excise endometriosis. His results are similar to his outcomes with laser excision, the advantage being cost containment (hospital charges are one-fifth the charges with laser) with no sacrifice of results.

The other new ultrasound device, the cavitational ultrasonic surgical aspirator (CUSA), has been used in neurosurgery and cancer surgery. The hollow tip on the CUSA probe used through the laparoscope vibrates so fast that it produces an ultrasonic wave that destroys cells. Both these devices are currently being studied for endometriosis surgery. The association newsletter will carry additional information as it becomes available.

Surgical Techniques Used Through the Laparoscope

The surgical techniques used in operative laparoscopy include, of course, those used in major abdominal surgery:

Excision: Cutting out of tissue.

Vaporization: Destruction of tissue by instant boiling of the cellular water with a high-power density laser or high-power density metal electrosurgical tool.

Coagulation: A term defined by clotting (the process of changing a liquid, especially blood, into a solid) but used to mean desiccation and other processes involved in cellular death. Desiccation is the heating and drying of tissue that results in cellular death.

Ablation: Destruction by any surgical means.

Fulguration: Superficial burning with a spark of electricity from the electrosurgical tool to the tissue.

All these techniques except fulguration must be available to the surgeon so he or she can adequately handle endometriosis surgery. The new treatment methods being used laparoscopically (mechanical, electrosurgical, laser, ultrasonic) have varying abilities to handle these basic surgical techniques. In addition, some techniques are more effective in certain parts of the pelvis, and some may be more successful than others with different types of endo.

As noted in *Endometriosis*, edited by Emery A. Wilson, "[The surgeon] must be well versed in all modalities available for the operating laparoscope—even though he may choose to vaporize endometriosis with the carbon dioxide laser, use of the bipolar or unipolar cautery may be necessary to control unexpected bleeding."

Dr. Dan Martin, Memphis, Tennessee, in *Laparoscopic Appearances of Endometriosis*, volume 1, states it another way: "Bipolar coagulators, unipolar knives, thermal coagulators, and lasers have been used to ablate (coagulate, vaporize, or excise) endometriosis. A combination of these techniques is superior to concentrating on one of them."

The fine points of the various techniques are debated hotly at surgical and research conferences, and new research and improvements in equipment are becoming available all the time. (Watch the association newsletter for information on future developments.) All of this make decisions difficult for women facing surgery today, but it's reassuring to know all this activity will probably eventually produce conclusive proof of the best surgical techniques, equipment, and adjustments for each location, type, and depth of endo.

A Turning Point

The availability of lasers was the main turning point in more and more endometriosis surgeries being done through the laparoscope. James Daniell, a Nashville surgeon who pioneered both electrocauterization and laser techniques through the laparoscope, writes in an article on the KTP laser, "the use of laser has tremendously changed my personal patterns of gynecologic surgery." Dr. Daniell presents data showing how lasers have influenced his ability to carry out more and more procedures through the laparoscope over the years.

Dr. Victor Gomel, the well-known Vancouver, British Columbia, microsurgeon cited earlier, writes: "Laparoscopic surgery is being used increasingly to treat more advanced stages of endometriosis that require ablation [destruction] or excision of large endometriomas [cysts] and frequently significant adhesiolysis [cutting of adhesions]. This movement was spearheaded largely by those employing lasers, especially CO_2 and argon."

When the association's first article on lasers appeared in 1983, the possibility of doing major surgery through the laparoscope seemed like a fantasy. By 1985, when we introduced members to the "one-day wonder" surgery Dr. Camran Nezhat of Atlanta had pioneered by combining laser, laparoscope, and video monitoring techniques (videolaseroscopy), now standard in operative laparoscopy of all types, it was clear the dream was coming true. But still, in 1985, precious few surgeons were able to do the new surgeries. Today not only are more technologies available, but also it is becoming widely acknowledged that surgery through the laparoscope is generally best. Patients, rather than hoping for easy one-day surgeries, are now demanding them.

In the United States, laser and electrosurgical technology are commonly available for laparoscopic surgery for endometriosis. Surgeons are even beginning to experiment with tiny laparoscopes that allow the use of local anesthesia and laparoscopy in the physician's office! In Canada, because of limits on hospital budgets to purchase equipment and other factors, the new technology is not as available yet, but that is changing. Association advisor Dr. Kay Lie, Toronto, has had long waiting lists for surgery with the CO_2 laser. In Europe, the surgical revolution was slower (except where leaders pioneered, such as Dr. Kurt Semm in Germany and Dr. Maurice Bruhat in France). And in some countries, such as Japan, there is limited surgery for endometriosis even for diagnosis. Wherever surgery is practiced for endometriosis, patients and endo specialists have pushed for the new surgeries once they became aware of the advantages over laparotomy (see Glossary).

Surgical Treatment of Different Types and Locations of Endo

Endometriosis is often a surgical challenge. All different types of tissue, on varying organs, in difficult-to-reach and sensitive areas must be addressed. The traditional training of most gynecological surgeons, with its focus on cesarean sections and hysterectomies, does not address the new understanding of this disease, or the technologies available. Endometriosis surgery is becoming a field for specialists, which should mean better treatment for women with endo in the future. So, how do specialists address different types of endo surgery?

Implants

Implants can be excised, vaporized, or coagulated. The key to the treatment of endometrial implants is to get below the level of endometriosis. The area around the implants is also vaporized by some surgeons to destroy possible microscopic implants around the larger ones.

Some experts believe excision is better than vaporization to ensure that the entire implant is removed and also because it can then be sent to the lab for study. The vaporization process can obscure the deep extent of an implant, making it difficult to be sure all the endo is removed. More research is needed on the best approaches.

When there are dozens of implants, larger implants are excised and smaller implants are vaporized or coagulated. On occasion lesions can be so diffuse that distortion of tissue occurs and interferes with safe and complete resection.

Cysts

Cysts can be excised or vaporized, varying with physician preference. Dr. Miller generally excises cysts larger than 2 centimeters, and vaporizes those below 2 centimeters.

Vaporizing larger cysts becomes very tedious. Moreover, there is concern that the cyst could be treated inadequately if vaporization is not to the desired depth. Removing the cyst allows a microscopic study of the tissue to be performed and certainty as to the type and nature of the cyst.

Highly specialized techniques have been developed for endometrial cysts. David Olive, M.D., New Haven, Connecticut, notes in the chapter on conservative surgery in *Endo-*

metriosis: Contemporary Concepts in Clinical Management that simple aspiration of the fluid in cysts has been found to result in a 40 percent recurrence rate, so most surgeons believe removing the cyst is more appropriate.

The disadvantage of removing cysts is that it also removes healthy ovary. With large or multiple cysts, this may mean damaging hormone production and future fertility. Removal of multiple or large cysts can lead to premature menopause.

Cul-de-Sac

Superficial implants in the cul-de-sac can be handled similarly to other superficial implants. Deeper implants in the cul-de-sac provide a greater challenge. Laparoscopy can sometimes provide better visibility of the cul-de-sac than laparotomy.

The surgeon most known for his surgical techniques for endometriosis in the cul-de-sac is Dr. Harry Reich, a Kingston, Pennsylvania, surgeon. Dr. Reich has carried out operative laparoscopy, complemented by vaginal incision when necessary, even when extensive, fibrous endometriosis and adhesions were present. Some have questioned whether it's wise to keep the patient under general anesthesia for the long time necessary for operative laparoscopy in these sites. Ongoing research is needed. For the most part, women with endometriosis will not have the option of operative laparoscopy in this situation, since few surgeons are willing at this time to take the accompanying risks.

Additional Surgical Techniques for Operative Laparoscopy

Near-Contact Laparoscopy: Much endometriosis is missed if the surgeon is unaware of the numerous visual appearances of endometriosis. Obviously disease that isn't recognized can't be surgically treated. One of the important techniques developed by Dr. David Redwine, an association advisor who has done much work to make people aware of the varying appearances of endometriosis, is near-contact laparoscopy. He has found that bringing the laparoscope to within one centimeter of the peritoneum (lining of the pelvis) is important to seeing all the subtle types of endometriosis.

Aquadissection/Hydrodissection: Dr. Kurt Semm, operative laparoscopy pioneer from Germany, developed a surgical pump called an Aqua-Purator, which is used for putting fluids into the abdomen during surgery and for removing them as well as for suctioning out debris, laser smoke, etc. Dr. Harry Reich was among the first to use the Aqua-Purator to push fluid under pressure into areas in the abdomen to separate adhesions and adhered organs (such as ovary and tube or bowel). The pressurized fluid provides a gentle way to handle sensitive areas. Drs. Camran and Farr Nezhat have described injection of fluid under the peritoneum to lift it from sensitive areas such as the bladder and allow safe removal or vaporization of endo. They call the technique *hydrodissection* (see illustration).

Adhesions

Adhesions are very common with endometriosis. Adhesions *must* be treated since they can cause much pain and contribute to infertility. Many surgeons simply cut the adhesion, but association advisor Dr. David Olive notes that it's important to remove the entire adhesion rather than just cut it because cutting it leaves behind tags of tissue that die off and may contribute to adhesion formation. He also notes that active endo implants have been found in pelvic adhesions and these implants will be left behind if the adhesion is simply cut rather than being removed completely. See the article "Adhesions and Endometriosis: The Puzzle Continues" at the end of this chapter.

Deep Disease

Deep implants generally are excised. Deep disease is suspected when pelvic examination finds nodularity or tenderness at a specific point ("focal tenderness"). This idea is noted by Dr. Dan Martin in his research publications on depth of infiltration of endometriosis. He notes that palpation is carried out with a blunt probe during laparoscopy or, if a major

The pelvic organs can be seen in this illustration. Hydrodissection is a technique developed by Drs. Camran and Farr Nezhat, Atlanta.

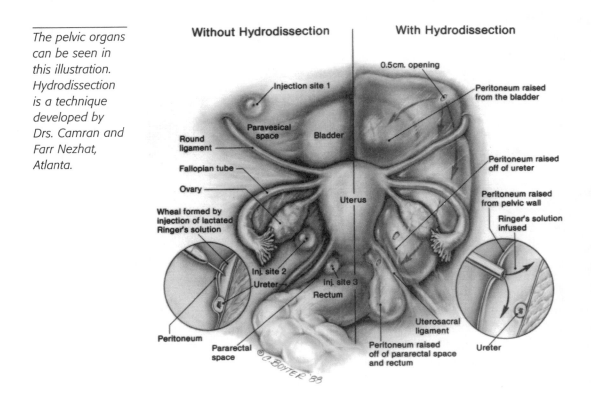

surgery is needed, manually. Palpation is important because it's often easier to feel the deep lesion than to see it.

Peritoneum over Sensitive Areas (Bladder, Ureters)

Endo in sensitive areas covered with peritoneum is often vaporized or excised. Excision of endo from these areas is delicate and requires skill and experience. Dr. Redwine has developed techniques that involve tenting the peritoneum up, nicking a pleat in it, and then using a combination of incising and gently pulling/separating/teasing the diseased areas away from the underlying healthy tissue. Laser vaporization is the technique most surgeons would use in these areas as well as with the uterosacral ligaments, where damage to the ureter or vessels going to the uterus is a danger.

Bowel Endo

Dr. Redwine and his colleague Dr. Dean Sharpe, a bowel surgeon, have developed techniques to remove endo on or in the bowel through the laparoscope. They state that endo on the bowels can often be removed without removing a small wedge of bowel, and only rarely is a bowel resection (cutting and removing an entire section of diseased bowel) needed.

Dr. Robert Franklin, Baylor College of Medicine, Texas, has also done pioneering work on severe bowel endo. He works with a general surgeon to remove part of the bowel wall when endo infiltrates deeply.

One of the most exciting revolutions in laparoscopic surgery is the development of new methods of bowel resection. In the past bowel resection nearly always required a laparotomy. Now laparotomy can be avoided with the aid of bowel surgeons and a whole array of instruments and skills not used by laparoscopists in the past.

The instruments include a sigmoidoscope, basically a scope like the laparoscope that is inserted through the anus and used to check sutures, and mechanical circular staplers that allow the instant complete cutting of the bowel and complete end-to-end stapling. This eliminates the difficulty of suturing intestine through the laparoscope. The airtight suture prevents leakage of bowel contents that can cause serious infection and rarely, if unattended to, death.

In one new technique, Drs. Redwine and Sharpe pull the diseased portion of the intestines through a colpotomy incision (in the wall of the vagina) and resect it, and then the two ends are sutured.

New bowel techniques have also been developed by Thierry Vancaillie, M.D., and Morris Franklin, M.D., of the Texas Endosurgery Institute in San Antonio, and Drs. Camran and Farr Nezhat with bowel surgeon Dr. Earl Pennington of Atlanta. Drs. Nezhat perform a somewhat different technique in which the endometriosis-affected part of the colon is allowed to prolapse (to fall or slide) through the anus. The diseased part of the colon is

---

New Surgical Frontiers in Treating Endometriosis: Highlights

• Surgery for endometriosis has been revolutionized. No longer do most women with endometriosis have to face several major surgeries, at least not if they are aware of and can seek up-to-date help.

• No longer is the laparoscope just a diagnostic tool. Now the surgeon can treat the endo right away—as long as the surgeon is a specialist.

• By combining various surgical tools with the laparoscope, most of the procedures done in the past in major abdominal surgeries can now be done through the laparoscope.

• Some of the surgical tools being married to the laparoscope are

traditional scissors and forceps

laser (various types with various properties)

magnification, brilliant lighting, video cameras, and high-resolution video screens (these have made excellent visibility possible, even better than with major surgery for some areas of the pelvis)

• New techniques for stopping bleeding (endocoagulation) and new materials applied during and after surgery are being used to help prevent adhesions.

• The new technologies are saving women not only much pain but also time (no long hospital stays or recuperations at home) and money!

• Choosing a surgeon is hard! Lack of credentialing by professional groups leaves those with the disease on their own. Claims and counterclaims and lack of long-term studies muddy the waters.

---

removed, the mechanical stapler used to close the two parts of the intestine back together, and the rectum put back in its normal position inside the body during visualization through the laparoscope. The suture is tested with air pushed into the rectum—the absence of air bubbles in the cul-de-sac, which is filled with saline, shows it is airtight. Remarkably, patients are able to take in clear liquids the day after surgery and can be discharged from the hospital on the second day after surgery. This technique is especially useful when endo occurs very low in the colon.

Remember that these techniques are new. Proceed with caution in choosing a surgeon, and make sure that a colorectal surgeon is involved with your gynecologic surgeon if you're considering such surgery. The interest of colorectal surgeons in what they call *laparoscopic-guided colon resections* is growing. As with operative laparoscopy, the new techniques have not caught on yet in most other countries (France and Germany are exceptions) but are sure to do so since patients want and benefit from minimally invasive surgeries.

The group from the Texas Endosurgery Institute in San Antonio exemplifies a new concept that is evolving from general surgeons and gynecologic surgeons working together. At the institute gynecologists, general surgeons, urologists, orthopedic surgeons, and gastroenterologists work together on the many new types of endoscopic surgery evolving today. (Endoscopic surgery is surgery through an endoscope, an illuminated optical instrument for visualizing the interior of a body cavity or organ. The laparoscope is the endoscope best known to those with endometriosis.) Hopefully, with the growing interest of general surgeons in operative laparoscopy, more contributions from general surgeons and other surgical fields to endometriosis surgery will occur.

Urinary Tract Endo

New techniques are evolving for dealing with tough urinary tract endo through the laparoscope also. Dr. Camran Nezhat and other leading surgeons have developed techniques for resecting parts of ureters that are involved with endo as well as endometriosis of the bladder. Here again teams of gynecologists and urologists are forming. While the leading surgeons in our field can handle even the toughest endo even when found on non-gynecological organs, few in the rank and file of gynecology can. Without specialists to help the gynecologist deal with endo in areas such as the urinary tract, there may be the temptation either to ignore the endo in these areas or to attempt dangerous procedures that the gynecologist does not have the expertise to handle.

Peritoneal Pockets

Peritoneal pockets are defects that form a little pouch, or pocket, in the peritoneum. Endo is sometimes found inside the pocket. Dr. Redwine pulls the pocket inside out during operative laparoscopy to determine if endo is present and excises it if it is.

Results of Operative Laparoscopy

Reporting on the success rates of the various surgical techniques is a very difficult endeavor for several reasons. First, very few physicians have reported results on more than one surgical method. For example, surgeons performing studies using endocoagulation techniques do not report studies with laser. Thus, the technical expertise of the surgeon is not standardized.

Second, the patient population can never be standardized. In an effort to overcome this, various classifications of endometriosis and adhesions have been devised. Over the last several years the Society of Reproductive Surgeons, within the American Society for Reproductive Medicine (formerly the American Fertility Society), has sought to devise a classification system, but without understanding the cause and typical course of endo this is very difficult. In addition, at least in relation to fertility, no one knows the precise reasons for fertility problems with endo.

Finally, it's easy to find surgeons vehemently arguing the merits of the various technologies at conferences and in private sessions with patients. To protect ourselves, it's important that we understand some of the basics and remember that those advocating one technique only or implying they have a proven cure must be regarded skeptically.

Those caveats aside, a comparative chart presented by Drs. Luciano and Manzi in a 1992 medical text indicates that in seven studies pregnancy rates ranged from 26 percent to 72 percent in mild disease and from 25 percent to 67 percent in severe disease. Obviously such a broad range of rates doesn't really tell us what any one woman will face. Also, remember these comparisons are limited by heterogeneous patient populations, variability in prior treatment, length of follow-up, and varying surgical techniques. Some comparisons have shown that, when other infertility factors are weighed in statistically, the preg-

Open Laparoscopy

With the development of the newer operative laparoscopy techniques, many women with endo are now having multiple laparoscopies over the years because of the ongoing, chronic nature of the disease. This is at least better than the multiple laparotomies—major open abdominal surgeries—that we used to endure.

But with the multiple surgeries comes a danger of scar tissue right under the navel, where the surgeon introduces the laparoscope into the abdomen. If the intestines are adhered up to the navel, it can mean that the surgeon could puncture the intestines (or a blood vessel) on the way in for a laparoscopy. Hitting a blood vessel on the way in is a risk, in fact, even without scar tissue adhering things together at the navel.

For these situations, as well as in very heavy women in whom laparoscopy is more difficult because the instruments are sometimes not long enough to reach into the pelvic cavity and the amount of body tissue can make it hard to keep tissue out of the way, new techniques have been developed. In open laparoscopy, rather than forcibly thrusting a sharp instrument called a *trocar* into the abdomen, a small incision is made in the navel area. In addition, new instruments allow the surgeon to see tissues on the way into the abdomen. This may lessen the risk of injury.

So, if you've been told you can't have a laparoscopy because of too many prior surgeries or because you're heavy, you could seek out a skilled surgeon who uses open techniques—especially valuable in those with scar tissue, since open laparoscopy can allow a surgeon to get in to cut the adhesions without a laparotomy, which might result in more adhesions.

Surgery, especially major surgery, is also riskier for heavy women, so again these techniques allowing heavier women to have a laparoscopy are beneficial. In fact, these approaches may be safer across the board for everyone with endometriosis.

As with other more advanced techniques, seek an advanced laparoscopist who has done hundreds of cases if you have these special risks.

nancy rates tend to be quite close. (Just one more example of how statistics fail to tell the whole story!)

Data regarding pain relief after different laparoscopic surgical methods is somewhat more certain. In a 1980 study 77 percent of 43 women treated with electrocautery experienced relief. In a 1986 study 61 percent of 31 patients undergoing electrocautery and excision of ovarian cysts achieved pain relief. Of 50 patients treated by Dr. William Keye reported in 1987, 92 percent of patients reported pain reduction. Of 270 patients with pelvic pain, as reported by Dr. Camran Nezhat in 1989, 210 (77 percent) were still pain-free after one year. In more than 500 patients with pelvic pain, as reported by Dr. David Redwine in 1995, patients reported dramatic improvement in nonmenstrual pelvic pain, tenderness on pelvic exam, pain with sex, and painful bowel movements one year after surgery.

And in a randomized double-blind (meaning neither the patient nor the nurse assessing results knew who had what procedure) controlled study in which one group of patients had laser destruction of their endometriosis and of nerves to the uterus and another group had only a diagnostic laparoscopy, Dr. Christopher Sutton showed statistically significant pain relief in the laser laparoscopy group six months after surgery. Sixty-two and a half percent of the patients in the laser treatment group reported improvement or resolution of painful menstruation, pelvic pain, or pain with sex. (Patients found at the diagnostic laparoscopy to have severe endo were not included in the study and were immediately treated with laser destruction of their endometriosis because the hospital Ethics Committee felt that it was unethical to withhold treatment from patients in severe pain due to stage IV disease. Patients who were in the no-treatment arm of the study were offered the opportunity for laser laparoscopy six months after their diagnostic laparoscopy. This study was carried out in England. In the United States and Canada, patients have been unwilling to participate in studies such as this one because of unwillingness to undergo two surgical procedures, greater awareness of the efficacy of operative laparoscopy, and the desire for immediate pain relief. Two large-scale similar studies in North America had to be dropped because of inability to recruit patients.)

■ *Dr. Charles E. Miller* *is the medical director, Center for Human Reproduction, Chicago, Illinois, and an association advisor.*

Other Procedures That Can Be Done in Operative Laparoscopy

By Mary Lou Ballweg

Laparoscopic Removal of Ovaries: A development that has helped many women with endo who have had a hysterectomy but kept an ovary (or both ovaries) and then had continuation of the disease is the ability to remove the remaining ovary (or ovaries) through the laparoscope. Drs. Kurt Semm and Liselotte Mettler first reported the technique for removing ovaries laparoscopically. And Dr. Harry Reich developed techniques for removing ovaries laparoscopically even when stuck with adhesions on the side of the pelvis. He described a technique involving a vaginal incision to remove the ovary where it is too large to be removed through the incision in the navel (or in cases where the ovary needs to be removed whole for lab study).

These techniques make it easier for women with endo to consider retaining their healthier ovary (or ovaries) at hysterectomy, knowing that they could have it/them removed if necessary through laparoscopy rather than major abdominal surgery, as was required in the past. (For more on the many issues related to hysterectomy and removal of the ovaries, see the articles on hysterectomy in this chapter.) For even more assurance that they could stay healthy in the future, women can now have ultrasound to locate and treat any small and/or deep cysts in the remaining ovary or ovaries. See description under "Ultrasound."

Laparoscopy/Colpotomy: Dr. Dan Martin has described a combination of two techniques for removing endo nodule(s) in the cul-de-sac. By using a forceps and laser through the scope, he is able to dissect deep nodules, first on one side through the scope and then on the other side through the vaginal incision. This type of endo has been very difficult to remove in any type of surgery (including major open abdominal surgery) for a number of technical reasons. The combination procedure seems very promising for women with endo who have suffered from this type of nodule and the painful sex that can occur with it. Only a very skilled endo specialist could (or should!) attempt this.

Laparoscopically Assisted Vaginal Hysterectomy and Laparoscopic Hysterectomy: Doing an extensive operative laparoscopy first to remove all endometriosis, adhesions, and possibly ovaries now allows some women with endo to have a vaginal hysterectomy instead of the more invasive, painful abdominal hysterectomy. Vaginal hysterectomy involves removal of the uterus through the vagina and suturing at the top of the vagina.

In addition, some surgeons are now removing the uterus through the laparoscope (laparoscopic hysterectomy). When Dr. Harry Reich first presented his technique for laparoscopic hysterectomy, he was roundly criticized—the technique was thought too far out for most to attempt. But the technique caught on quickly. Clearly even hysterectomy, one of the most frequently done abdominal surgeries, is going the route of minimally invasive surgery, and that's good for women with endo.

As Dr. C. Y. Liu of Chattanooga, Tennessee, notes, "Laparoscopic hysterectomy provides almost all the advantages of the abdominal hysterectomy, yet with decreased morbidity, blood loss, postoperative discomfort, and pain and shorter hospitalization and recovery."

Remember, a laparoscopic hysterectomy is still a hysterectomy with all the long-lasting implications of hysterectomy. It's not appropriate surgery simply because it's easier on the patient than previously, unless you're out of options and have made the decision to have a hysterectomy. (While easier on the patient, the procedure, like others done at operative laparoscopy, requires the surgeon to develop new skills. Choosing an experienced surgeon is important.)

Supracervical Hysterectomy: Another development in hysterectomy has been the return to the pre-1940 practice of leaving the cervix in place in some patients at hysterectomy. Some surgeons destroy the inside lining of the cervix to prevent periodic bleeding that can occur in a small number of patients who retain their cervix. Proponents of leaving the cervix argue that it improves sexual functioning and pelvic floor support. Dr. Harrith Hasson, Chicago, states that significant nerves affecting sexual function are lost when the cervix is removed. Complications of bladder and bowel dysfunction that can follow hysterectomy in a small number of cases may also be related to the loss of these nerves, according to Dr. Hasson. Few surgeons are currently leaving the cervix on a routine basis, but surgical leaders interviewed for this article said they would honor a woman's wishes if she wished to retain her cervix.

Hysteroscopy: A procedure in which a scope is put into the uterus through the vagina under anesthesia for diagnosis of problems in the uterus and for surgical procedures. It, like laparoscopy, is combined with video monitoring so the surgeon can see the inside of the uterus on a video screen.

Presacral Neurectomy: A procedure severing the nerves at the back of the uterus to help provide pain relief.

Uterosacral Neurectomy: Also called *Doyle procedure* and *LUNA*, which stands for "laparoscopic uterine nerve ablation," this procedure cuts the same nerves as in presacral neurectomy but cuts them closer to the uterus. The procedure sometimes results in good pain relief. Complications are possible—again, a technically accomplished surgeon is needed. It is also possible for the nerves to regrow.

Ultrasound: Ultrasound is a procedure in which sound waves at a frequency higher than a human ear can detect are projected through a portion of a person's body, creating an image on a video monitor. Ultrasound can be done either abdominally or with a transvaginal probe, a small ultrasound device inserted into the vagina.

Using this instrument, physicians can detect small and/or deep cysts inside the ovary that would have been missed at laparoscopy. In addition, ultrasound done before laparoscopy makes it possible for surgeons to be quite sure that cysts are not malignant and to aspirate them and perform other surgical procedures without the worry that the procedures could possibly spread cancer cells if the cyst had been malignant. (They note that United States cancer data indicates this is rare—they could expect to find an ovarian tumor in only 4.5 cases per 100,000.)

Emerging Principles of Surgery for Endometriosis

By Mary Lou Ballweg

1. Operative laparoscopy appears to offer better results than major abdominal surgery. Laparoscopy has been shown to lead to significantly fewer adhesions.

2. Some experts believe that excision gives better results than vaporization. In one study, as the use of excisional techniques increased, the accuracy of endometriosis identification increased. (This means the results may have improved in part because the surgeons using excision increase their skill in identifying and removing more and more endometriosis.) Also, excision allows the entire lesion to be removed, whereas vaporization and coagulation can remove part of the lesion and cover or obscure the rest, leaving part behind.

3. Experts seem to be coming to agreement that removing *all* the endometriosis may offer the best potential for leaving the woman pain-free and that attempts to remove adhesions are necessary to relieve pain and increase fertility.

4. Recognizing all of the visual manifestations of the disease is considered very important. Magnification, close-up laparoscopy techniques, and palpation of deep lesions and implants in certain areas of the pelvis are steps used by experts to recognize and treat all the endo possible.

5. Sending tissue to the lab for confirmation of diagnosis is becoming more and more the norm. Research has shown not only that there are many more visual manifestations of endometriosis than suspected or understood in the past but also that a number of abnormalities in the pelvis can appear to be endometriosis but are not, as well as different types of cysts that could be mistaken for endometrial cysts. To know what was treated, documentation is necessary. This will also improve the quality of research results and treatment outcomes over time.

6. Steps to prevent adhesions are important. Operative laparoscopy itself (vs. open abdominal surgery) as well as gentle handling of tissue and complete control of bleeding have all been established as important in preventing adhesions.

7. Finally, there is an emerging sense that operative laparoscopy for endometriosis is a specialty surgical field. A Belgian study published in the June 1990 issue of *Fertility and Sterility* found, for instance, "that the ability to detect endometriotic lesions increases with experience of both the surgeon and the pathologist."

A Life-Threatening Complication of Surgery in Women

By Mary Lou Ballweg

At a hearing called by the United States Office of Research on Women's Health in June 1991, Dr. Cosmo L. Fraser, assistant professor of medicine, Veterans Administration Medical Center, University of California, San Francisco, presented testimony on a serious complication of surgery in women. This complication has been overlooked and considered unimportant or incidental because the research studies on the condition have been carried out in men or in male animals rather than in women or female animals. In males the condition is usually not serious.

The condition is called *hyponatremia* or *low blood sodium*. Dr. Fraser testified that the reasons patients develop hyponatremia are quite complicated but are essentially due to normal events gone awry and to a lack of understanding by medical personnel of these changes in affected patients: "Vasopressin (Antidiuretic Hormone), the hormone which is principally responsible for water handling by the kidney, is markedly elevated after surgery. Thus, the administration of an improper amount and type of intravenous fluids will result in water retention and dilution of the patient's sodium (hyponatremia). If the patient is unable to compensate for this water load, and the condition is not recognized by the medical team, she will most likely develop brain swelling that could eventually lead to death."

Dr. Fraser notes that in men testosterone appears to help the brain adapt to hyponatremia and prevents brain swelling. In women the hormones estrogen and progesterone

A week later. . .

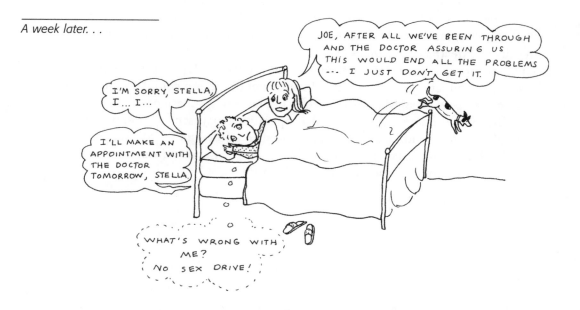

appear to prevent adaptation and allow brain swelling to occur. His studies have found that "with the same degree of hyponatremia, a young woman has greater than 25 times the chance of dying from hyponatremia than does a man of any age.

"As a result of work done in our laboratory, it became clear that the patients who were at increased risk of dying from hyponatremia were primarily premenopausal women and, to a lesser degree, postmenopausal women on hormone replacement (age range 22–66 years; 90 percent were under 50 years of age and have had a menstrual period within a month). At first this idea was greeted with skepticism by the largely male-dominated research field. However, it has now become quite clear that the complications from rapidly developing hyponatremia in women represent a major public health concern."

Dr. Fraser noted in his testimony that "women continue to be needlessly put at risk after successful, uncomplicated surgery" because of lack of understanding of the differences between men and women developing hyponatremia. Perhaps we can help protect ourselves when having surgery for endometriosis by giving our surgeons copies of Dr. Fraser's studies.* In addition, Dr. Fraser wrote to the association:

> Fortunately for the affected patients, they usually develop symptoms that are warning signs that should alert them and their physicians that something is wrong. All of the patients we described developed progressive headache, nausea, and vomiting after their operation. These symptoms increased in severity despite the administration of medication that would normally cause them to abate.
>
> As recommendations, I would inform female patients and their families that they should report the above symptoms to their physicians or nurses. They should also tell their surgeons and anesthesiologist that they do not want to be given plain dextrose and water intravenously after surgery. If intravenous fluids are indeed required, they should be given either lactated ringers or normal saline.

Don't delay reporting any such symptoms to your doctor—sometimes we take for granted discomforts after surgery and simply wait for them to go away. But if it was by chance hyponatremia, any delay could be deadly. In one of Dr. Fraser's studies he notes that the patients who developed the symptoms about 32 hours after the surgical procedure went from alertness to respiratory arrest in less than one hour.

---

*"Fatal Central Diabetes Mellitus and Insipidus Resulting from Untreated Hyponatremia: A New Syndrome," *Annals of Internal Medicine*, 112, no. 2 (Jan. 15, 1990); A. I. Arieff, "Hyponatremia Associated with Permanent Brain Damage," *Advances in Internal Medicine*, 32 (1987): 325–44; J. C. Ayus, R. K. Krothapalli, and A. I. Arieff, "Sexual Difference in Survival with Severe Symptomatic Hyponatremia," *Kidney International*, 33 (1988): 180; "Sex Differences Result in Increased Morbidity from Hyponatremia in Female Rats," American Physiological Society, 1989; "Na+-K+-ATPase Pump Function in Rat Brain Synaptosomes Is Different in Males and Females," American Physiological Society, 1989; A. I. Arieff, "Hyponatremia, Convulsions, Respiratory Arrest, and Permanent Brain Damage After Elective Surgery in Healthy Women," *New England Journal of Medicine*, 314 (1986): 1529–35.

Pain Maps: A Tool for Surgeon and Patient

By Mary Lou Ballweg

As this surgical series was being prepared, one of our new staff members asked a question that has probably occurred to every woman with endo facing surgery: How do you know what kind of surgery you'll need (for instance, whether you have bowel endo and might need a general surgeon to assist the gynecologic surgeon)?

Basically, you don't know, because you don't know exactly what will be found in surgery, especially with your first surgery. But a number of things can help. First, of course, you want to choose a surgeon who is going to be able to handle a variety of endo problems. Since the surgeon doesn't know what will be encountered in surgery either, you want a surgeon who is fully prepared for whatever is found. As Dr. Jim Wheeler writes, "For most endometriosis cases, only a few of the pelviscopy instruments are usually needed. Unfortunately, one rarely knows how severe the case is likely to be prior to diagnostic laparoscopy; thus, we do request the full complement of pelviscopic instruments when endometriosis or adhesions are suspected."[1]

Second, to help reduce the unknowns when preparing for surgery, do a very careful job of recording your symptoms, preferably over three months. This will give you and the surgeon lots of hints as to where the problems might be. In this article we've reproduced a symptom chart developed by Dr. Arnold Kresch, Stanford University Medical Center, Palo Alto, California.

Third, some surgeons are now using a helpful tool called a *pain map*. This simple body grid, on which you record the precise locations of your pain, can suggest areas for the surgeon to especially focus on. Dr. Kresch, who developed the pain map, has used it extensively with patients and notes that it's uncanny how accurate patients are in pinpointing the sites of disease.

Using the pain map: Put numbers *1, 2, 3*, etc. (with the highest number representing the most pain and

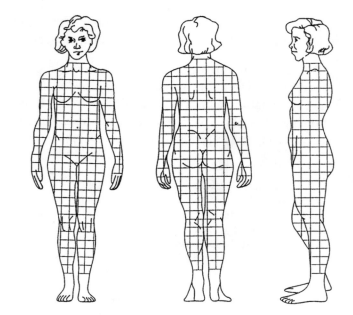

lower numbers representing least pain) in the boxes to show the location of your pain. Also, write a short description of the pain, what makes it worse and better, and your use of pain medications. Give this to your surgeon along with a copy of your symptom chart.

Symptom chart: If you have other symptoms besides the ones listed here, write them in on the side of the chart and mark the days for that symptom with a colored *X*. An additional symptom chart, which provides a more long-term view of symptoms, is provided in the association diagnostic kit, available from headquarters. (See page 15 for address and toll-free number.)

Note

1. J. M. Wheeler, "Macro- and Microsurgical Treatment of Endometriosis," *Modern Approaches to Endometriosis* (United Kingdom: Kluwer Academic Publishers, 1991), 189.

Day of Cycle	1	2	3	4	5	6	7	8	9	10	11	12	13	14	15	16	17	18	19	20	21	22	23	24	25	26	27	28	29	30	31
Date																															
Menses																															
Medications:																															
Cramps - Pelvic																															
Cramps - Other																															
Backache																															
Pelvic pain - Left																															
Pelvic pain - Right																															
Pelvic pain - Low middle																															
Pelvic pain - Other																															
Painful Bowel Movement																															
A. Before																															
B. During																															
C. After																															
Painful Sexual Intercourse																															
A. During																															
B. After																															
Urinary Problems																															
A. Pain																															
B. Urgency																															
C. Frequency																															
General Aches/Pains																															
Feeling the Blues																															
Feeling Depressed																															

Menses:
X = Menses
S = Spotting

For medications, list the initials and medications used:
_____ = _____
_____ = _____
_____ = _____

Grading of Symptoms and/or Complaints:
1 = Mild, but does not interfere with activities.
2 = Moderate and interferes with activities but not disabling.
3 = Severe and disabling, unable to function.

KRESCH Pain Analysis and Mapping

Choosing a Laparoscopic Surgeon

By Mary Lou Ballweg

Treating endometriosis through the laparoscope "takes a lot more surgical skill to perform than many gynecologists realize," notes an article in *Ob/Gyn News* citing experts Dr. Joseph Feste, an infertility specialist in private practice in Houston, and Dr. Camran Nezhat, Center for Special Pelvic Surgery in Atlanta. The two doctors discussed the issue at the Second International Symposium on Endometriosis in the spring of 1989.

Dr. Feste said there appears to be a relatively large pool of physicians who have an unrealistically high assessment of their own surgical expertise when it comes to endoscopy.

At one hospital only 10 of 50 ob.gyns. who indicated they thought they were ready to perform advanced operative laparoscopy qualified for privileges, according to the medical center's evaluation. In a similar survey at another institution, only 5 of 58 physicians who wanted to do the same met the standards necessary for using operative laparoscopy in the advanced stages.

TRH: testosterone replacement hormone

Another leading operative laparoscopist, Dr. Dan Martin, discusses a similar point:

> Laparoscopic laser techniques of excision have required significant time and effort to develop. The first case in this series [combining laparoscopy and colpotomy] was the author's 509th case of laser laparoscopy. With experience comes an increased ability to visualize a lesion throughout the dissection.

Dr. Martin goes on to indicate that without experience even recognition of the different types of tissue is not a given:

> Fibrotic endometriosis is whiter and has a firmer texture than does fat, which is yellow and soft. Loose connective tissue is easily dissected with a blunt probe. The recognition of these differences in tissue types has become easier with experience.

In spite of the extensive skill needed in the new technologies as well as a great understanding of endometriosis (including the varying visual appearances), professional groups have only recently begun addressing the issue of certifying or credentialing surgeons. This leaves laypeople in the distinctly uncomfortable position of attempting to evaluate surgeons themselves. Given the barrage of marketing information on the new technologies, practice-building information coming from many surgeons, and general confusion about endo itself, this is an uncomfortable position for all of us.

Added to all of these are the understandable fear and emotion involved in any surgical procedure (reasonable responses because any surgery, including operative laparoscopy, carries with it risks of complication, injury, or even death). We want desperately, of course, to trust our surgeon, and given the difficulty of evaluating a surgeon's skill, some women opt for total trust. Unfortunately, this has never worked very well in endometriosis!

Our suggestions for choosing the best surgeon for your endometriosis include, for starters, the following:

- Realize that you are dealing with a difficult area, not only in terms of the information you must come to grips with but also in terms of your own emotions, which are likely to make it harder to learn what you need to learn before proceeding with surgery. Give yourself time to do your homework. Ask for help from your association support group or chapter to feed back information and sort out fact and emotion. (Other women with endo have been there, and some will be extremely good at helping you with this!) Ask your partner or a trusted family member to assist you in this also.
- Ask questions! It is your right to ask as many questions as you need to feel comfortable before allowing an invasive procedure—after all, it is *your* body!
- Don't make snap decisions if at all possible. Women with endo who are not immediately facing surgery should learn as much as possible, because chances are all too good that they will face surgery in the future. The longer you have to prepare, the better.

- Remember that professionals share information from their own beliefs, training, and experience. Some results are in on the new techniques and are shared in this chapter, but many results are not in yet. Anyone who proclaims a real cure for endo must be regarded skeptically at this time.
- Two surgeons involved as members and supporters of the association (neither named in this chapter) put the preceding caution even more strongly: "It remains patently clear that, either as a result of misguided enthusiasm for particular treatment modalities or because of more venal, self-serving reasons, there exists misapplication of technology and medical therapy in the treatment of endometriosis. Exclusion by some practitioners of therapeutic approaches that may be equally or even more effective than those favored by a physician unwilling to objectively reassess his position is an exploitation of women that is to be deplored.
- "As we have discussed together before, too many of our colleagues take a two- or three-day course, laser a tongue or grapefruit, stick a laser laparoscope into a bunny rabbit for 15 minutes, and become experts."

Here are questions you need to ask about any surgeon you're considering for operative laparoscopy for endometriosis. There are many sources for this information: talks given by the surgeon or others from his or her practice to local association groups, flyers and brochures from the surgeon's practice, research studies in which the surgeon has participated, the surgeon's surgical nurse or office staff, other members of the association who know the practices of surgeons in the area, and association newsletters. If you are unable to obtain this information, by all means question the prospective surgeon. After all, it's *your* body going "under the knife."

1. *What surgical technologies does the surgeon use for endo?* Be aware that no one technology addresses all the needs in endometriosis, so if the surgeon describes only one approach, you need to be prepared to ask further questions. If the surgeon suggests use of medication to "clean up" what's left, are you comfortable with the fact that this almost certainly cannot eradicate all the endometriosis?

2. *What surgical* techniques *does the surgeon think are best for endo?* If your prospective surgeon uses a laser, be aware that excision is more difficult to learn than vaporizing/coagulating, and the technique described can give you a clue to the expertise of the surgeon. Besides becoming something of the preferred method for the removal of endo (not, of course, in all the implants), extensive use of excision can also tell you the surgeon is probably more skilled with the laser.

3. *Does the surgeon routinely send the removed implants to the pathology lab?* This indicates excisional techniques are being used where possible, and studies have shown that surgeons who routinely do this improve their recognition of the many appearances of endometriosis over time.

4. *Does the surgeon remove* all *the endo if at all possible?*

5. *How does the surgeon plan to treat lots of tiny implants on the peritoneum?* If he or she says that those small implants won't cause you any problems or says it takes too long to get them all, get another surgeon. Research shows that it's these implants that produce the most prostaglandin, which is strongly linked to the pain of endo. If the surgeon is not willing to spend the time to treat the disease, why bother having surgery?

6. *Does the surgeon think it is too dangerous to treat endo on bladder, bowels, etc.?* If the answer is yes, either the surgeon does not have the appropriate technology available or the surgeon is just beginning to learn the technology. The reason for great excitement about laser and other new technologies is precisely the ability to treat endo in these sensitive areas that for the most part cannot be treated with the older techniques.

7. *Is the surgeon aware of the work in recent years on the many appearances of endometriosis?* You might be able to ask what appearances he or she sees most often as an indirect way to get at this. Does the surgeon belittle these concepts? Find yourself a different surgeon! No surgeon willing to read the literature is likely to believe that the different appearances of endo do not matter.

8. *How many cases of endo with the surgical techniques the surgeon has described has he or she performed? Over what period of time has he or she performed these procedures?* Note whether the surgeon speaks enthusiastically about his or her work in this area—usually people who are good at what they do are enthusiastic about it. Dr. Camran Nezhat in the association's first book, *Overcoming Endometriosis*, states: "It takes at least one year of continuous practice of an average two to three cases a week (a total of 150 cases) before one is comfortable in videolaseroscopic or laser laparoscopic treatment of the disease."

9. *How long does the surgical approach typically take?* Depending on the procedures involved, there will be a range.

10. *May I have a copy of the surgeon's résumé or curriculum vitae?* This will outline the surgeon's training, credentialing, if any, special course work done with the new technologies, and research publications. Typically a surgeon who does primarily medical work will not have the extensive research publications that an academic physician or surgeon will have, so do not judge a potential surgeon solely on this basis. In fact, research publications are not proof of a surgeon's skill unless, perhaps, the physician's surgeries are being reported on in the publications. Even then, the surgeon's being published often depends on how well-known he or she is or on whom he or she knows, so again some caution is in order. Check for membership in professional organizations that have been at the forefront of the new research on surgical techniques for endometriosis. Leading in this area is the American Association of Gynecologic Laparoscopists. (Despite its name, it's a strongly international group.) Other groups include the Society of Reproductive Surgeons and the Gynecologic Laser Society, International Society for Gynecologic Endoscopy, and the American Board of Laser Surgery, Inc. In addition, membership in the Endometriosis Association helps show that the surgeon has a special interest in endometriosis.

11. *Has the surgeon done follow-up on his or her prior surgeries and for how long after the surgeries?* Ask detailed questions about the results related to pain relief and infertility. Again, be cautious, since numbers are extremely difficult to interpret in this field.

12. *How does the hospital, surgical center, and surgeon guarantee enough time for a case if it turns out to be a difficult one?* If enough time isn't allotted by either the hospital or the surgeon, the surgeon may feel great pressure to skip some of the endo or leave other loose ends (figuratively speaking) so that the next surgeon can get into the operating room. Or your own surgeon may need to get on to the next case or back to the office where patients are waiting. As Dr. David Redwine notes, "A typical case can take from one to four hours to accomplish, and a busy obstetrical practice can interfere with the time needed to treat endometriosis well."

13. *Does the surgeon provide the patient a written report, photographs, and/or a copy of a videotape of her surgery, and how complete is that videotape?* Be aware that most videotapes of surgeries are likely to be incomplete and/or edited. Still, a videotape record of the extent of the disease and procedures performed is a protection for you—you will be able to see the disease for yourself, see it treated for yourself, and have a permanent record for comparisons in the future.

14. *What measures does the surgeon take to help prevent adhesion formation?* See the article on adhesions at the end of this chapter for more information.

If you have preliminarily chosen a surgeon based on satisfactory answers to your questions, continue to evaluate the surgeon as you move along toward surgery:

1. *Did you feel the prospective surgeon listened carefully to you?* If not, you cannot be sure that he or she has clearly heard all symptoms and made notes on what those symptoms might mean surgically or understood completely your fertility wishes, concerns related to future treatment, or desires related to going on to (or *not* going on to) laparotomy in case of disease the surgeon may not be able to handle through the laparoscope.

2. *Did the prospective surgeon do a* very *thorough pelvic exam?* If not, you have to wonder if he or she is as concerned about deep nodules as you are or will be prepared to address them if found.

3. *Was your prospective surgeon as gentle as possible?* Despite the need for thoroughness, it is possible to be reasonably gentle in the pelvic exam. Of course, with endo and tender nodules, it *will* hurt, but a distinction can be made between this and a sloppy, roughshod approach. If the latter is used, you might well wonder if similar rough handling of tissues might occur during surgery, leading to more adhesion potential.

4. *Where does the surgeon think the endo is in your case and how would he or she handle it?* Pay particular attention to the manner in which the surgeon addresses sensitive areas such as the bladder, uterosacral ligaments, and the bowel. If endo is present on the bowels, does the surgeon work with a bowel surgeon if the endo goes deep? What kind of preliminary work-ups will be done to determine if the endo does go deep or to determine the nature of endo in sensitive areas?

A New Aid for Coping with the Emotions of Surgery

By Mary Lou Ballweg

So far in these articles on surgery we've covered mainly the new techniques, equipment, and procedures, and other medical aspects of the new surgeries for endometriosis. But in preparing these articles, I kept thinking about the emotional elements of coping with surgery. Facing surgery is hard! It's difficult to put into words the anxiety that most of us feel when facing surgery, even when we're well prepared and feel confident in our surgeon. In the weeks before surgery a certain anxious gloom pervades the mind at least part of the time, and it grows in the days just before the procedure. When I was facing surgery again (my fifth for endo), I was fortunate to find an aid that made this surgery far more emotionally manageable than my earlier surgeries.

At the American Association of Gynecologic Laparoscopists' annual meeting in November 1990, a study from the University of Massachusetts Medical School and the Fertility Institute of Western Massachusetts was presented on special relaxation audiotapes. In the study one group of patients used the tapes before going to the hospital, while under anesthesia, and in the recovery room, while another group of patients did not use the tapes. All the patients underwent diagnostic or operative laparoscopy. The patients using the tapes had significantly less pain and nausea following the operation, required less medication following the operation, and returned to full activity sooner than the other group.

According to the researchers, the tapes "consist of blended and sequenced sound patterns that promote 'whole brain thinking' or focused consciousness. The tapes are designed to create a condition in which portions of the electrical wave patterns (EEG) of both the left and right hemispheres of the brain are simultaneously equal in frequency and amplitude. This synchronicity is believed to enhance receptivity and relaxation." Another study reported in *The Lancet* 2, no. 8609 (August 27, 1988, p. 491) found that patients who listened to a relaxation tape during hysterectomy recovered more quickly with less fever and significantly fewer gastrointestinal problems than patients who listened to a blank tape.

Other studies have suggested that operating room sounds may be registered in the brain even though the patient is under general anesthesia and that these sounds may influence recovery. So, part of the effect of the tapes, besides putting positive, affirming, reassuring thoughts in the patient's head, may be that they block out operating room sounds and statements that could be disturbing. Because of these studies, some anesthesiologists now make gentle suggestions to the patient, such as telling her, still under anesthesia, that the operation is over and was a complete success and that she will be waking soon and will do well.

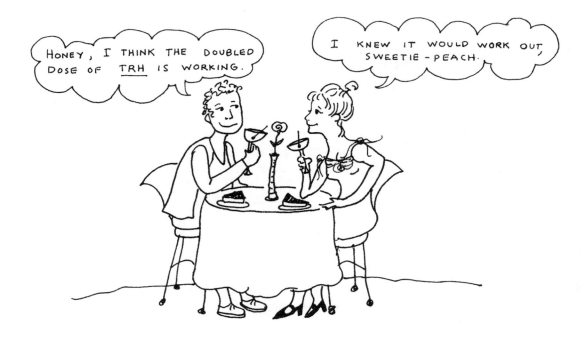

When I decided to try out the tapes used in the Massachusetts study and share the experiences with our members, who face so many operative laparoscopies, my doctor (my general practitioner) was supportive and gave me another article on the subject. I then contacted the Monroe Institute in Lovington, Virginia, a nonprofit educational and research organization devoted to understanding human consciousness and practical applications of this understanding, which produces the specialized tapes.

The set, called *Surgical Support Tapes*, included one tape for use before surgery, one for use during surgery, one for the recovery room, one for recuperation from surgery, one called *Energy Walk*, and one called *Surf*, recorded surf sounds. The brochure in the cassette holder said the series was "designed to assist individuals through a physical crisis such as major illness, traumatic injury, or surgery." It does so using the blended, sequenced sound patterns that are the result of research by Robert Monroe and colleagues at the institute. Their work has identified specific signals, called *binaural beats*, that are fed into each ear through stereo earphones to produce the synchronization of the left and right hemispheres of the brain mentioned earlier (which Monroe Institute calls *hemi-sync*). These audio signals help reduce "that constant psychological turmoil that people go through" with surgery, says one surgeon who has used them for his patients.

Binaural beats are not the same as the subliminal messages that some tapes advertise. *Subliminal* means that the message is not audible. On these tapes, in addition to the special modulated frequencies to control brain waves, the voice, if one is present, is audible. The voice on the Monroe Institute tapes is a very soothing one that encourages the listener to relax.

In tape one, the preop tape, the narrator takes the listener step by step through conscious relaxation, head to toe: *"First, let your jaw, let your jaw go limp and relax, let the muscles and nerves of your jaw go limp and relax. Now, your eyelids. Let your eyelids relax and go limp. Now, let your lips, let the muscles and nerves in your lips relax, relax easily and go limp. Now, the muscles in your forehead. . . ."* Chances are that by the end of this tape you're asleep or at the least very relaxed and no longer anxious. The instructions note that you should use the preop tape as many times as possible prior to surgery, both before and after admission to the hospital. I found this tape unbelievably soothing and used it many times. One night when I was finding it hard to sleep—I was anxious, and the foghorn sounding out on Lake Michigan bothered me—I started the tape in the hope that it would knock out the sound. It didn't, but it made me feel so good and so relaxed that I wasn't bothered by the foghorn anymore. After the surgery I realized that the tape did the same thing with the pain and discomfort—it was still there, but it didn't bother me, just as the tape said.

As I wrote at the time (Shirley Bliley of the Institute had suggested I keep notes on my use of the tapes):

> Several times anxiety hits me, and I listen to the preop or, a couple times, the intraop tape and find despite my thoughts still being somewhat anxious, I'm surprisingly calm and feel an inner peace. After a disconcerting doctor visit and as anxiety builds the night before, the tapes help.
>
> The morning of the surgery I listen to them at 5:15 A.M. on the way to the hospital. I listen waiting to be taken down to surgery and in the preop area. I discussed them with the anesthesiologist—he's very interested and more than willing to help by being sure the earphones stay on during surgery and replacing the intraop tape with the recovery room tape when I go into the recovery room.
>
> I woke in the recovery room to the soothing sounds of the recovery tape: *"Let the others help you restore your balance. . . .*
>
> *"You accept the green, blue, and purple healing energy that they are bringing to you; the bright, healing, warm energy they are giving to you. . . . The nerve signals of pain flow through you and do not register during this period now. . . ."*

It's a far better way to wake than my previous four surgeries, when I remember waking either to searing pain (in the laparotomies) or the dread feeling of not quite knowing where I was and being in a haze. The tape made me feel that although I was feeling pain, I would be able to manage it, and I was! It helped me feel I could manage until my blood pressure came up a little and they could give me an injection of Demerol.

Tuesday, the day after surgery: On the recuperation tape the soothing voice says that for now the pain signals are unimportant—helping you tone them down and hopefully sleep. I like that very much—it's a way to be aware of what's happening to your body so you can take necessary pain meds or rest or not try to do too much, yet at the same time not let the pain and discomfort messages take over. It helps impart or put you in touch with a wonderful sense of equilibrium.

Wednesday, the second day after surgery: I feel better but then become restless, a little blue, irritable about the music and voices upstairs—is this the third-day blues? I put the recuperation tape on and, despite my restlessness and inability to sleep, find a sense of peace and relaxation. It's amazing how effective these tapes are. As one woman wrote about her spleen surgery in the Monroe Institute newsletter—"Every sound and word took on a special therapeutic meaning."

Fifth day after surgery: So sore—I overdid yesterday! I felt so good I forgot I wasn't really ready to be out more than three hours or so. I feel *good*, though sore—just no energy. I want to read but just don't have the energy, not really tired enough to sleep, so I sew instead while listening to the postop tape. The soothing voice on *Energy Walk* guides me to imagine being on a beach, a grassy meadow, looking at my favorite tree at the end of the meadow. It's really quite beautiful.

These tapes seem to be designed by people who have been through this—I didn't know this is what I would need after the recuperation tape, but here it is and perfect for what I need today:

"You step into the grass, and you feel it soft and cool under your feet. You feel the living green of the grass, the energy of the grass; the green energy is very special. You need to feel much more of this balancing energy, of the green in the grass, so you drop down and lie in the cool green grass, lie down in the cool green grass, roll in it and feel a balancing freshening energy in the grass, feel it move throughout your entire self."

The tapes are also very useful in pain management. The recuperation tape is also sold separately under the title *Pain Control*. For information on purchasing the tapes, contact the association. (See "Additional Resources" at the back of the book.)

For surgical use of the tapes, be sure to use a handheld tape player or battery-operated headphones with automatic reverse so that the tape can keep playing no matter how long the surgery or recovery time.

Ethical Guidelines on Surgery for Endometriosis

By Veasy C. Buttram, Jr., M.D.

The integrity of the vast majority of infertility surgeons is beyond reproach. Most are honorable, honest individuals who use their skills to help patients with problems associated with the inability to bear children. However, a few surgeons are creating a major concern for all practitioners and their patients. This concern has been expressed at professional meetings and in editorials in medical journals. In fact the American Society for Reproductive Medicine (formerly the American Fertility Society) has formed a practice committee to consider such problems. Although unethical practices undoubtedly occur in other aspects of infertility surgery, some experiences reported by my patients suggest that violations of ethics are occurring in the treatment of endometriosis:

• An infertile woman who came to me shortly after laparoscopic laser surgery reported that her gynecologist had told her she had been treated for severe endometriosis. Subsequent review of her operative report showed clearly that her disease had been mild.

• Another infertile patient reported that her surgery for endometriosis had been performed by a gynecologist who claimed to be an infertility specialist when, in fact, he had no specialized training in infertility.

• In another patient laparoscopy had revealed the presence of endometriosis, but because the surgeon had been unable to perform the laparoscopic surgery, he referred her to a surgeon qualified to provide definitive treatment. Thus a second laparoscopy was required to deal with endometriosis that was easily eradicated.

• A fourth woman had been told she had a 90 percent chance of conception after major conservative surgery for endometriosis and pelvic adhesive disease. The surgeon had charged a fee of $8,000 and the assistant surgeon $1,600. The patient was told that the charges were increased because laser technology was used. Unfortunately, when the woman, still unable to conceive, underwent repeat laparoscopy by another surgeon, she was found to have extensive pelvic adhesions.

What can be done about those few surgeons whose unethical behavior jeopardizes the reputation of their peers and may actually harm the patient? It was to meet the need for guidelines for practice that the American Society for Reproductive Medicine board of directors formed the Practice Committee. To ensure that such guidelines help to resolve many of these problems, the committee will need input and support from all members, affiliated societies, and special interest groups.

In a lecture called "Principles of Conservative Surgery for Endometriosis" presented at the Second International Symposium on Endometriosis, I proposed five guidelines related specifically to treatment of the disease:

1. No surgeon should misrepresent his or her credentials or qualifications. No surgeon should even attempt to perform laparoscopy or laparotomy without having the skills to accomplish the surgery safely and to avoid unnecessary risk of adversely affecting the patient's future fertility.
2. No surgeon should perform a laparoscopy without the skills and surgical tools to resolve all cases of minimal and most cases of mild endometriosis that might be found.
3. No surgeon unable to successfully remove endometriosis at the time of laparoscopy or laparotomy should overstate the results of his or her attempts to resolve the problem.
4. No surgeon should *overstage* endometriosis or claim that it has reached a more severe stage than it has, to make his or her results appear more impressive.
5. No surgeon should charge exorbitant fees for endometriosis surgery. The additional training required to become skilled in the surgical treatment of endometriosis does not justify extraordinary fees.

These guidelines pertain only to one aspect of fertility surgery. The newly formed Practice Committee, to be successful, must address all areas of infertility surgery and gain the support of all society members.

■ *Dr. Veasy (Bill) Buttram, Jr.,* Houston, Texas, has been a leader in the field of endometriosis. Now retired, he was an active leader in the American Fertility Society and a member of the clinical faculty at Baylor College of Medicine.

Decision Making on Surgery

By Mary Lou Ballweg

Recently I had the opportunity (even though it was not initially perceived as one!) to test the results of my work with the Endometriosis Association. What I learned was tremendously gratifying—that because of the sharing among association members and our research, we now have options and information previously unavailable.

In 1982 I had decided on a hysterectomy and removal of my remaining ovary because I'd exhausted all other options. My "miracle" child was 6 months old, and I wasn't willing to let endo, which had made me bedridden before, destroy my ability to care for and enjoy her. Following that surgery, I had 8½ years of endo relief (although I struggled with candidiasis and related problems) before joint pain and other problems led to an increase in my estrogen dose to a still-low .625 milligram in the summer of 1990. By November some unwelcome, familiar symptoms had become part of my life.

Because of all that I had learned from the Endometriosis Association, I knew that the disease could return and I knew I would have to act. (If we could just teach surgeons to remove the endo too when a hysterectomy and removal of the ovaries is done for severe disease, we could prevent some of this!) In the process of making my decisions, it was very rewarding to learn that what we've taught all along worked well in my own situation.

The importance of paying attention to your body and believing in your ability to read your own body was reinforced. As much as I wanted to believe it couldn't be happening again, I knew my years of listening to women with endometriosis—as well as my own past experiences—were going to force me to pay attention. So I sought the help of a new general physician who I knew was open to acting as a consultant, working *with* the patient, reinforcing her own sense of her body and providing technical help and encouragement rather than simply telling her what to do. When I hoped against hope that the various tests would show something other than endo, he reminded me that I already knew, from paying attention to my body and from having done my homework, what was most important and that the tests were not likely to give us new information. He was exactly right.

The importance of doing your homework now *and not waiting for a crisis.* I was shocked at how quickly my symptoms reemerged and at the speed with which some alarming bowel dysfunction arose. Only the combination of my past reading and talking with women with endo, close attention to my own endo history, and ruthless honesty with myself about what was happening enabled me to move as quickly as I did. If I had not already done that "homework," I would have experienced delays while I tried to obtain needed background and information from my medical records, from the EA, and from doctors.

In fact, if I hadn't been well informed, I might not have known what types of medical helpers I needed, what tests were likely to be needed, and which of my past medical records were needed. I could not have predicted the way things would flare up, and only because of the broad range of endo stories I've heard could I make sense out of my symptoms.

Go to local meetings, focus on the needs you have now, but also try to learn what happens to others with endo. You never know when that information will help you in the future as endo follows its poorly understood course. Read our books, special and collected articles and newsletters, and listen to our conference audiotapes even if you think some of the topics don't apply to you. Again, you never know when important bits of information are going to give you just the clue you need for your own situation.

Had I not done my homework in advance, I could easily have been a victim of disastrous medical advice. I could have been subjected to a whole new round of "in your head" approaches—since I'm so many years posthysterectomy, most doctors would never believe my symptoms could be endo again, and, as is so often the case, when other tests prove normal, the doctors often imply that the symptoms are not related to endo or perhaps are not really even happening. Also, without my own knowledge base to help guide my physicians and me through the process, I could have ended up going through totally pointless surgical procedures.

My greatest fear, once I realized what was going on, was that my symptoms might lead to an emergency surgery involving people who are not endo specialists and might not recognize the endo—in other words, a needless surgery. Only my own homework on endo and surgery for the disease done before the crisis occurred provided that important information.

I could not have predicted what would happen, but I was ready—I strongly encourage you, too, not to assume your own endo will follow certain paths but to prepare yourself for a variety of possibilities. One of the best ways to do this, besides following the association's education materials, is to listen to the stories of other women with endo: attend local meetings, be part of a correspondence network, order a contact list of other members and get to know some of them (see "Additional Resources" at the back of the book). You'll be surprised at the many roads endo takes, and you'll prepare yourself by thinking through what you would do if your endo took a particular course.

The importance of **individually** *coming to the best decision for yourself, a concept* *we have emphasized since our beginnings in 1980.* My symptoms emerged in a peculiar way (pain and intestinal bleeding when going off hormones and feeling I was having a period with all the nausea, cramping, hot/cold flushes, and "sickening" feeling I remembered!) but with new twists—bloating, nausea, days without intestinal function or bowel movements, lumps in my abdomen at night; a sick, blocked feeling when on hormones. (Some of these problems I now believe were caused not only by the irritation of the endo but also by a malfunctioning thyroid—due to Hashimoto's thyroiditis—and to severe food allergies. With almost a year of treatment these problems have been greatly alleviated.) Because of my particular symptoms and other needs related to hormone replacement (being so many years posthysterectomy, I felt doing without replacement hormones was not a good option), I decided to move quickly to surgery to remove the endo. I chose a surgeon based on the surgeon's ability to do extensive bowel work through the scope if necessary to avoid possible bowel adhesions, which tend to occur with bowel surgery done with laparotomy.

Also, I was determined that this fifth surgery for my endo would be my last. So, I was very concerned that the surgeon I chose be acutely aware of the various appearances of endo, which in my case might be neither typical nor in the typically recognized locations (or the locations on which many fertility-oriented specialists seem to focus). And I wanted someone *committed* to removing it all. From the many women with endo I talk with and whose letters I read, I knew all too well that many surgeons convince themselves that endo in locations they were not trained to address can be or has to be left! We simply must teach those doing surgery for endo that they must prepare themselves to deal with all of the endo, wherever it is, or be willing to refer. These very specific requirements made choosing a surgeon much easier—I knew what questions to ask. (Fortunately for me, I did not require invasive bowel surgery. Lesions on my colon and in my cul-de-sac were handled through the scope.)

This time around was much easier than in the early eighties because my health insurance was no longer an HMO. Once again, the extreme importance that women with endo not have restricted insurance coverage was brought home to me! (In the United States, this means not accepting HMO coverage or other plans that require you to see a particular group of physicians—and don't be swayed by the promises that "if you need it" you'll be referred to specialists. The need for specialists for endo is not yet well recognized—most gynecologists believe they can treat endo and resist women going to the surgeons and others who have experience with hundreds of patients with endo, which is what it seems to take to begin to get a handle on this puzzling disease! In Canada and other countries with government payment plans this means continuing efforts to allow women to go outside their provinces or areas when needed!)

I also was not destitute as I had been when long bouts of being bedridden had drained my savings in 1980. Having the financial resources to take care of myself made everything more tolerable.

I realized that my choice was completely individualized, and that's exactly what the EA has taught—that each of us is the best person to make decisions about our own body as long as we do our homework and work through a careful decision-making process. We should not make decisions based on what others do or even on what our physician wishes, especially if the physician has a particular way of treating endo. So, please don't call us and ask what surgeon I chose—there is no one-size-fits-all approach to endo! Your own situation must determine your decisions.

How to Donate Your Own Blood
for Use in Surgery

"The chances of contracting AIDS through a transfusion of blood are statistically the same as those of being struck by lightning," said Ron Franzmeier, former director of blood service operations of the Blood Center of Southeastern Wisconsin. Still, some women with endo are taking no chances at all and donating their own blood for use during or after surgery.

According to the blood center, the first step is to tell your doctor that you want to donate your own blood to be used, if necessary, during surgery. The doctor must call the blood center with (1) the date of surgery, (2) the number of units requested, and (3) whether whole blood or packed red blood cells are needed.

Accordingly an appointment is set up for the blood donation at the blood bank. The blood volume in your body is quickly replaced, but it is probably wise to give the blood a couple weeks ahead of the surgery rather than a couple days ahead. As described in our first book in the articles "Overview of Surgery in the Treatment for Endometriosis" and "Coping with the Hospital Experience," you probably should prepare for the stress of surgery with nutritious food, plenty of rest, exercise if possible, and quitting smoking if possible (because it may increase the risks associated with anesthesia). Planning your self-donation of blood well in advance is another logical part of this preparation.

The blood can be kept for 35 to 42 days after donation in the hospital blood bank where surgery will take place. If for some reason surgery has to be rescheduled you'll have to redonate. Even if you cannot donate to others because of some condition like a prior case of hepatitis, you can self-donate.

The same procedures would apply in most other parts of North America, but to make sure of the procedure in your own area, it is best to check with your doctor—and the closest *nonprofit* blood bank or the Red Cross. You must use a nonprofit blood bank or blood center because of the necessity for a doctor's authorization. Plasma centers will charge and will not bank your blood for your procedure or surgery.

Hysterectomy and Endometriosis: Overview

By Mary Lou Ballweg

"*A*fter four surgeries within a period of a year and a half, I feel I have finally reached some level of being able to cope with the disease. I consented to a hysterectomy with right oopherectomy. Six months after the surgery I began feeling the constant pain I had experienced prior to the hysterectomy. After three minor operations and one major surgery, I felt I needed to seek advice from an expert in the field. Upon examination, he found a mass on my left side and proceeded with surgery. I had severe pelvic adhesions, and endometriosis was found in various areas of the pelvic cavity.*

"*I felt very disappointed that I had undergone major surgery in the hopes that it would cure the disease. I must encourage those who have been diagnosed with endo to seek expert medical advice. There are many avenues to explore before undergoing major surgery for endometriosis. Hysterectomy is definitely not a cure. I strongly recommend those with endometriosis educate themselves about the disease, explore and evaluate all possible treatments available.*"

Sue, California

"*T*he Endometriosis Association has been a great help to me. I wish I had known so much more before than I did when my troubles came to crisis. I would like to share my horrors with you, and then tell you what I have been able to do to cope.*

"*I am 43 and had terrible menstrual cramps from about a year after menarche (14). For 28 years I was told the usual 'You are a woman, so of course you have to suffer,' was told nothing was the matter, was told to get more exercise (didn't help), etc. In 1987 my right ovary was found to be very enlarged, and I accepted that it had to be removed. My gynecologist said there were several possible reasons for its condition and warned me that if I had cancer she would do a complete hysterectomy and remove the other ovary as well. She skated over the possibility of endo, but thanks to your wonderful newsletters I now know that I had every symptom of endo and that it ought to have been diagnosed and treated years ago.*

"*When I woke from the anesthetic for the surgery (in agony!), I learned that she had removed both ovaries and done a complete hysterectomy—without consulting me. I was totally unprepared in body, mind, or spirit. I now know that I could have been treated with drugs first and then if necessary submitted to surgery as a last resort. The last year has been the worst of my life. I must add that I have a new gynecologist!*

"*My six postoperative months with no replacement hormones were ghastly, but I certainly didn't want my endo back again. At the end of the six months I was prescribed estrogen and progesterone in the usual cycle of 25 days for the former and 11 days for the latter.*

Being forced back into a pseudo-menstrual cycle was very unpleasant (PMS, depression, bloating, etc.), and I decided that this would not do.

"During the course of the year I talked several times with a friend who is a gynecologist and who had had endo resulting in the same surgery. She suggested that I get my gynecologist to prescribe methyltestosterone, since ovaries make testosterone as well as the 'female' hormones we all know about and that if I could tolerate it (she hadn't been able to stand the 'acne' she developed), it would give me a great boost.

"I had a great battle to get methyltestosterone, but I won. (Why, why, why do we have to know more about the subject than the physicians do?) It has changed my life. It is wonderful. I take 10 milligrams daily. And I persuaded my gynecologist to let me take estrogen daily (.625 milligram) and progesterone daily (2.5 milligrams) as well. I could see no sense (and neither did she eventually) in forcing my body into a senseless cycle. This way I have no unpleasant effects from the progesterone, but I am protected from breast cancer (if that study is right) by having the estrogen opposed by the progesterone. And the testosterone gives me energy and physical strength. My dry skin is gone, my sex drive back to normal. I sleep much better. I have had none of the side effects that I was warned about, such as growing more hair or having my voice deepen. I have never been a hairy person—another reason for wondering if my testosterone level was low before. It is really great. I feel for the first time in a long time that all of my 'switches' are working and on. I hope that other women who have undergone surgical menopause can persuade their physicians to let them take the three hormones. I don't know how to say strongly enough that I feel completely different from how I felt before I got onto this regime. . . ."

Ellen, Rhode Island

EDITOR'S NOTE: We do not know if continuous estrogen and progesterone use is a good approach for women with endo. We share Ellen's letter as an example of someone adapting her hormone protocol to her individual needs.

"November will be the fifth anniversary of my hysterectomy and removal of my ovaries because of endometriosis. I suffered daily with the disease for five years up to that point. What began as a catch in my side blossomed into a full-fledged, incapacitating illness. When it became bad enough to seek help, I went from doctor to doctor, explaining it as a ripping pain in my side. The responses I received varied from 'How's your home life?' to 'Wait until it gets worse.' I finally found a doctor who knew what the problem was. I was so relieved—I thought my problems would be over. Then I started researching, and the more I read, the more I realized what an incurable disease I had.

"I had laparoscopies to gauge the extent of the disease—implants on the rectum, bladder, ovaries, intestines, and uterus. I tried the birth control pill route—I never could take them; the side effects were too strong (fluid, mood changes, so uncomfortable). I tried six

months of danazol therapy—probably the second-worst six months of my life. All it did was postpone the inevitable.

"I was 25 when the symptoms had progressed to the point where I sought help. . . . My doctor told me something had to be done. The endometriosis was on my cervix. He even let me look at it with a mirror—it looked like a large blood blister. I told him I would try birth control pills again, but he told me it might be too late for that. I insisted, and after one month of symptoms I realized it was time for my decision. I read everything I could—pro and con. I wished I could keep even just a piece of my ovary, but I knew that I couldn't if I wanted to be free of the disease.

"My doctor spent an hour one evening with me and my husband answering all our questions, and I was scheduled for the surgery two days before Thanksgiving.

"I have to backtrack and say that my husband and I had decided not to have children, so that was not an issue. I am so glad we made that decision, because I think it had already been made for us even when we were first married. Throughout everything we maintained a good relationship, although I must admit that I could feel him losing patience with me as the disease wore on.

"So I had a hysterectomy. Eighteen days after the surgery my world fell apart. That must have been when my estrogen level dropped. I had prepared myself, but I never expected the strength of both the physical and mental consequences of my decision.

"I shook, I cried, I felt light-headed, my skin crawled—I felt like I couldn't survive another minute, let alone the rest of my life. I'd [be] calm for a few minutes, and then I'd have those spells again. The next six months were a nightmare with hot flashes and anxiety attacks.

"I survived. I learned to act. I took antidepressants, which seemed to help. I went back to work, and I suffered the humiliation of incapacitating hot flashes when my face would turn beet red and my eyes would burn. I understood hot flashes—I read anything I could get my hands on. I really learned to hide all that I felt inside, but I couldn't disguise the flush.

"I hid my problems so well that I even got a promotion to a supervisory job. Only my family and close friends knew I was still having problems. . . . I'm almost 35 now, but mentally I feel much older. When I was suffering, I used to look older, but now I'm looking better. I've lost 30 pounds (I didn't gain any after surgery—this weight was what I put on when I was inactive). I have more energy and ambition. . . . I resent the disease and aftermath for stealing time from me. My only hope is that from now on I will be healthy and at peace with my body.

"I am happy with my decision to have the hysterectomy even though it brought its own problems. It seems the surgery shifted the pain from physical to mental. . . .

"Although I no longer suffer with the disease, I still feel its effects, and that's why I joined your association. I wish you had been there years ago. Thanks for listening."

Linda, New York

"This letter is in response to your request to hear from those of us who have taken estrogen replacement with androgens. I began taking Premarin immediately after hysterectomy and removal of the ovaries. The first 1.25-milligram tablet literally appeared on my food tray the day after surgery along with my clear broth. I continued to take 1.25 milligrams of Premarin daily for 26 months.

"The first year I felt great. Then I began experiencing hematuria [blood in the urine], very light at first, then heavier. I felt no pain, and after about six months the intermittent hematuria disappeared. Five months later it came back with a vengeance and this time with that old familiar pain of endometriosis. An outpatient surgical procedure confirmed that I did indeed have endometriosis in the bladder; some implants were "zapped," providing very temporary relief. Within a few weeks the hematuria became gross with large clots and incredible pain. I stopped the Premarin, and after about a week the hematuria subsided.

"That was last October. Since that time no estrogen has entered this body, and no pain or hematuria has been experienced. At age 39 I am cheerfully enduring surgical menopause. Advice I would have for other members: never, never consent to estrogen replacement therapy without first giving your body plenty of time after hysterectomy."

Gail, Texas

Seldom in the history of the association has a topic been as hard to write about and edit as this one. Paula Zimlicki, past president of the Boston chapter, and I slaved over these articles—researching, interviewing, drafting, revising, going back and forth to references time and again on the hormones, and carrying on endless discussions on the topics covered as we tried to sort everything out.

Why was this topic so difficult? The reason saddened me: in the area of hysterectomy, removal of the ovaries, surgical menopause, and hormone replacement, women with endo are unique. A lot of information is available, but it is almost totally inapplicable to women with endo, so it creates far more confusion than exists even in other areas related to endo. So much of the research literature, for instance, is quoted in books written for laypeople (often by doctors) without even clearly indicating whether the women in particular studies had their ovaries removed.

In addition, people use their personal biases about hysterectomy and their lack of understanding of endo to create even more turmoil and pain for women with endo. For instance, those who do not understand the lifelong repercussions of hysterectomy and removal of the ovaries will learn that the only hope for a (supposedly) definitive end to endo, when all else has failed, is hysterectomy and removal of the ovaries and then inquire why a woman who has been severely affected with endo doesn't just go have a hysterectomy. The agony of making that last-resort decision seems hard for some people to understand. (Maybe sharing "Joe with Endo," the young male cartoon character who faces castration, might help some of these people understand.)

Others are very much attuned to the seriousness of hysterectomy and removal of the ovaries as well as the very many unnecessary hysterectomies performed for reasons ranging from fibroids and prolapse of the uterus to overgrowth of the inside lining of the uterus. But they seem so intent on believing there is *no* reason, short of a life-threatening problem such as cancer, for having a hysterectomy that they apply this thinking to endo without ever understanding the tremendous devastation endo can cause in women's lives. As one woman who opted for hysterectomy said, with endo she didn't *have* a life. Both sides take such a simplistic approach to endo and the hysterectomy issue that it made me feel all over again the lonely struggle of women with endo to be understood. How much we women with endo need each other!

Because I agree so wholeheartedly with those who are struggling to end unnecessary hysterectomy, I find it particularly frustrating to see the lack of understanding of endo by those working in this important area of women's health. One of the most disappointing examples in this regard is the book *No More Hysterectomies* by Vickie Hufnagel, M.D. (New York: NAL Penguin, 1988). We appreciate Dr. Hufnagel's work in promoting the concept of reconstructive surgery of the female organs rather than just removing them, in helping to compile a very valuable report on hysterectomy produced by the U.S. Department of Health and Human Services, and in getting a pioneering law in place in California. The law requires California surgeons to inform hysterectomy patients of the risks due to hysterectomy and of alternatives. But when it comes to her chapter on endometriosis, I nearly cried. She states that the number of hysterectomies for endo has increased 176 percent from 1965 to 1984 (no mention is made of the greatly increased diagnoses of endo during that time) "despite the fact that successful surgical techniques and drugs which can conserve organs have been developed during the last 20 years."

Statements like these imply that there now are truly successful treatments for endometriosis that end the disease and that hysterectomy for endo is no longer necessary. (If *only* it *were* true!) These statements also give little sense of the difficulty involved in many of the treatments for endometriosis and imply that danazol and other drug therapies are easy to tolerate and a woman with endo can just take them and be done with the endo, like taking antibiotics for an infection. It makes the treatment and control of endo seem so simplistic that friends and family of women with endo reading this chapter are likely to think that stubborn continuation of the disease and difficulties tolerating danazol and other hormones are peculiarities of that woman or, worse yet, evidence of a tendency to hypochondria on her part rather than typical of stubborn symptomatic endometriosis.

The author does discuss doing a laparoscopy six months to a year after initial surgery and lasering implants at that time, as well as repeating drug therapy if necessary, so it seems she has encountered the stubborn nature of endo in at least some patients. And Dr. Hufnagel does list and recommend folic acid (a B vitamin), vitamin B_6, essential fatty acids, evening primrose oil, and other minerals and herbs. We hope she continues to recommend and use these substances, which we described in greater detail in our first book, *Overcom-*

ing Endometriosis. But the overall tone of the chapter is that hysterectomy for endo is not necessary. This is a terrible burden for women with endo who have been through every possible current treatment, not once but many times, and who can no longer engage in the work of their choice, have sex without pain, plan social lives, dig themselves out of poverty, or get on with their lives and their dreams.

I agree so completely with her conclusions about hysterectomy in general that it's hard to have to disagree with this author on her endo chapter. But it's just this experience—of finding that even people on "our" side, who really care about women and their health, don't understand endo—that makes the endo experience and especially hysterectomy related to it so lonely.

Another reason for the sadness is the overwhelming frustration in the realization, brought home once again, of just how far short hysterectomy and removal of the ovaries falls even as a last resort. How do we get the message across that even at the point of hysterectomy women with endo need top-notch endometriosis specialists? You may hear the thinking that any trained gynecologist can go in and remove a uterus and ovaries, and that's true. But if that's all that's done for you, chances are all too great you'll still have endo, especially if you take hormones right away.

We've learned too many times, from the heartbreak of our members, that endo is a stubborn, persistent disease. To leave traces of endo behind on the peritoneum, cul-de-sac, bowel, and so on, and think they will just disappear because the ovaries are gone is wishful thinking. And to blithely reassure the patient "I got it all" without having done, as one doctor in the next article describes as a "religious" examination, is also wishful (and ignorant) thinking.

To tell a patient with endo that she needs hormones right away because of the risk of osteoporosis—before being sure the endo is gone—is like telling someone recovering from skin cancer to expose herself to sunlight to get the vitamin D to prevent rickets! Women with endo whose ovaries are removed early are indeed at serious risk for osteoporosis, and the greatest bone loss occurs in the five or six years following menopause. But, based on the tragic stories of some of our members, not completely ridding the body of all endo first actually *increases* the risk for osteoporosis. This is because, if the endo continues or returns, the woman will face double estrogen depletion. She will more than likely not only be taken off estrogen but also be put on an estrogen-depleting or blocking drug such as danazol. She could, in the worst-case scenario, end up with both endo and osteoporosis.

Finally, the best surgeon possible is necessary, first to remove all endo possible and second because careless surgical techniques, such as poor placement of the sutures closing the vagina where the cervix used to be or shortening the length of the vagina, can mean painful intercourse even for women who didn't have it before. See the surgery articles earlier in this chapter for information on the new laparoscopically-assisted hysterectomy surgical techniques.

The only way women with endo can protect themselves at this point is to learn all they can about endo—not just from books but also from other women with endo; to choose the very best endo specialist they can (we know all too well the limits insurance places on this); and perhaps to forgo estrogen replacement for a short time after hysterectomy and removal of the ovaries. The last is a protection against the microscopic traces of disease that may have been unrecognized or endo on the bowel and bladder that the gynecological surgeon was not prepared to handle. (For more on bowel endo, see Chapter 4; on urinary tract endo, see Chapter 5.)

Still, there are signs of progress and hope. For some lucky women who are not too far away from menopause and who have endo that is not too severely symptomatic, laparoscopic techniques used by endo specialists offer the hope of buying time every few years, if necessary, up to menopause. Also, the truth is finally being told about hysterectomy so those facing it have a better handle on what they may be facing. The biggest change in this area has been on the subject of sexuality after hysterectomy, something that was long a closed-door subject. When our former advisor, medical sociologist Susanne Morgan, published her book *Coping with a Hysterectomy* in 1982, she included a chapter on sexuality that acknowledged that many, if not most, women experienced distinct changes, often negative, after hysterectomy. This was a breakthrough, the first time the truth was told in a book. The fact that she dared label removal of the ovaries castration (the medical term for removal of the testicles or ovaries) was also a breakthrough. Now quite a number of books have elaborated on this, and women are more open on the subject. (Books before that, some written by doctors, assured women that any change in their sexuality, even after removal of the ovaries, was purely psychological!)

Thinking about what would be needed *now, today*, to avoid hysterectomy for endo was also one of the things that made preparing this chapter so hard. For ultimately the crux of the issue is that we simply are not diagnosing endo soon enough to avoid hysterectomy today. In all too many cases, by the time the endo is diagnosed, the disease has been active for 10 to 15 years or more and is so entrenched that the woman is already well on her way to a hysterectomy. Because any hope of controlling the disease with current methods of treatment (which cannot yet cure) is to gain the upper hand *before* massive involvement occurs, adhesions proliferate, the stubborn cycle of inflammation and symptoms is in place, and distorted anatomy has taken its toll, only earlier diagnosis will provide any possibility of avoiding hysterectomy.

And yet that appears to be the toughest problem of all. If only we could diagnose the disease at 15, when symptoms are beginning for those who are probably going to have the most severe disease, perhaps the woman would not be infertile at 25 and facing hysterectomy and removal of the ovaries in her thirties.

How many women have hysterectomies due to endo? According to a report from the U.S. Department of Health and Human Services, hysterectomies for endometriosis rose 176 percent from 1965 to 1984 and 120 percent from 1970 to 1984. The terrible impact on young women can be seen in the fact that there has been an even greater increase in hysterectomies for endo among them: a 250 percent increase for females aged 15 to 24 between 1965 and 1984 and a 186 percent increase for women aged 25 to 34 in those years. (Analysis of data on younger women was provided by Dr. Gary Berger, Chapel Hill, North Carolina.)

While medical reports on this study have found this jump unexplainable, it seems perfectly logical to us, given the lack of attention to and diagnosis of endo in the 1960s and 1970s. In fact, until the widespread use of the laparoscope in the late 1970s (even when the association was getting started in the early eighties, it was not used by some gynecologists), diagnosis of endo was far more difficult to obtain than today. (And we know how hard it can be to get diagnosed even today!) Frequently a woman wasn't diagnosed at all unless the disease was affecting her job so severely that she was willing to go into major surgery, which might result in a hysterectomy, before finding out what was wrong.

In terms of actual *numbers* of hysterectomies for endometriosis, nearly 1.5 million hysterectomies were performed for endo from 1970 through 1984 in the United States! Why has this disease been neglected for so long?! Nearly 10 million (9.8 million) hysterectomies were performed for all reasons from 1970 to 1984.*

A further breakdown shows 136,000 women had hysterectomies for endo in the years 1965 to 1967; 202,000 in 1970 to 1972; 263,000 in 1973 to 1975; 289,000 in 1976 to 1978; 321,000 in 1979 to 1981; and 375,000 in 1982 to 1984, the last years for which data is analyzed. However, even more telling is that endo as the reason for hysterectomy increased from 9.8 percent of hysterectomies in 1965 to 1967 to 18.7 percent of hysterectomies in 1982 to 1984. To truly know whether the rate of hysterectomy for endo is increasing we would need good comparable data on diagnosis for the same years. Unfortunately, as the authors of this study point out, gathering the data on endo was the most difficult because it was found in four different diagnostic coding systems, one of which also included adenomyosis (a disorder in which the inside lining of the uterus grows into the wall of the uterus, sometimes causing heavy, painful periods). So we still need far better data to be sure of what is happening—as usual with endo.

Are there unnecessary hysterectomies for endo? Unfortunately, yes, but not usually for the reason people opposed to hysterectomy think. It's not that the woman having a hysterectomy today for endo hasn't had other treatments that failed. Rather, it's that if only she had been diagnosed *earlier* and treated adequately by a physician who understood the nature of endo (which at this point seems to be something only a few doctors in any major city do), she *might* not be having that hysterectomy today. (It would still take some luck on top of that good care, though.) We spend years being told our symptoms and problems are in our heads and then, within a few years of diagnosis, are told the very same symptoms are so severe that there's nothing left to do about them except have a hysterectomy and removal of the ovaries. Obviously, all women with endo and those who care about them need to keep working and supporting our efforts to change this!

---

* An interesting footnote: The highest rate of hysterectomy was in the southern United States, where women who had hysterectomies were likely to have had them at an earlier age.

Hysterectomy: The Loneliest Decision of All

By Paula M. Zimlicki

Hysterectomy—the very word conjures up dreadful images for most women with endometriosis. Many women wonder how a hysterectomy will affect their sexuality, their emotional state, whether one ovary should be left in, whether hormone replacement therapy is necessary. These are just a few of the questions women ask.

When a woman is diagnosed with endometriosis, she experiences some degree of loss of control over her life. When a woman chooses to have a hysterectomy, it is usually because her endo pain has taken over her life. In many cases having a hysterectomy is the only means by which she can get on with living. Hysterectomies are most often contemplated by women who have tried surgery, hormonal therapy, pain medications, and alternative treatments, all without success.

The medical definition of hysterectomy is surgical removal of the uterus. Many women with endometriosis also have their ovaries and fallopian tubes removed, a procedure referred to as *hysterectomy with bilateral salpingo-oophorectomy.*

Of all the decisions women with endometriosis have to face, one of the loneliest is deciding whether to have a hysterectomy and removal of the ovaries. Women facing this decision enter the unknown to a certain degree because the operation affects persons in different ways and you will not know until after surgery exactly how it has affected your body.

Two questions seem to be asked most frequently of a woman who has opted for a hysterectomy: how did she decide, and how was she affected sexually? How do you know when you're ready for a hysterectomy? Are you ever totally prepared? In the fall of 1987 the association published in its newsletter a request that women who have had hysterectomies write and tell their stories. The quotes in this article are taken from the responses we received.

Althea, a woman who lives in the Northeast, in her midthirties at the time, recalls that her pain increased to the point where she missed several days of work each month. Advancement in her career was impossible.

She writes, "I am very lucky that I am good at what I do, have achieved some notoriety, and would be hard to replace. Even so, the situation with missing so much time and being sick when I was there was getting sticky, along with my life being miserable, so I realized it was either my uterus or me.

"In other words, I had to lose the battle to win the war. The agony for me was reaching this decision and closing the book on children. After the fact I feel relieved, liberated."

Most women have found it is their responsibility to inform themselves as much as possible about the issues when facing a hysterectomy. If you are faced with this decision, try to research all of its dimensions. Many women have found they cannot, unfortunately, rely on their physicians to do this for them. A common theme that runs through the stories of women with endo facing hysterectomy is the often-conflicting information doctors give women and what they read on their own.

Elise, from the Midwest, writes, "My appointment with the gynecologist was a nightmare. After a brief description of the history of a painful left ovary at a certain time of the month for many years, the recent vaginal pain with intercourse, and the recurrence of bleeding after intercourse, plus the current cyst on my right ovary, he diagnosed me as having endometriosis, which required drug treatment with bad side effects or a hysterectomy.

"Needless to say, I was overwhelmed! I had never even heard of endometriosis. Drugs? Hysterectomy? I was only 30 years old!"

As Elise discovered, being told you may need a hysterectomy is a shock. No woman should have a hysterectomy as a treatment of first choice. Surgery and/or drug treatments should be tried first. A hysterectomy should be only a last resort.

Making the decision to have one is the issue that concerns most women who have unrelenting endometriosis. If you are fortunate, your gynecologist presents you with many options before you ever reach the stage of having a hysterectomy. Women who are able to make this decision for themselves, rather than waking from surgery and discovering the physician made the choice for them, recover better from a hysterectomy.

Dr. Dub Howard of Carrollton, Texas, one of the association's advisors, said in an interview that women have to cross that "invisible barrier" of knowing emotionally they have reached the end of their tolerance in dealing with this disease and of knowing also that they can have a good quality of life after surgery.

As president of the Boston chapter, I spoke to hundreds of women, and it has been my experience that the women who are happiest with their decision to have a hysterectomy are those who have tried whatever surgeries and treatments are available but whose endo has always returned full-force. These women have informed themselves of all the facts concerning their disease.

Althea, the 34-year-old woman quoted earlier, says, "I think anyone contemplating a hysterectomy needs to make the decision alone and not be pressured into it. For me, I had to hit bottom before I would do it. I think when one is ready to let go and then does so, she can live with the consequences."

Althea makes an important point about "hitting bottom." If you have to ask yourself if you are ready to have a hysterectomy, chances are you are not. You will know when you have reached the end of your tolerance. For myself the moment of crystal clarity came when I was on a business trip 800 miles from home and found myself passing blood clots on the bathroom floor of a hotel room at one o'clock in the morning. Until that moment it hadn't mattered that I was existing on Tylenol with codeine to get through each day or that all of my vacation time was spent in the hospital having surgery. I wanted a child, and that is why I had avoided having a hysterectomy for so long. But as I felt I was going to pass out on the bathroom floor, I decided I wanted my life back again.

One important issue in making the decision to have a hysterectomy is how much your life is compromised by the disease. Many women find they have incapacitating pain at times other than their period, and this pain interferes with their careers and their personal lives. Many women become what is known as pelvic cripples in which all the reproductive organs are "glued" together. This is what happened to me. Like me, many women hang on because they want to have a child. The issue of fertility seems to be the most difficult one to resolve—not only for women with partners but also for single women who want to preserve their fertility.

Robin, a woman from California whose doctor has been advising her to have a hysterectomy for several years, writes, "I have withheld doing so for the fact that I deeply want a child. I just can't put an end to that hope. However, there are some months when the pain and my emotions are [so] out of hand that I think of giving in, but I can't. Sometimes I think my bigger problem is that I can't come to terms with never being able to have a baby."

Many women first look at all the negatives in having a hysterectomy, which is a healthy thing to do. However, we should not lose sight of the positives. For the first time in years I can now have a bowel movement without feeling as though my insides are coming apart. I no longer have to worry about whether sex will hurt, because it doesn't. My husband and I are free to plan vacations and business trips. I can fly on airplanes without being consumed by the fear of having an attack of excruciating pain and wondering what I will do when I am 25,000 feet up in the air.

Roxanne, a 36-year-old woman from New York, writes, "I realize that a total abdominal hysterectomy is not the answer for everyone. It was the hardest decision I have ever made in my entire life. Every day now I thank God for what I have been given. I feel especially grateful after finding out the pathology results. Had I not had the surgery, I would have gone on in endless pain. Happy birthday to me." The pathology reports showed she also had adenomyosis. In one research study 13 percent of patients who had a hysterectomy for adenomyosis also had endometriosis, so at least in some women both conditions occur.

It is true that when you have a hysterectomy, you put to rest forever some dreams you may have. But you open up your life to many other possibilities. For a positive view of hysterectomy, read "Hysterectomy: A Positive Story" following this article.

Having a hysterectomy frees a woman from dealing with the pain of endometriosis in many cases, but it does not free her from thinking of her health. Women who have their ovaries removed have special issues to consider: surgical menopause, osteoporosis, heart disease. If the only reason you want a hysterectomy is that you're tired of making difficult health decisions you should not have this surgery, because you will still be facing serious health decisions as well as potentially serious psychological issues. Some women are so buried in the physical pain and difficulties of endo that they cannot deal with the psychological aspects and then are surprised to find themselves faced after hysterectomy (sometimes immediately and sometimes not until one to two years postop) with this emotional baggage.

One of the issues of most concern when you are researching all aspects of hysterectomy's effect on your body is whether one or both ovaries should be removed. Although this is still a tough decision, it is easier today to opt for keeping one or both ovaries because they can be removed laparoscopically if the disease continues. In the past removing the ovaries later would have meant another major surgery.

A review of the medical literature and discussions with doctors leads to conflicting conclusions on whether or not to keep some ovarian tissue. Studies cited in medical texts on endo have found that the disease recurs in such a broad range (from no recurrence up to 85 percent recurrence if the ovaries are retained) as to be almost useless to the woman trying to decide what the chances of recurrence might be for her. However, according to the text *Endometriosis: Contemporary Concepts in Clinical Management*, edited by Dr. Robert S. Schenken, several studies have found higher recurrence or reoperation rates associated with more severe disease. One study (dating back to 1951 unfortunately) found only a 4 percent recurrence rate in women with stage I or stage II disease but a 44 percent recurrence rate in women with stage III or stage IV disease (using a classification system roughly paralleling the currently used American Society for Reproductive Medicine system). All the women in this study had a hysterectomy but kept some ovarian tissue.

In a study that followed women with bowel endometriosis there was a 33 percent recurrence rate when one or both ovaries were conserved. "These studies suggest that, for mild or moderate endometriosis, the ovaries can be conserved with a low rate of symptomatic recurrence, but with advanced pelvic or intestinal endometriosis, at least one third may develop recurrences if oophorectomy is not performed," note the authors in the Schenken text. A similar pattern of recurrence, especially where bowel or bladder endo had been involved, was found in the study of endo following hysterectomy sponsored by the Endometriosis Association (see the report on the study in the article "Does Hysterectomy and Removal of the Ovaries Offer a Cure for Endometriosis?" later in this chapter).

Other sources indicate different perspectives on the ovaries in/ovaries out question. "Bilateral oophorectomy is essential to deprive the ectopic endometrium of the cyclic estrogen that sustains and stimulates its proliferation and growth. . . . In patients who have completed their family and have enough pain to justify hysterectomy, we strongly recommend concomitant removal of both ovaries, regardless of age, as the best hope for a permanent cure," write Drs. Luciano and Manzi in the 1992 text *Infertility and Reproductive Medicine Clinics of North America: Endometriosis*. And a 1991 text (*Modern Approaches to Endometriosis*, edited by Drs. Eric Thomas and John Rock) states: ". . . in the woman with endometriosis of sufficient severity to indicate TAH [total abdominal hysterectomy], many surgeons suggest complete removal of the adnexa [ovaries and fallopian tubes]. Others suggest that the perfectly normal adnexum may be conserved in the young woman (the age threshold varies between surgeons from 35 to 40 years). . . ."

Of the 51 responses received in our request for information, 34 of them were useful for information pertaining to the ovaries in/ovaries out issue. Of the 34, 18 had their ovaries removed at the initial surgery *and* waited a minimum of several months before beginning estrogen replacement therapy. Of the 18, no endo has yet occurred in 14; four had the endo continue or return.

Of the same 34, 11 women did not have their ovaries removed at the initial hysterectomy. Nine have had a recurrence of the disease, and two have not. Five of the women had their ovaries removed, but estrogen replacement therapy was begun immediately, and endo continued or returned in all five.

For women who have had hysterectomies with removal of both ovaries and a return of endometriosis, hormone replacement is stopped and the same treatments used before hysterectomy and removal of the ovaries, hormonal and surgical, are often tried. Of course, women who had a hysterectomy and removal of the ovaries have usually already been through all these treatments and still had the endo recur, so it's not surprising that these women often feel frustrated, frightened, and hopeless.

In an interview that touched on this issue, Dr. David Redwine of Bend, Oregon, said he feels that the ovaries do not necessarily have to be removed and that the decision to excise them depends on what the woman wants and on the extent of her endometriosis. "I do try to educate a woman on the pros and cons," said Dr. Redwine. "If a woman has little endo in her pelvis and the ovaries aren't involved, it's frequently a good bet to leave the ovaries in." One of the reasons Dr. Redwine feels the ovaries can be left in is that he is a firm believer in his ability to remove all of the endometriosis. Even in the cases of severe disease Dr. Redwine feels a surgeon should be able to remove all of the endo.

Dr. Redwine believes that endometriosis is a congenital condition, not a progressive disease, and that the amount of endo remains the same from the teenage years on, although it changes in appearance. Therefore, he believes he can remove it all and no further disease will develop, so the ovaries can remain. (Many others do not agree with this assessment.)

Nancy Petersen, R.N., with the St. Charles Medical Center in Bend, clarified the conditions they feel are necessary for leaving the ovaries in: (1) the doctor has to operate under magnification, and (2) the doctor has to perform a "religious examination" of the entire pelvic area and the peritoneum. These conditions would hopefully help prevent inadvertently leaving disease behind. (However, endometriosis can be microscopic and can occur in areas that appear normal, so that it may be difficult to guarantee all disease can be removed.)

Another advisor to the association, Dr. Camran Nezhat of Atlanta, believes that if at all possible it is preferable not to remove the ovaries. He too follows scrupulous procedures to remove *all* the endometriosis, wherever it is. It is unlikely, however, that most gynecologists, even those quite skilled at surgery, can duplicate the results of the top endo specialists with their experience with thousands of cases.

Ultimately the decision to have your ovaries removed at the time of your hysterectomy is yours to make. It is true that if your ovaries are left you will not have to experience surgical menopause. But the risk you run is that the endometriosis will continue or return. The worst nightmare is when this happens, as it did to Diane, a 39-year-old woman from Texas who had a hysterectomy when she was 24.

She writes, "I had this operation leaving one ovary, then started taking estrogen after I experienced depression for no reason and hot flashes until age 32, when I experienced the same symptoms of endo, which required me to have an oophorectomy because endo had taken over my last ovary and part of my colon plus many other lesions throughout the abdominal cavity."

Diane writes that her physician then "burned" these lesions but was not successful in removing the endo from her bowel, explaining to her after the surgery that to do so ". . . would have caused death." [**EDITOR'S NOTE:** Laser and other new tools, used by a skilled and experienced surgeon, with techniques described in Chapters 2 and 4, can safely remove endo on the bowel where cautery, burning, cannot.] After this surgery she was pain-free for two months, "then it recurred suddenly [with] excruciating pain. The doctor said, 'yes,' I had it again but could not understand why. He put me on mild birth control pills and Stresstabs instead of the estrogen I was taking."

Diane has not been on any hormones since the age of 33 but writes that she now follows a balanced, nutritional diet supplemented with calcium and potassium pills with lots of rest and daily exercise. She is still in pain. (Magnesium should also be supplemented with the calcium.)

Another important decision that must be made concerns hormone replacement therapy. As with the ovaries in/ovaries out issue, much controversy surrounds hormone replacement therapy, and once again, there are no clear-cut answers.

For instance, the same surgeons who state in the text quoted earlier that "bilateral oophorectomy is essential to deprive the ectopic endometrium of the cyclic estrogen that sustains and stimulates its proliferation and growth" declare that hormone replacement therapy is "associated with only a small risk of disease recurrence." This seems paradoxical—to remove the ovaries one day so as to remove hormonal stimulation and then to immediately return some of those hormones to the body. These surgeons do state that the minimum dose of hormone replacement therapy should be used and that the amount of estrogen required to induce growth and proliferation of endometriosis appears to be higher than the amount needed to prevent osteoporosis. (However, the amount needed to sustain endometriosis already in place is not known.) This argument seems to be similar to the "estrogen window" concept currently being studied related to the use of addback therapies with GnRH drugs (see the articles on GnRH drug treatment in Chapter 3). It is not known if such a window really exists.

Drs. Luciano and Manzi note, as support for their belief that the ovaries should be removed and that hormone replacement therapy can be used, a study in which only one patient had a recurrence of her disease while on estrogen replacement after hysterectomy and removal of the ovaries. (In contrast, 25 percent of the women with comparable disease who kept some ovarian tissue required further surgery for disease recurrence.)

If Drs. Luciano and Manzi have patients in whom they are unable to remove all disease, they use progestins instead of estrogen for the first three months after surgery and then switch to combined estrogen and progestin for the first year after surgery. Then they use just estrogen. "We have found that a single intramuscular injection of 100 milligrams of medroxyprogesterone acetate (Depo-Provera), administered on the second postoperative day, suppresses hot flashes for up to 12 weeks and, in conjunction with the hypoestrogenemia [state of reduced estrogen] that follows castration, results in regression of residual implants." Oral Provera is also effective according to the authors. (We need to be aware, however, that, just as with medical therapy generally, not all implants have estrogen or progesterone receptors and thus may not all be responsive to medical therapy. In addition, note in the study by Lamb and others later in this chapter that four women who were on progesterone alone had their endo recur. It is not clear what form of progesterone was used.)

The awareness that disease is often left behind at hysterectomy and removal of the ovaries and the many reports to the association of continuing endo after this surgery have led some association members over the years to go without hormone replacement for some months after surgery in the hope of increasing their chances of clearing their bodies of stray endometrial tissue. One study using monkeys with surgically induced endometriosis, for instance, found that, after castration (removal of the ovaries), implants of disease were still active four weeks after surgery but at 12 weeks after surgery only "burned out" tissue remained. Weigh the risk of bone loss in your decision and be sure to consult your doctor on this issue. Remembering that the symptoms of surgical menopause are perhaps the best proof you have of diminishing estrogen in your body and that the lack of estrogen should hopefully eliminate any traces of endo that remain may help you feel better about tolerating the hot flashes and other problems.

Obviously, much more study on this important issue is needed. Meanwhile, as with so much involved with endo, it is up to each woman to weigh the information available and the facts and issues involved in her own situation to make the best decision.

Separate from the endo recurrence problem, there are important reasons why young women who have had their ovaries removed generally cannot go without hormone replacement indefinitely. A study published in the April 30, 1987, issue of the *New England Journal of Medicine* found that hysterectomy with bilateral oophorectomy increases the risk of coronary heart disease for instance. However, the study also found that this increased risk appears to be prevented by estrogen replacement therapy.

In addition, the risk of osteoporosis greatly increases with early menopause, and this too is counteracted, at least in part, by hormone replacement. Not to be overlooked are critical quality-of-life issues—sex drive and functioning, energy levels, mood (women off hormones sometimes report difficulties with depression)—that can be improved with hormone replacement.

If a woman has a total abdominal hysterectomy with both ovaries removed, she will experience surgical menopause, which is more abrupt and severe than natural menopause. The long-term physiological consequences for a young woman whose ovaries are removed are now being documented in the medical literature.

What makes surgical menopause so difficult is the severe drop in hormones a woman experiences. One day she has her ovaries, and the next day she does not. In addition, young women have *higher* levels of hormones than women at the age of natural menopause. Most women report the start of hormonal imbalance about three to four days postop. When a woman goes through natural menopause, her ovaries begin slowing down their hormonal production over several years, giving her body a chance to adjust. Surgical menopause does not give a woman that grace period. Even after natural menopause, a woman's ovaries continue to excrete estrogen and testosterone.

Women who go through menopause at a much earlier age than normal are at a higher risk of developing osteoporosis as well as heart disease. This is because estrogen protects against bone loss and aids in preventing cardiovascular problems in women. A substance produced by the uterus, prostacyclin, is also thought to play a protective role in preventing heart disease in women.

What can you expect if you experience surgical menopause? During the months when you are not on estrogen, you can expect to have hot flashes, night sweats, dry vagina, and mood swings. Perhaps the best definition of surgical menopause is supplied by Susanne Morgan in *Coping with a Hysterectomy*. Morgan calls the experience "menostop" because of the suddenness of the onset of menopausal symptoms.

Surgical menopause is not fun, but you can survive it. Having a good support system with a partner, family, and friends helps, as does having a positive attitude. You should be gentle with yourself and recognize that having a hysterectomy and removal of the ovaries is a major step. Major hormonal changes will be taking place in your body. Take time to recover physically and emotionally.

The reactions of women to their hysterectomies and to surgical menopause differ. Following are quotes from three women, two positive and one negative.

Anna, a 35-year-old woman from California, writes, "Before the day came, I decided to read all I could about hysterectomies and menopause. A lot of people gave me advice, including some scary stories about menopause. Take it all with a grain of salt—menopause isn't so bad and you won't go crazy! It's sure better than severe pain and heavy periods. I only wish I had done it sooner."

Many women who choose to have their ovaries removed find that dealing with surgical menopause is not as difficult as dealing with the debilitating pain of endo. Donna, from

Michigan, writes, "So now at age 33 I do not consider my surgical menopause to be anywhere near the psychological problem that trying to deal with my endo was."

However, Mary, from South Carolina, writes, "About a year ago I had a hysterectomy—the worst decision of my life. For the past 12 months my doctor has tried pills, injections, patches, but to no avail. I still have hot flashes several times every day. My hair gets totally drenched. I sweat like I am burning up, and my skin is as cold as ice."

> **EDITOR'S NOTE:** One sourcebook used for this article states that estrogen with testosterone controls symptoms like Mary's that are not controlled by estrogen alone.

Donna and Mary write from two completely different points of view about having a hysterectomy. Their stories show how differently our bodies react to the abruptness of surgical menopause.

Regardless of the physical consequences, or perhaps because of them, there is some emotional baggage we need to explore. Allow yourself to grieve, not only for the loss of your fertility (if that is an issue for you) but also for the loss of your body parts. A sense of humor helps. Try to reach out emotionally to family and friends. Many women find it difficult to be vulnerable in front of others because many times the same persons were not supportive during the bouts with endometriosis. However, it has been my experience that these people react more supportively to your experience during menopause (perhaps because they know what menopause is).

What also helps is knowing that if you decide to take hormone replacement your menopausal symptoms should abate. In the meantime, wear clothes made of natural fabrics such as wool and cotton because they absorb perspiration, and synthetics do not. See the suggestions for coping with menopausal effects in the GnRH drug articles in Chapter 3. Also, following Morgan's prescription for "home brew estrogen" from _Coping with a Hysterectomy_ will help, and some herbalists and alternative practitioners can suggest herbs and supplements that can help. (See _Women and the Crisis in Sex Hormones_ by Barbara Seaman and Gideon Seaman, M.D., New York: Bantam Books, 1977, for suggestions.)

Home-brew estrogen consists of taking a series of steps: exercise, good nutrition, vitamin and mineral supplements, and regular sexual activity. What also plays a major part in successful home-brew estrogen is reducing the amount of stress we put on our bodies, according to Morgan. To make home-brew estrogen, we need to help our adrenal glands (which produce small amounts of estrogen) to function at their most efficient level.

Morgan writes, "If we do not ask our bodies to deal with substances such as alcohol, sugar, salt, and coffee, we will be enduring much less stress. Not only will that make us feel better, function better, and rest better, but also it will free our adrenal glands from dealing with some of the stress and strengthen it for helping to produce more home brew estrogen."

Debra, a 30-year-old woman from Pennsylvania, consented to a hysterectomy with removal of her remaining ovary because she hoped it would be the answer to "this never-ending cycle of pills, pain, and surgery." Immediately after her hysterectomy she was started on estrogen replacement therapy. Debra writes, "This decision was never discussed with me in any way; rather my surgeon arrived in my hospital room one night and put an estrogen patch on my hip. The months that followed were difficult. I was beginning to realize that no one had truly explained to me what it meant to be thrown into a surgical menopause, nor were the pros and cons of estrogen replacement ever discussed.

"I thought I had educated myself well about my endometriosis, a hysterectomy, menopause, etc., but I soon found that when you know absolutely nothing about something, it is hard to know if you are asking all the right questions. At this point I was so exhausted and worn out that I trusted my doctor's judgment."

Six months after the surgery Debra began to suspect something was wrong, "very wrong." Her endometriosis had returned. She writes, "We will probably never know for sure why my endometriosis returned. With so many surgeries and complicating adhesions, it is possible that a small piece of one of my ovaries was left behind, or more probably, it may have been that the estrogen replacement was started too soon and thus activated any remaining cells of endometriosis."

Finding as many answers as possible regarding the impact of hysterectomy on sexuality is yet another part of crossing that "invisible barrier" mentioned earlier. The issue of sexuality has traditionally been secretive and not discussed between doctor and patient, but hopefully that is changing. Unfortunately, you do not know how your body will respond sexually until after your uterus and/or ovaries are removed.

Most women who have had hysterectomies agree that the surgery changed their sexual response, either in the amount of time it takes for lubrication, in the intensity of their orgasm, or in a decrease in their libido. For some of these women how they respond sexually is a moot point because they were in so much pain before surgery that pleasurable sexual intercourse, sometimes sex in any form, was impossible.

Rhonda, a 31-year-old woman from Washington, had a positive sexual response after her hysterectomy with removal of both ovaries. She writes, "The good news is that I feel more sexual and more responsive than I have for a number of years. The first time we made love I cried from deep inside, it was such a relief to feel my body respond easily and without pain! The feeling of congestion, tension, and pain is gone. I feel in touch with my body again. Lubrication and basic responses pose no problems to speak of."

She goes on, "The changes are there, however. Orgasms are good, better even in some ways, but definitely different. Some old favorite positions aren't quite as satisfying, but others are better than before. I feel like I still have some learning and exploring to do; that should be OK, though. Intercourse feels better than it ever did!"

However, Rhonda says that oral sex is not as satisfying as it was before her hysterectomy, that she needs "more vaginal stimulation to make that work. However, I have a strong feeling that oral sex worked as well as it did *before* the surgery mainly because it was the only thing we could do that didn't hurt! *Nothing* sexual hurts anymore, so sometimes I feel like I'm starting over."

Janet, from Michigan, writes, "And I still have not had a deep climax as before. I guess there's nothing there to deep-climax with, but sex is still a lot of fun. It's a small price to pay with considering what endo had done to my insides."

Anne, a 34-year-old woman from Massachusetts, was 30 at the time of her hysterectomy. Both of her ovaries were removed. She writes that the major drawback has been a decrease in lubrication but notes that is rectified by using vaginal lubricants that are available without prescription at drugstores.

Anne's orgasms have changed, mainly in their intensity. "I feel that my uterus played a big role in my physical pleasure during orgasm. I still have orgasms, but they peak more quickly, and their intensity is more shallow. But I have noticed I feel pleasure from parts of my body I never noticed before. For example, my face gets an intense flush that is extremely pleasurable." Oral sex is as pleasurable for Anne now as it was before her hysterectomy.

The downside for Anne is a decrease in her libido, which affects the physical intimacy she and her husband share. Other women report the same. One woman writes, "He [the doctor] said the loss of libido was only temporary and asked me if I wanted Valium. (It's only temporary—till I die.)" She goes on to say, "I feel so much better on a daily basis. But the loss of libido is killing me inside, and not doing much for my marriage either!"

A decrease in libido is most likely due to a lack of testosterone, a hormone secreted by the ovaries but not replaced by estrogen replacement therapy. One older study described in Susanne Morgan's book notes that doctors had prescribed testosterone pellets inserted under the skin, with apparently good results, and writes that women who have used the pellets successfully say they make a great difference in their sexual response. For more information on testosterone replacement, see "The Thorny Issue of Hormone Replacement for Endo: Estrogen, Progesterone, Testosterone" following this article.

A factor that seems to be equally important to how a woman feels after a hysterectomy is the attitude and knowledge of her physician. Roxanne, a 37-year-old woman from New York, writes about discussing her decision with her doctor. "He let me know that a positive attitude was very important, that it would even help with the recovery. I now know that he was absolutely 100 percent correct."

You should give yourself time to heal, both emotionally and physically. Peggy, a 34-year-old woman from Wisconsin, recognized this. She writes, "It has been two years now. I feel wonderful. I've gotten my life back into control. Even my seven-year-old daughter remembers seeing Mommy in so much pain and has told me, 'I love to see you not sick, Mommy.'"

Peggy continues, "I would recommend hysterectomy for any seriously complicated endometriosis. The surgery recuperation suffering is nothing compared to the toll endo takes on your body. You have to weigh yourself what you want the quality of your life to be!"

Some women who responded to our request for information feel cheated (as they should) because their surgeons were not fully informed. This happened to Kim, a 31-year-old woman who had her uterus plus one ovary removed when she was 24 years old.

Kim writes that her physician diagnosed her problem as pelvic inflammatory disease and discovered endometriosis only when he performed her hysterectomy. Two months later, when her pain returned, the surgeon performed another laparoscopy to cauterize the endo and then put her on danazol.

Kim ended up having a third surgery during which the physician removed her remaining ovary. Immediately afterward he put her on estrogen replacement therapy (ERT) because he "didn't want me to suffer from menopausal symptoms or develop osteoporosis." Kim has a strong family history of osteoporosis.

When Kim developed pain again, her doctor took her off the ERT and put her back on danazol. She changed doctors. "The physician that I saw there said my pelvic pain was due to referred pain from my bladder that was atrophied from lack of estrogen. I was then put on Premarin (a replacement estrogen) and told that I would not have endometriosis again and that I may not have ever had it."

> **EDITOR'S NOTE:** Kim actually did have endometriosis, as one of her doctors noted the classic "powder burns" during a laparoscopy. We included this quote here to show the emotional stress a doctor's offhanded comment can cause.

The next several years were a nightmare for Kim, who consulted another physician, who told her "if I had the right attitude, the pain shouldn't bother me too much." Finally Kim found a gynecologist who knew how to treat endometriosis and surgical menopause. But because of the years in which she was not on ERT, Kim had developed osteoporosis.

Kim was being treated at a major medical center. What happened to her should not have happened.

When women call me and ask about hysterectomy, I try to give them information that will help them make the best decision for them and their lives. It's a weighty decision—don't rush it. Take the time to feel sure it's the right decision for you.

There is one thing we must not forget, and that is not to alienate each other. In some of the support groups I have led, women who have not had a hysterectomy cannot understand why those of us who have chosen this route did so. Like them, those of us who have had hysterectomies also said at one time we'd *never* have a hysterectomy. But when all treatments have been tried and one is still in pain (and association members know that the treatments themselves are not easy to tolerate), what do you do?

Recent years have seen tremendous strides in new treatments for endo. Other new treatments and increased understanding of endometriosis are sure to occur due to the work of the association and the people it has interested in the disease. Unfortunately for some of us, those treatments won't come soon enough.

Those of us who have had hysterectomies must remember not to get caught in the "what if" syndrome. What if we had held out longer? The finest gift we can give to ourselves is to accept that we made the best decision at the time with as much available information as we could.

Roxanne, introduced earlier, writes, "One woman I spoke to told me that whatever decision I make, I have to believe that it is the best decision for me and to be willing to accept the consequences, no matter what, good or bad. I have done that. Acceptance and faith go a long way. They make everything a whole lot more bearable."

Of all the women who responded to our request for information, one woman in particular said something that struck me as being the most enlightening way to end this article, not only for women who have had hysterectomies but also for every woman with endometriosis. Jeannine, from California, writes, "You must learn to recognize the power that you have within yourself, and you will be surprised just how much you can help yourself. . . ."

■ *Paula M. Zimlicki, Baton Rouge, Louisiana, is an award-winning medical writer who specializes in women's health. Zimlicki is the author of a book on menopause.*

Hysterectomy: A Positive Story

Dear Endometriosis Association,

I am pleased to announce a birth, not the birth of a baby, but the birth of a newly developing woman—me!

After suffering for several years with incapacitating dysmenorrhea, PMS, chronic fatigue due to anemia secondary to hemorrhaging every month, lack of mobility due to adhesions, and so on, I finally decided to have a hysterectomy. The irony of the whole situation is that what I envisioned as my own free choice became a necessity, as another ovarian mass was diagnosed by ultrasound.

Society, my family, and my own internal values told me I wasn't really a woman until I produced a child. I can't count the number of family gatherings at which I heard, "When are you going to be married and have a baby?" It was like I was a second-class citizen until I fulfilled their expectations, becoming the 'model' woman. How it hurt to hear, "You'd make such a good mother," knowing that I was sterile as a result of endometriosis. I never let them know just how deeply their remarks hurt, mostly because I wasn't aware myself until the decision was made to undergo a total hysterectomy.

Through the pain of this disease I gave birth to an incredibly strong woman. Since my hysterectomy I have found that there is life beyond the menstrual cycle. Also a woman's role in today's society is only as limiting as I choose to make it.

I have always wanted to give birth to a person who would not have existed if it weren't for me. Someone I could love and nurture, guide and protect. Someone I could look upon and say, "Yes, that is my child." These and many other reasons were the basis of my decision to have a baby. As an aside, I also wanted a baby shower, but this I am reluctant to add. Looking honestly now, the reasons seem self-centered, though at the time they were very important.

After having the hysterectomy, I needed to grieve the loss of my unborn child. It was not a very happy time; actually it was quite painful, requiring much work on my part to stay alive and functioning. I view this time as my own labor and delivery of my new self.

I had discovered many personal issues, which were buried under the guise of PMS, that needed attention. Under the guidance of therapists, support of many friends, and the Endometriosis Association, I found understanding and acceptance of myself. I am no longer chronically fatigued, depressed, pain-filled, and my life is no longer menstrual cycle–centered. I can run without pain for the first time in years!

Through therapy and the support of the EA, I have learned I am not alone in my struggle. One particularly moving article, regarding infertility in young women, started the flow of tears, allowing the healing process to begin. The positive aspects of this time are too numerous to list, which in itself is a miracle.

I am starting back to school this fall to learn what I want just for fun. Did I say fun? I had forgotten what that was like. This fall is being met with joy and anticipation. I am healthy, emotionally and physically. I am finding there is much living to do even if my original goal was to have a baby. The future is so bright and so different from what I had envisioned two years ago when I had my hysterectomy.

I feel life is just beginning for me. I wanted to send out birth announcements, but I don't feel the average population would understand. So I am sharing my joy with the people who will understand. Hopefully for the other women needing to make major decisions I can present options. I know that after surgery many complications do arise. I was fortunate; however, there are positives to both sides. I wanted to share mine with you.

Thank you all for your support, love, and acceptance. I am sending positive, gentle energy to you.

In Love,
Judy, Wisconsin

Hysterectomy: A Negative Story

Dear Endo Association,

I was very glad to receive your newsletter on endometriosis and the bowel. I am posthysterectomy and oophorectomy six months, and my gynecologist left "a little spot" of endo on my bowel after three hours of surgery, which was supposed to be conservative surgery. I have been battling my endo the past three years, with the last year the most aggressive and most frustrating. I have also been living a hormonal nightmare the past year and a half.

I was advised by one doctor to have surgery or get pregnant. My cycles were down to 19 days with 10 days of bleeding and severe pain three days, with moderate pain the rest of the time. My hematocrit [percentage of red cells in whole blood] was getting low, down into the transfusion range. Since I wasn't finished having my family yet, I chose pregnancy. . . . After three months the pain was worse. . . . [The gynecologist said it] was the worst he's ever seen. The adhesions and scar tissue were so thick he couldn't even see one of my ovaries, and only part of the other one was visible. He videoed it for me so I could see how bad it was. It reminded me of a dark cave full of spiderwebs.

I was placed on danazol with hopes of pregnancy after conservative surgery to be performed after six months of therapy.

At the end of six months I returned to OR for conservative surgery. I awoke after three hours of surgery with a hysterectomy and bilateral oophorectomy. I felt (and still feel) I have been castrated. There's no other term for it. I really liked "Joe with Endo" in your book because it expressed my feelings so well. My doctor decided my endo was so severe the hysterectomy was needed, so he called my husband from OR, and they decided it was best. After the surgery my doctor told me the ERT would make me feel wonderful. He said, "My mother swears by it." I felt like saying, "But I'm only 35, and I'm not your mother."

I tried to wait three to six months to start ERT, but by two weeks postop the hot flashes, insomnia, chills, and crawly skin were more than I could bear. I started on Premarin .625 milligram and cycled it with Provera 10 milligram the last part of the month, with one week off. I couldn't handle the last week off, so I was put on a regimen of Premarin .625 milligram and Provera 25 milligram daily with no time off. I would do OK for three weeks, then have all the feelings of a period the last week except the bleeding. I am six months posthysterectomy, and my menopausal symptoms keep recurring about every three weeks with the endo symptoms. . . . I also have had abdominal pain and fullness again the past two months and bowel symptoms. Sometimes I can't even sit because of pain, and I have the feeling of needing to have a BM without having anything there. I have had a lot of constipation and gas, but so far the diarrhea hasn't returned. My gynecologist doesn't think it's endo. My family doctor referred me to a psychiatrist who is female and has been helping me cope. She has helped me start to like myself again and has helped me research endo and ERT after oophorectomy. . . .

My gynecologists haven't given me any answers, and I feel like a hypochrondiac. My psychiatrist assures me I'm not crazy and has helped me look for answers. I am an R.N. in women's health, so I have access to medical literature, but your literature has by far been the best.

I sat in on a hysterectomy class at the hospital where I work after my hysterectomy. The teacher was giving everyone the impression a hysterectomy was the answer to all their problems. I didn't feel she covered the emotional aspects and brought this to her attention. She made me feel I was abnormal for my feelings. Yet after the class two of the four women in the class were having misgivings and spoke to me about their upcoming hysterectomies.

My endo has been my nightmare. I'm trying to go back to school to get a Ph.D. to enable me to help others to cope with female problems. Most of the time I do OK. Other times I have a very hard time due to pain and discouragement. I wish I could have been in on the decision about my hysterectomy more; I would have put it off as long as I could. I feel I've traded one nightmare for another. . . .

The . . . membership fee has helped me much more than my $10,000+ in medical bills. Thanks for caring.

Sincerely,
Susan, Utah

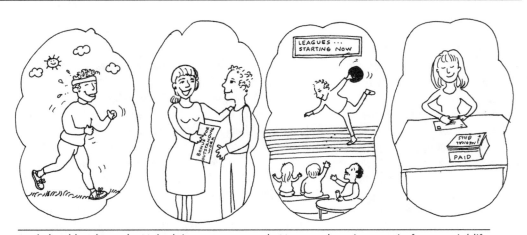

Joe's health rebounds. He's doing great at work. He even has time again for a social life. It appears his bad experiences with endo are going to become just a memory.

The Thorny Issue of Hormone Replacement for Endo—Progesterone and Testosterone

By Mary Lou Ballweg

Loss of sex drive (libido) is one of the most devastating consequences of removal of the ovaries noted by many women. Doctors frequently assure the woman that replacing the estrogen produced by the ovaries should take care of the problem, but research shows that testosterone is the key hormone involved in sex drive. Testosterone is produced by the ovaries and adrenal glands (a pair of endocrine organs located on top of each kidney), but the ovaries are the more important source according to Dr. Vickie Hufnagel in the book *No More Hysterectomies.*

In women who go through natural menopause the ovaries continue to produce testosterone and a related hormone (both are called *androgens*). In fact, according to *Understanding Your Body,* by Felicia Stewart (New York: Bantam Books, 1987), the ovary produces even more testosterone *after* menopause than before. Naturally, without the ovaries, this testosterone is also gone along with the estrogen and progesterone and is not replaced by estrogen replacement therapy or estrogen-progesterone therapy.

"Testosterone depletion can also be devastating," according to Hufnagel. She notes that a British study of 100 women found a greater incidence of depression, painful intercourse, and loss of libido with oophorectomy.

So why don't physicians suggest that the testosterone produced by the ovaries be replaced? Studies have clearly documented the effects of testosterone on sexuality, and in one study testosterone pellets implanted in women after removal of the ovaries resulted in the women reporting a restoration of their lost libido. The reason the suggestion is seldom made or the subject even broached seems to be the lack of understanding of the importance of testosterone in women and the belief that testosterone is a "male" hormone. Actually all the hormones are made by both men and women—just in different ratios in each.

Dr. Hufnagel addresses this topic:

> There is a belief today that women neither make nor need testosterone. And women fear the 'male' hormones. The misuse of these labels frightens us needlessly, for all the hormones produced in a woman's body are 'female.' They are all necessary for normal cyclic functioning and the integrity of our other organs. It's the balance that's important.
>
> Time after time, I've administered minute amounts of testosterone to women complaining of loss of libido after menopause, surgical removal of the ovaries, or hysterectomy, and watched these patients spring back to life. Their energies and sexual activities returned to normal, and their marriages were saved.

Testosterone replacement is a popular idea in Canada according to an article in the June 27, 1988, issue of *Medical World News*, but in the United States testosterone fell out of favor in the 1960s and has yet to make a comeback. A mix of the two hormones in injection form has been used in Canada for the last 20 years according to the article. Psychologist Barbara B. Sherwin says it's indicated especially for a woman whose primary complaints are loss of libido and decreased energy, according to the article. She and Dr. Morrie L. Gelfand, both of McGill University in Montreal, "studied women injected every 4 to 8 weeks with estrogen and testosterone following hysterectomy and bilateral salpingo-oophorectomy. In a small but carefully controlled study, they found that 'castrated women receiving androgen and estrogen reported fewer somatic and psychological symptoms than those getting estrogen alone,' reported Dr. Gelfand."

Estrogen-testosterone preparations are available in the United States as a cream, an injection, a pellet, and a pill. One of these is Estratest, a combination of .625 milligram of estrogen and 1.25 milligrams of methyltestosterone in the half-strength pill. The full-strength capsule contains 1.25 milligrams of estrogen and 2.5 milligrams of methyltestosterone. Another preparation available is Premarin with methyltestosterone, which has .625 milligram of estrogen and 5 milligrams of testosterone. Obviously the Estratest is a lower-dose way to try the testosterone and watch for potential side effects.

Testosterone replacement may also help in maintaining bones. "Recent studies have shown that anabolic steroids or androgens can slow down bone loss in a manner similar to that of estrogens," according to *Stand Tall! The Informed Woman's Guide to Preventing Osteoporosis* by Morris Notelovitz, M.D., and Marsha Ware. "Investigators have reported that the incidence of adverse side affects (unwanted growth of facial and body hair, acne, and deepening of the voice) can be almost totally eliminated by administering either drug on a '3 weeks on, 1 week off' schedule. Studies of the long-term benefits and risks of anabolic steroids and androgens have not been performed. Until they are, these preparations should be viewed as a viable alternative for women osteoporotics who cannot take estrogens."

In Dr. Robert W. Kistner's gynecology textbook entitled *Gynecology: Principles and Practice*, androgens such as testosterone are noted as inhibiting the bone loss of a hypoestrogenic state (less than the normal amount of estrogen). Just as with all the hormones, however, we are a long way from knowing the long-term effects or all the many subtle ways in which they work. Another researcher quoted in the *Medical World News* article notes that there are "preliminary data indicating that it [testosterone supplementation] might reverse the beneficial effects of estrogen on bone," but she appears to be talking about the effects in women with ovaries.

How can various studies produce such contradictory results? First, be aware that studies have to be checked carefully to be sure that the subjects are women without ovaries. Second, all of the hormones are constantly being interconverted, and fat tissue in particular has the ability to convert hormones, with subtle influences that are probably different in pre- and postmenopausal women, into other hormones. For instance, the androgens produced by the adrenal glands are converted into estrogen. As Dr. Penny Budoff says in her book *No More Hot Flashes and Other Good News* (New York: G. P. Putnam's Sons, 1983), as she refers to diagrams of testosterone and estradiol (the most active form of estrogen):

> I think it is fascinating to see from the following diagrams of male and female hormones how little difference there is between what we hold to be the sacred distinction between male and female. Once you have seen these structures, it is easy to understand how readily they can be converted into one another. And they are constantly being interconverted. Progesterone is often the precursor for either male or female hormones; estradiol can be converted to estrone [a less active form of estrogen] and vice versa; and testosterone can be converted into female hormone and vice versa. Male and female physiologies are not all that exclusive.

Actually, trying to sort out the issues related to testosterone is 100 times easier than for progesterone because progesterone is the true mystery hormone at this time, particularly in women with endometriosis. According to *Women and the Crisis in Sex Hormones*, "Progesterone is a most mysterious hormone, and its influence on sexual behavior could fill a textbook. Yet scientists remain uncertain whether to assign progesterone . . . as a male or female hormone. Testosterone, a male hormone produced by both sexes, stimulates sex drive; estrogen, a female hormone produced by both, stimulates it under some conditions. Progesterone, a hormone chiefly connected with pregnancy or preparation for pregnancy in the female (although in some ways it has more in common chemically with testosterone than estrogen), often has an adverse effect on sex. Ordinarily in the female, progesterone levels are low for most of the monthly cycle."

And, according to Dr. Budoff, "Although there are tremendous amounts of data on the clinical effects of estrogen in women, trying to dig out data on the clinical effects of natural or synthetic progesterone is nearly impossible. The problem is that the progesterone data are always mixed up with the data from estrogen, because the information comes from studies on birth-control pills that contain both hormones. I have spoken to pharmaceutical manufacturers as well as to the Food and Drug Administration, and they agree that true data, that is, data that refer only to progestational agents, are almost impossible to come by." (Progesterone is the hormone produced by the woman's own ovaries. Synthetic hormone is derived from either progesterone or derivatives of testosterone, which can impact the type of side effects experienced. Natural progesterone, often made from soy, is available from certain pharmacies and may be tolerated better by women with endo than synthetic.)

The recent movement toward replacing progesterone along with estrogen came about because of the risk of cancer with so-called "unopposed" estrogen given to menopausal women who still had their uterus. Obviously this condition does not apply to women who've undergone surgical menopause due to removal of the uterus and ovaries for endometriosis. The question of continuous unopposed estrogen stimulation of breast tissue is also an important one. A study published in the January 9, 1987, issue of the *Journal of the American Medical Association* reported that overall the risk of breast cancer did not appear to increase appreciably with increasing ERT duration or latency, even for time periods of 20 years or longer. It is possible that not taking estrogen *continuously* could accomplish the same goal as using progesterone to oppose the estrogen.

Progesterone in some forms also has the ability, it seems, to reverse some of the good effects of estrogen and testosterone. It can create adverse effects on blood lipids, an important factor in prevention of heart disease. According to an article in the June 1988 issue of *Medical Times* by Brian W. Walsh and Isaac Schiff, both of Harvard: "Since progestins adversely affect lipoproteins and thus increase cardiovascular mortality, the use of progestins in women without a uterus is unnecessary and possibly detrimental."

Adding progesterone does not interfere with the beneficial effects of estrogens on bone, however. In fact, progesterone may stimulate formation of new bone according to several studies. This could be a great plus for women who've lost bone and are at great risk for osteoporosis. The role of progesterone related to continuation of endometriosis is also a big question. A good summary of this issue occurs in the gynecology textbook *Endometriosis*, by Emery A. Wilson, M.D. (New York: Alan R. Liss, Inc., 1987). "Laboratory models of experimental endometriosis in the rat and rabbit indicate that estrogen stimulates the growth of endometriotic tissue and androgens tend to induce atrophy in endometriotic implants. The role of progesterone in the regulation of endometriotic tissue is controversial. Progesterone alone may actually support the growth of endometriotic tissue. However, the synthetic progestogens, many of which have androgenic properties, appear to inhibit the growth of endometriotic tissue."

According to Kistner's *Gynecology: Principles and Practice*, "In experimental endometriosis in monkeys, the most extensive growth has been obtained by the cyclic administration and withdrawal of estrogen and progesterone." Kistner also writes, "The use of estrogen-progestin combinations given in 20-day cycles or sequential estrogen-progestin preparations, however, has been shown to reactivate endometriosis. These preparations should never be used in a patient who has had a hysterectomy and bilateral salpingo-oophorectomy."

However, the authors of an article on malignancy arising in endometriosis in the March 1988 issue of *Obstetrics & Gynecology* argue *for* using progesterone in these patients. The only reason they cite is that, according to them, no cases of malignancy (cancer) have been documented to arise with combined replacement. They appear to mean *proven* related to progesterone, however, as they cite one case in their article in which the woman developed cancer arising from endometriosis in the rectovaginal septum three months after starting progesterone (and previously she had been treated with estrogen plus progestins for nine months).

The article does not discuss the issues for women with endo related to recurring or continuing endo and thus seems limited in its conclusions. It does serve to remind us of the risk of cancer when any endometriosis is left behind. Just as estrogen increases the risk of cancer in the endometrial lining of the uterus in postmenopausal women, it has the same effect on any stray endometriosis. The only good solution, again, seems to be to remove all endo and perhaps to go through surgical menopause to allow any tissue inadvertently left behind to die out. (A discussion of cancer and endometriosis can be found in Chapter 15 of our first book, *Overcoming Endometriosis*.)

Progesterone appears to play some important role related to the immune system, but of course this raises more questions than it answers. Certainly we know that it is involved with candidiasis since *Candida albicans* has progesterone receptors on its cell walls. But what this means for women with endometriosis is certainly not yet clear. (See *Overcoming Endometriosis* for information on candidiasis.)

Since the majority of women with endometriosis seem to have their most difficult problems with the disease in the second two weeks of the cycle, when progesterone is predominant, it might be easy to conclude that progesterone is more problematic for us than estrogen. Of course, we have no way of knowing this without understanding how endometriosis develops. Ultimately we will need feedback from our members and readers who are utilizing progesterone replacement to learn about their experiences and what might be the best hormone replacement overall. So, readers, please keep writing to us—together we can learn so much!

Does Hysterectomy and Removal of the Ovaries Offer a Cure for Endometriosis?
An Exploratory Study

By Karen Lamb, R.N., Ph.D., Lyle J. Breitkopf, M.D., and Karen J. Hamilton, M.D.

EDITOR'S NOTE: When the association began, it was commonly noted in the medical community that hysterectomy and removal of the ovaries resulted in a cure of endometriosis in 95 percent or more of cases. We were surprised then that from our earliest days there seemed to be so many women who had had this procedure and still had endo. In the mid-1980s we asked Karen Lamb, director of the Endometriosis Association Research Registry, to explore the question of whether hysterectomy and removal of the ovaries cured endo, utilizing the registry. She did, and we're pleased to present her study here. The study is written in scientific language, but the information is so important that we felt members would want it in spite of the technical language. We've tried to provide definitions and explanations to help readers.

This study must be viewed as a preliminary one in that it raises as many questions as it answers. One question is whether more women would have had a successful outcome if disease on the bowel and bladder had been removed. There were a large number of women with bowel/bladder involvement in the study. At the time of the study, and all too commonly now, it has been typical to leave the disease behind on bowel and bladder.

Tragically, the bowel and bladder involvement may have been the reason for many women resorting to hysterectomy because other treatments available up until recently did not address disease of these areas very well. Only recently have a few surgeons developed good techniques for removing endo of these areas. For more on surgeries for endometriosis (not hysterectomy), see the surgery articles earlier in this chapter. For more on bowel involvement, see Chapter 4. For more on endometriosis involving the bladder, see Chapter 5.

Introduction

The U.S. National Center for Health Statistics[1] reports that about 12.5 million hysterectomies were conducted between 1965 and 1984. Of 97 million females aged 15 years and older, alive in 1985, approximately 19.5 percent had undergone hysterectomy. Roughly 670,000 hysterectomies were performed in 1985.

Between 1970 and 1984 cancer accounted for 10.7 percent of all hysterectomies; fibroids was the most common diagnosis, an estimated 27 percent of all hysterectomies.

Endometriosis accounted for 14.7 percent. Among all diagnoses, only endometriosis demonstrated a sharp increase: a 121 percent overall increase between 1965 to 1967 and 1982 to 1984. (Cancer and fibroids increased 2.1 and -7.2 percent, respectively.)

Although bilateral oophorectomy is relatively uncommon, 305,000 procedures were performed in 1984, 88.5 percent in conjunction with hysterectomy. Data were not reported specifically for endometriosis.

Several reasons were postulated for the dramatic increase in the number of hysterectomies for endometriosis. The authors speculated that endometriosis may be more common, or severe, as women delay childbearing and the use of oral contraceptives falls. While the prevalence may not have increased, improved technology, notably use of the laparoscope, has led to improved diagnosis. (Prevalence, in epidemiology, is the number of all new and old cases of a disease or occurrences of an event during a particular period of time.) Finally, the authors noted changes in medical practice—most notably, physicians' willingness to perform hysterectomy may account for rate changes.

The enormous variation in surgical procedures for endometriosis has been referred to as a "blue plate special." Cauterization, microsurgical dissection, laser surgery, removal of implants and adhesions, and excision of endometrial cysts are a few descriptions applied to the procedures performed. For many patients no surgery carries more anxiety than the one procedure touted in the past to offer a cure: total hysterectomy, TAH/BSO (total abdominal hysterectomy/bilateral salpingo-oophorectomy—removal of the uterus, fallopian tubes, and ovaries).

Common medical practice uses estrogen replacement. The question arises as to whether hormonal replacement to offset surgically induced menopause causes a recurrence of endometriosis or endometriosislike symptoms. A review of *Index Medicus* (an index of medical and research journals), 1984–1987, showed no assessment of recurrence rates with estrogen administration; a computerized search spanning 1966 to April 1989 yielded no answers.

Questions raised include: Are there factors in the natural history characterizing patients proceeding to hysterectomy? Related to estrogen replacement therapy (ERT), does estrogen used alone or in combination with progesterone affect surgical outcome?

Factors in the natural history include the occurrence of classical symptoms, including dysmenorrhea and pelvic pain and disability, which is the inability to perform routine daily functions. Medical treatment with danazol, oral contraceptives (OCs), and/or surgical intervention prior to hysterectomy were compared between groups; and, patients' experiences with hysterectomy, with and without ERT, were evaluated.

Methods

The study group was composed of patients having hysterectomy for endometriosis seeking assistance from the Endometriosis Association from 1980 to 1987. (Because of this time frame, many in the study were treated with danazol, the most commonly used hormonal treatment at the time. The GnRH drugs, Synarel and Lupron, were not yet available.) Many complained that endometriosis had recurred or they had experienced a return of symptoms.

The data registry of the association has been housed at the Medical College of Wisconsin. The survey instrument covers medical, surgical, pregnancy, and psychosocial information. Approximately 3,000 case histories have been furnished by some members and have been analyzed.

For patients having had hysterectomies, attention focused on these questions: If you had a hysterectomy, did you receive estrogen replacement therapy? Did surgery relieve or cure the endometriosis? If ERT was used, have you experienced any return of symptoms?

Because of the categorical nature of responses, data were analyzed, primarily, using chi-square (X^2) measures.*

Results

The data set consisted of 2,655 patients who have undergone laparoscopy or laparotomy, who have received firm diagnoses, and for whom complete demographic data were available. Of these, 238 (9.0 percent) had hysterectomies, although 43 (18.1 percent of patients having hysterectomies) did not have both ovaries removed and were therefore not subject to ERT; parts of any ovary were not removed in 7 cases (2.9 percent).

For the remaining 189 patients (7.1 percent) the uterus, both ovaries, and the fallopian tubes were removed. Of these, 161 (85.2 percent) received ERT; 28 (14.8 percent) did not. For brevity the study group consists of these cases and is referred to as the *hysterectomy group, HYST GR,* or *HYST* patients. Estrogen replacement therapy is abbreviated *ERT; NO ERT* is used for its absence.

Respondents' ages averaged 36.8 years; range: 21 to 62. Seven of 10 (70.4 percent) were married; 38.2 percent were college educated. The median family income was $35,000 per year.

Examination of demographic variables between the HYST GR and remaining registry patients showed no statistically significant differences in any demographic variable except

---

* When an investigator examines an array of data, a picture of two events (or variables) occurring together, he or she always asks, "How often could this picture have occurred simply by chance alone?" Chi-square is a measure of statistical significance, or a measure of probability—the probability of this picture occurring by chance. For example, a chi-square probability value p of 0.01 indicates that the picture (the relationship between two or more variables) could have occurred 1 out of 100 times based on chance alone. This result, which would be pretty rare, indicates to the investigator that "something" is happening here that is probably *not* based on chance alone.

In this study we have cited the actual value of chi-square and the d.f. (degrees of freedom). The lay reader can disregard these numbers. What one continues to need to focus on is the p value, the probability that this event could have occurred by chance. A p value of less than 0.05 is considered statistically significant, rarely occurring by chance.

Table 1. Demographic Characteristics of Patients with Endometriosis Having Hysterectomies (N=189)

Age of Respondents	36.8 years (s = 7.2 yrs)
	Percent (%)
Married	70.4
White race/ethnicity	92.6
College educated	38.2
Median family income	$ 35,000
Hysterectomy Status	
Estrogen Replacement (ERT)	85.2
NO ERT	14.8

N = number of patients
s = standard deviation

age. HYST GR patients were older: 36.8 years vs. 31.5 (X^2) = 112.241; d.f. = 3; p = <0.001. For hysterectomy patients there was no relationship between age and educational status, nor any statistical relationship between whether a woman was married and the age that hysterectomy was performed.

The Severity Index

Lacking data on size of implants and extent of adhesions, a simple severity index (SI) based on Acosta's and his colleagues'[2] criterion of endometriosis involvement of the urinary bladder and/or intestinal tract was devised. In other words patients who had endo of the bladder or bowel were classed as having severe disease. By this measure patients undergoing hysterectomy were more seriously ill (Table 2). Almost 62 percent of the HYST GR were characterized as having severe endometriosis by virtue of bowel and/or bladder involvement vs. 36.1 percent of the remaining registry respondents (X^2) = 48.312; d.f. = 1; p = <0.001.

The Natural History

For brevity patients' symptoms, pain profiles, and disability levels from patients' case histories are not included in table format. However, examination of data on the HYST GR vs. remaining registry patients showed 8 of 11 symptom complexes demonstrated statistically significant differences. (X^2 probabilities range between 0.02 and 0.001.)

Table 2. Severity Index Based on Urinary Bladder and/or Intestinal Involvement

	Hyst Patients (N=188)[a]		Registry Respondents (N=2393)[b]	
	f.	%	f.	%
Severe—Bladder and/or Bowel Involvement	116	61.7	865	36.1
Less Severe—No Bladder and/or Bowel Involvement	72	38.3	1528	63.9

[a] Missing = (0.5%) $X^2 = 48.312$; d.f. = 1; p = <0.001
[b] Missing = 73 (2.7%)   f = frequency or number of patients

Striking were the proportions in both groups experiencing symptoms, yet in every instance, excepting complaints of infertility, the HYST GR demonstrated higher rates. For example, they offered more complaints of dysmenorrhea and pelvic pain; fatigue, exhaustion, and low energy; dyspareunia (pain with sex); nausea and gastric upset at menses; complaints of low-grade fevers; low resistance to infection; but lower rates of infertility as noted.

All HYST patients reported symptoms prior to diagnosis (2.9 percent of registry patients reported no physical symptoms). Symptom complexes: heavy or irregular bleeding; dizziness and/or headache; diarrhea, painful bowel movements, or other intestinal upsets with menses were not statistically different.

The severity index was unrelated to most symptom complexes. However, complaints of infertility (p = 0.05); fatigue and low energy (p = 0.02); and symptom complex—diarrhea, painful bowel movements, and other intestinal upsets (p = <0.002)—were statistically different. The latter, perhaps we're repeating needlessly here, could be expected to correlate with bowel/bladder involvement. All were in the expected direction.

The majority of both groups complained of pain throughout the menstrual cycle, not simply at menses (p = 0.02). However, HYST patients fell more heavily into this category. So too, these patients classified pain levels as more severe (p = <0.001). The severity index was unrelated to pain profiles.

Disability measures showed HYST patients were incapacitated longer. Both the proportion disabled and the length of time disabled, ranging from days to weeks, were statistically significant at the 0.01 probability level or less. The severity index was unrelated to the extent of disability.

Treatment Before Hysterectomy

Provocatively, fewer HYST patients had been treated with danazol (Danocrine). Of 189 HYST patients only 91 (48.1 percent) had used danazol vs. 1,610 (65.3 percent) of 2,466 registry patients (X^2 = 22.44; d.f. = 1; p = <0.001).

Approximately two of three patients in the registry have been treated with danazol; less than half of the HYST GR were treated. The variable, time on danazol, showed a trend for HYST patients to have used danazol for shorter periods; however, results were not statistically different. (The severity index was not related to this variable, to the length of time since hysterectomy was performed, or to age at hysterectomy.)

Because of the implication that HYST patients had had less medical therapy a thorough examination of events surrounding hysterectomy was conducted. Particular interest lay in patients' ages at hysterectomy, the time between diagnosis and hysterectomy, and the treatment modalities used before hysterectomy.

Results showed the time between diagnosis and hysterectomy averaged 2.98 ± 4.27 years* (184 cases). Diagnosis preceded hysterectomy for some by 11 to 18 years. Yet, and more important, *at least* 37 (20.1 percent) were diagnosed *simultaneously* with removal of the uterus.

Diagnosis at Hysterectomy: Case Descriptions

Of 37 patients diagnosed at hysterectomy, 27 (73 percent) were classed with severe disease by virtue of bowel and/or bladder involvement, perhaps justifying hysterectomy in the eyes of many practitioners. Ten (27 percent) were classed as less severe. Historically, none of the 37 had had prior surgical or medical treatment, including use of OCs. Severe cases' ages ranged between 28 and 56 (mean = 38.148; ± 6.34);† the majority were in their thirties and forties.

Among 10 patients classed as less severe, ages ranged from 21 to 62 (mean = 36.1; ± 12.34). Three were 21, 24, and 25. None had received prior medical/surgical intervention. None reported bowel or bladder involvement. We classed these as questionable surgeries.

Anomalously, two cases were diagnosed simultaneously at hysterectomy, but both had prior treatment. One, a 28-year-old, had had several surgeries and danazol prescribed, yet diagnosis remained elusive. A 36-year-old had a prior surgery; both had bowel/bladder involvement.

---

* The most important number for the lay reader here is the statistical mean or "average," which is the first number.

† The most important number to focus on is the mean or average. The number following the plus-or-minus refers to the standard deviation: the distance to the first standard deviation on each side of the mean. Readers interested in exploring the standard deviation should check a statistics textbook and study the area under a normal bell curve.

An additional four cases, diagnosed at hysterectomy, had used only OCs; however, it could not be determined if OCs were used for pseudo-pregnancy or pregnancy prevention. No other modality had been used; all were between 34 and 39, yet only one was classified as having severe disease.

For thoroughness, we examined 16 cases (8.7 percent of the HYST GR) that, while there *had been* a time interval between diagnosis and hysterectomy (months to years), had received no treatment. Six had bowel and/or bladder involvement; 10 were classed as less severe. Summarizing 184 cases, at least 37 (20.1 percent), and perhaps as many as 43 (23.4 percent), were diagnosed at the time of hysterectomy, marking the extent of under-diagnosis of endometriosis. An additional 16 (8.7 percent) were not treated. Importantly, the remaining 125 (67.9 percent) patients with hysterectomy received a diagnosis of endometriosis prior to hysterectomy and did receive medical and/or surgical intervention before hysterectomy.

Extent of Medical Therapy

An analysis of 175 patients, for whom all data were available, examined use of medical modalities: oral contraceptives, danazol, both, or neither. Almost half (48.9 percent) of 45 patients who had a hysterectomy at ages younger than 30 had used both drugs; an additional 24.4 percent had been treated with danazol; 22.2 percent had used only OCs. Two (4.4 percent) had used neither.

For 130 patients, aged 30 or over at hysterectomy, 30 percent had used both danazol and OCs (vs. 48.9 percent of patients under 30); 10 percent had used only danazol. Over one in three (35.4 percent) had simply used OCs, and 24.6 percent used neither (X^2 = 17.318; d.f. = 3; p = <0.01).

The severity index revealed higher percentages of patients under 30 treated with danazol, or danazol and OCs: 74.1 and 72.1 percent for severe and less severe categories, respectively (Table 3). Percentages fell dramatically for patients operated on at 30 and older: 37.2 vs. 44.2 percent in the severe and less severe categories, respectively. Still, for patients 30 and older, about 4 in 10 were reached with danazol therapy (X^2 = 20.575; d.f. = 9; p = <0.02).

Outcome of Surgical Intervention with Hysterectomy

Only 6 of 189 HYST patients failed to respond to the question "Did surgery offer relief or cure of your endometriosis?" An analysis showed that of 183 cases 56.3 percent reported surgery had offered a relief or cure of endometriosis; 13.1 percent "didn't know yet" or thought it was "too early to tell." For about one-third (30.6 percent), hysterectomy offered neither relief nor cure.

Because the passage of time since hysterectomy is an important variable in questions of symptom recurrence, information was sought relating to when surgery was performed. Data were available for most cases and missing data occurred randomly. Estrogen replacement therapy may affect symptom recurrence. No statistical differences between use of

Table 3. Prior Medical Management in Patients with Hysterectomy by Age at Hysterectomy and Severity Index

Use of Hormonal Drugs	Severe Hysterectomy Age				Less Severe Hysterectomy Age			
	Under 30 (N = 27)		30 and over (N = 78)		Under 30 (N = 18)		30 and over (N = 52)	
	f.	%	f.	%	f.	%	f.	%
Danazol and OCs both	14	51.9	21	26.9	8	44.4	18	34.6
Danazol (Danocrine) only	6	22.2	8	10.3	5	27.7	5	9.6
Oral contraceptives only	7	25.9	27	34.6	3	16.7	19	36.5
Used neither	0	0.0	22	28.2	2	11.1	10	19.2

$X^2 = 20.575$; d.f. $= 9$; $p = <0.02$

Table 4. Estrogen Replacement Therapy by Time Since Hysterectomy

Time since hysterectomy	Estrogen Replacement Therapy		
	Yes %	No %	Total %
This year	11.3	23.1	13.1
One year ago	38.7	50.0	40.3
Two years ago	17.3	(11.5)*	16.5
Three through 4 years ago	18.7	15.4	18.2
Five through 8 years ago	14.0	—	11.9
Total	150	26	176

$X^2 = 7.27$; d.f. $= 4$; $p = $ NS†
* Parentheses indicate fewer than 5 patients fell into this category.
† NS = probability p is not statistically significant.

ERT and time since hysterectomy emerged ($X^2 = 7.27$; d.f. $= 4$; $p = 0.12$). In short, the decision to use ERT was not affected by time since the hysterectomy, and the decision to use estrogen seemed to be made about the time of the surgery.

Responses to the question "Did surgery offer relief or cure of your endometriosis?" were comparable between the ERT and NO ERT patients. Perhaps the most striking result (see Table 5) was that only about two of every three cases (65.2 to 66.7 percent) believed hysterectomy offered substantial relief or cure; 34.8 percent of the ERT group expressed a negative outcome; an almost identical percentage (33.3 percent) of the NO ERTs did so. Neither analysis was statistically significant.

Because the group without ERT was small, and the analyses excluded patients believing "it was too soon to tell" if surgery would offer relief, an additional examination was conducted. The best-case scenario would occur if all cases in the "too early" category fell into the column reflecting that hysterectomy did, in fact, offer relief or cure.

Once again, for ERT patients, surgery made no statistical difference in outcome; 30.5 percent still reported that surgery offered no relief or cure. Simultaneously, for those not undergoing the palliative effects of estrogen, surgery still did not offer cure for 26.9 percent. (Palliative means treatment designed to relieve or reduce intensity of uncomfortable symptoms but not produce a cure.)

Estrogen Replacement Therapy

The final two analyses are not without methodological problems. At the time the questionnaire was constructed only patients receiving ERT were invited to reply to the question "If you had a hysterectomy and received estrogen replacement, did your endometriosis symptoms recur?" This question was not asked of patients not treated with ERT. Data in Table 6 describe symptom recurrence for the ERT group alone on 152 of the 161 cases for whom data on all variables were available. Results demonstrated that symptoms of endometriosis recurred for 44.1 percent ($X^2 = 34.39$; d.f. = 8; p = <0.001).

Of 161 patients receiving ERT, 64 volunteered information about the kinds of estrogen received. With the caveat that this small group may not be representative of all patients

Table 5. Did Surgery Offer Relief or Cure of Your Endometriosis? Outcome by ERT Status

| | Did Surgery Offer Relief or Cure? | | | | | |
| | Estrogen Replacement Therapy | | | Estrogen Replacement Not Used | | |
Time since hysterectomy	Yes %	No %	Total %	Yes %	No %	Total %
Less than 2 years ago	54.7	47.5	52.2	64.3	71.4	66.7
Two years or more	45.3	52.5	47.8	35.7	(28.6)*	33.3
Total	75	40	115	14	7	21
Percent of total	65.2	34.8	100.0	66.7	33.3	100.0

* Parentheses indicate fewer than 5 patients.
$X^2 = 2.140$; d.f. = 3; p = NS

Table 6. Recurrence of Endometriosis Symptoms by the Time Since Hysterectomy (N=152 cases with ERT only) and Types of ERT Volunteered by 64 Cases

| | Symptom Recurrence | | | Total | |
Time since hysterectomy	Yes %	No %	Too early to tell %	%	f.
This year	(4.5)*	8.9	27.5	11.8	(18)
One year ago	25.4	42.2	57.5	38.8	(59)
Two years ago	23.9	15.6	(7.5)*	17.1	(26)
3–4 years ago	26.9	17.8	(5.0)*	18.4	(28)
5–8 years ago	19.4	15.6	(2.5)	13.8	(21)
Total	67	45	40	152	
Percent of total	44.1	29.6	26.3	100.0	

* Parentheses indicate fewer than 4 patients in these categories.
$X^2 = 34.39$; d.f. = 8; p = <0.001

| | Type of Hormonal Replacement (N=64) | |
	Number	Percent of Total
Estrogen alone	26	40.6
	%	
Symptoms returned	69.2 (18)	
Symptoms did not return	19.2 (5)	
Too early to tell	11.5 (3)	
Estrogen with Provera or Depo-Provera or progesterone	29	45.3
Symptoms returned	57.1 (16)	
Symptoms did not return	17.9 (5)	
Too early to tell	25.0 (7)†	
Other combinations*	9	14.1
Symptoms returned	100.0 (9)	
Total	64	100.0

* Progesterone alone (4 cases; endo recurred); birth control pills alone (2 cases; endo recurred); estrogen, progesterone, and birth control pills (1 case; endo recurred); progesterone and birth control pills (1 case; endo recurred); Megace (1 case; endo recurred).
† Missing data = 1

receiving ERT, results showed 69.2 percent experienced a recurrence. If three cases believing it was "too early to tell" (if symptoms would return) are excluded, the percentage increases to 78.3 percent.

For estrogen, in combination with Provera or Depo-Provera, the comparable percentage of patients experiencing symptoms was 57.1 percent; once more, excluding seven cases who responded "too early to tell," the percentage rises to 76.2 percent—a percentage close to the rate for estrogen used alone.

Discussion

Several needs prompted the examination of the prevalence of hysterectomy among members of the study group. First, the prevalence of hysterectomy, cited as 19.5 percent among patients of all ages over 15 by the National Center for Health Statistics, indicates that about one in five females in the United States will undergo hysterectomy during her lifetime. Incidence rates for endometriosis, ranging from 17 to 24 percent of new gynecological patients and surgical admissions, increase the risk of surgery.[3] The substantial prevalence, and perhaps the willingness to treat endometriosis with surgery, mandates an assessment of how "good" hysterectomy, with and without ERT, is as an accepted therapy.

Major interest lies in the question of whether total abdominal hysterectomy and bilateral salpingo-oophorectomy *with ERT* to offset menopausal symptoms causes a recurrence of endometriosis. Conversely, did the absence of ERT facilitate a cure or, at least, a substantial reduction in symptoms?

Here perhaps we raise more questions than provide answers. Results showed that about 1 in 10 patients (9.0 percent) completing the questionnaire between 1982 and 1987 had a hysterectomy, a figure below the national average for endometriosis of 14.7 percent for all patients over 15. However, the median age for the cases examined here was 36 years. The prevalence of total abdominal hysterectomy/bilateral salpingo-oophorectomy was 7.1 percent; 85.2 percent of these 161 cases received ERT.

Is this rate acceptable? Certainly, if total abdominal hysterectomy/bilateral salpingo-oophorectomy is accepted as the primary modality for cure of endometriosis, one would question why patients would continue to seek additional approaches for help. Although we found that radical surgery had been used on patients in their twenties, the median and mean ages (36 to 37 years) indicated that probably physicians were *not* eager to use hysterectomy as a treatment alternative. The severity index, unrelated to most variables, strongly differentiated patients in the HYST GR. Whether hysterectomy was justified for all these patients remains unanswered. However, we did find that the majority of these patients had disease involving the bladder and/or bowels, and they were older. That the severity index related to symptoms perhaps should lend greater credibility to patients' complaints of gastrointestinal and bladder problems. However, the relatively short period of time between diagnosis and hysterectomy to us indicated the problem was due more to underdiagnosis than to a willingness for physicians to use hysterectomy as a treatment for endometriosis per se.

Among factors supporting this contention was the finding that hysterectomy was used indiscriminately for married and single women. Age and education also were no respecters of surgery. Rich or poor, educated or not, with the exception of age (in that hysterectomy patients as a group are older), hysterectomy was an equal-opportunity technique.

We did find that among the HYST GR less than half (48.1 percent) had been treated with danazol (p <0.001). Given the widespread usage of synthetic androgens (e.g., danazol), we had to explore why this more conservative approach had not been used more often. Why was the attempt to medically manage endometriosis not tried for more than half of these patients? Was the condition of such severity that total hysterectomy was indicated? Given the longevity of symptoms, were the patients simply tired of illness? Are there remaining "schools of thought" that polarize medical vs. surgical therapy and preclude the use of less radical approaches? In short, it seems to be the "older" women (over 30) and the less severe cases who have slipped through the system. Abuses in hysterectomy, if any, and as measured by hysterectomy of women in their twenties without previous treatment, were found in the less severe category: only three cases.

However, the fact that only two of three (67.9 percent) were diagnosed and treated prior to hysterectomy was unexpected. The fact that over 20 percent, at a minimum, were diagnosed simultaneously at hysterectomy was also surprising. One is forced to ponder the lack of early intervention, both medically and surgically, and the use of less drastic treatment regimens.

Conclusions appear strong that HYST patients were more seriously ill, as measured on the majority of indicators of illness severity and the severity index used here. Several natural history factors were summarized, including the greater preponderance of dysmenorrhea and pelvic pain experienced throughout the menstrual cycle, fatigue and low energy, dyspareunia, nausea, and gastric complaints, among several factors studied. Two additional factors need comment in a discussion of disease severity. These support the conclusion that patients undergoing hysterectomy were, statistically speaking, more ill than their counterparts.

The pain profile and frequencies with which the HYST GR complained of severe pain—perhaps a rationale for surgery rather than prolonged medical management—is one factor. Second, disability data showed greater interference with daily lives and incapacitation for longer periods.

Does total hysterectomy, for many patients the most dreaded of procedures, cure endometriosis? Regretfully, as measured here, the conclusion reached is no, not always. According to these patients, 33 to 35 percent report surgery offered neither relief nor cure, and 44.1 percent of those receiving ERT have experienced a return of symptoms.

A limited analysis of volunteered information on estrogen therapy showed neither estrogen used alone, primarily as Premarin, nor estrogen in combination with progesterone made any difference in whether symptoms recurred. Progesterone alone was rarely used. Of four cases all experienced symptom recurrence.

We cannot answer whether total hysterectomy was used more often than warranted or whether patients were rushed to hysterectomy before more conservative medical measures were used. But according to many patients' experiences we strongly suspect that this procedure will neither relieve nor cure endometriosis. Perhaps earlier diagnosis will improve this risk. Data on medical management of patients under 30 was encouraging.

Whether the doctor and patient decide against estrogen—and decide to sweat out menopausal symptoms—for fear of provoking return of endometriosis seems paradoxical. Estrogen or no estrogen. For many, neither made a difference. Symptoms continued to recur, reinforcing that endometriosis remains among the most resistant of diseases.

The search for etiological factors, as well as cures, remains elusive. Cramer[4] suggests several avenues geared toward prevention. The plausibility of other research, for example the search for genetic[5-7] or congenital causes, and the growing possibility of underlying immunological disorders, such as reported by Dmowski and his colleagues,[8] must continue to be supported.

This is an exploratory study. Future research begs replication and evaluation of the serious questions raised here. Certainly the poor results offered by hysterectomy, with or without ERT, and for many women the discomfort of immediate surgical menopause without respite demand rigorous evaluation of treatment regimens offered to patients with endometriosis.

Notes

1. "Hysterectomies in the United States, 1965-84," *Vital and Health Statistics, U.S. Department of Health and Human Services, Public Health Service, Centers for Disease Control, National Center for Health Statistics,* Series 13, no. 92 (1987).
2. A. A. Acosta, V. C. Buttram, P. K. Besch, L. R. Malinak, R. R. Franklin, and J. D. Vanderheyden, "A Proposed Classification of Pelvic Endometriosis," *Obstetrics and Gynecology* 42, no. 1 (1973): 19–25.
3. Diana E. Houston, "Evidence for the Risk of Pelvic Endometriosis by Age, Race and Socioeconomic Status," *Epidemiological Reviews,* no. 6 (1984): 167–91.
4. D. W. Cramer, "Epidemiology of Endometriosis," *Endometriosis,* E. A. Wilson, ed. (New York: Alan R. Liss, 1987).
5. J. L. Simpson, J. Elias, L. R. Malinak, and V. C. Buttram, "Heritable Aspects of Endometriosis; I. Genetic Studies," *American Journal of Obstetrics and Gynecology* 137, no. 237 (1980).
6. L. R. Malinak, V. C. Buttram, S. Elias, and J. L. Simpson, "Heritable Aspects of Endometriosis; II. Clinical Characteristics of Familial Endometriosis," *American Journal of Obstetrics and Gynecology* 137, no. 332 (1980).
7. K. Lamb, R. G. Hoffmann, and T. R. Nichols, "Family Trait Analysis: A Case-Control Study of 43 Women with Endometriosis and Their Best Friends," *American Journal of Obstetrics and Gynecology* 154, no. 3 (1986): 596.
8. W. P. Dmowski, R. W. Steele, and G. F. Baker, "Deficient Cellular Immunity in Endometriosis," *American Journal of Obstetrics and Gynecology* 141, no. 377 (1981).

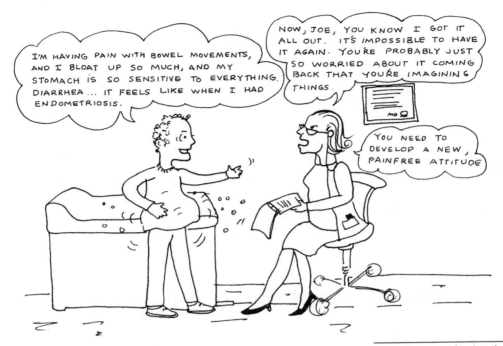

Unfortunately, the doubled dose of TRH has some consequences.

■ **Karen Lamb, R.N., Ph.D.,** *is the former director of the Endometriosis Association Research Registry and former director, Uihlein Family Health Program, Milwaukee, Wisconsin.* **Lyle J. Breitkopf, M.D.,** *is assistant professor of ob-gyn, New York University, and director of the Endometriosis Clinic, New York Downtown Hospital.* **Karen J. Hamilton, M.D.,** *was a volunteer at the time she assisted Dr. Lamb with this study. Originally trained as a laboratory technologist, Hamilton's struggles with infertility, pregnancy loss, and endometriosis contributed to her desire to become a physician. Currently training to become an ob-gyn, she feels she has found her calling in this field.*

This study was funded with philanthropic awards from Ms. Tracy H. Dickinson, New Jersey, and GeorgAnna and Joseph Uihlein, Jr., Wisconsin.

Adhesions and Endometriosis:
The Puzzle Continues

By Paula Zimlicki and Mary Lou Ballweg

"*I* have suffered with these (damn) adhesions for the past eight to nine years. . . .

"No doctor can help me, only take painkillers and when any vital organ is affected then they will operate, and more will grow after surgery. It is a horrible dilemma. . . .

"There are times when I feel if only I could die and be out of this misery, but on the other hand, I look at my family, which I am so blessed with, and think that life is so beautiful as well as nature, even though I am limited. . . ."

Veronica, Ontario

"*T*he results of the surgery were extensive adhesions involving the bowel, bladder, ovaries, tubes, uterus—you get the idea. There was endometriosis there, but from what I saw on the video there were more adhesions than disease. With me that has always been the case, and since this was my sixth surgery, I think the precedent is pretty well set. [The doctor's office] advised me to take Motrin around the clock to reduce inflammation because of the amount of surgery to the area. . . ."

Paula, New Hampshire

"*I* had a hysterectomy with lysis of adhesions. My uterus was so adhered to my bladder that some damage to that organ occurred.

"Fortunately the long-term effects have been minimal. Endo was still present in both ovaries at surgery even though I had continued on the danazol. The endo on my right ovary was cauterized, and my postop recovery progressed well. In fact, other than incisional pain, my postop pain was not much worse than my preop pain. I was placed on danazol for one month postop. I remained symptom-free for 10 months, then my pain returned. At that time I felt very betrayed by my body. My decision at that time was Depo-Provera. Six months on the Depo-Provera led to no improvement, so a second surgery was performed to remove my remaining ovary and again lyse [cut] the adhesions. Since that time I have been free of symptoms. . . .

"I do not for a minute regret my decision. I could not have continued on in the physical and emotional state I was in. . . ."

Donna, Michigan

Adhesions—bands of scar tissue that bind together surfaces and organs normally separate—can cause as many problems for women with endometriosis as active endo growths themselves. Dealing with adhesions can be perplexing and frustrating not only for the woman but also for her doctor because no one knows exactly how to prevent them or treat them.

So what exactly are adhesions? Essentially they are stretched-out scar tissue. When you injure your skin, with a cut, for instance, it can form a scar. Imagine what would happen if you had cuts or raw surfaces between two fingers and, during the time of healing, the two fingers were bound together so the cuts or raw surfaces were held next to each other. Under these conditions the two areas might grow together permanently with scar tissue.

Normally, of course, we are able to keep the two surfaces apart during healing when the surfaces are external. But when they're internal, such as inside our abdomen, the surfaces that are raw, cut, or inflamed from surgery or the inflammation that accompanies endometriosis can easily come into contact with each other. Because the pelvic organs are mobile, they may at times touch each other. Raw, cut, inflamed, or bleeding surfaces can then adhere to each other, and then, as the organs naturally shift and move, the surfaces can partially pull apart again, stretching the fibrous scar tissue between the organs. This stretched-out band of scar tissue is called an _adhesion_.

Another way to think of adhesions is to compare them to taffy, that sticky, stringy candy that, the more you pull it, the longer it gets and the more it adheres itself to your fingers. (See the illustration.)

Adhesions can have quite a variety of characteristics, as described by Dr. David L. Olive in the gynecological textbook _Endometriosis: Contemporary Concepts in Clinical Management_,[1] edited by Dr. Robert Schenken. He writes, "Adhesions may be thin, thick, transparent, or opaque and avascular or well vascularized. They com-

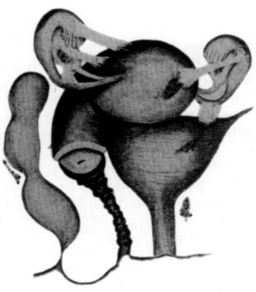

Adhesions can be seen in this picture stretching between the uterus and the ovary and fallopian tube on the left side, between the ovary and tube on the left side, between the uterus and tube on the right side, and between the tube and bladder on the right side. To the far left is part of the colon.

monly occur between structures of high mobility and in areas susceptible to endometriotic implantation. Pelvic structures most commonly involved include the ovaries, tubes, and posterior aspects of the broad ligaments."

They are also found on the front bladder peritoneum, the peritoneum over the front of the uterus, the sigmoid colon, and the posterior section of the vagina and the cervix, according to Dr. A. F. Haney, author of the chapter "Pathogenesis and Pathophysiology" in Dr. Emery A. Wilson's textbook *Endometriosis*.[2] He writes that the fallopian tubes and small bowel are most often spared. He also maintains that adhesions due to endometriosis are most common between immobile pelvic structures—just the opposite of Olive's comment noted earlier.

Experiences of members make it clear that adhesions, just as endometrial growths, can cause intense pain, impair fertility, result in bowel obstructions and bladder problems, and necessitate surgery. Adhesions can pull on internal organs and significantly distort one's anatomy, resulting in considerable pain and physical problems.

Symptoms caused by adhesions are similar to symptoms caused by active endo. Adhesions often seem to cause pain after activities that can stretch them such as exercise, intercourse, or pelvic and rectal exams.

Dr. Arnold Kresch of Palo Alto, California, has studied the words women use to describe abdominal pain and found there is a tendency to use certain words to describe the pain due to adhesions compared with the pain due to active endo. From hundreds of patients he selected 42 who had only adhesions or only active endo without adhesions. (He says many of the patients have both.) The adjectives more commonly used to describe adhesions were *stabbing, sharp, pulling, sickening, intense, nauseating*. The adjectives more commonly used to describe active endo were *burning, pinching, dull, heavy,* and *miserable*. There was some crossover in both sets of descriptive words. (Also, only one-quarter of the adhesions-only group had had endo. It seems likely that adhesions due to endo feel similar to adhesions due to other causes such as pelvic inflammatory disease, for example, but we don't know for sure.)

For some women with endo their pain may be due to adhesions, even if they've never had surgery, and may be the unsuspected cause of their problems. Esther, from Pennsylvania, learned this. She writes: "Dr. H. I. has been treating me since I was a teenager (I'm now 36). I'll spare you the gory details of the years of pain and medications we tried. I finally got to the point where I was ready for the laparoscopy. Dr. I. and his associate seemed to work a miracle on me by cutting adhesions. That was six years ago, and I have been a different person since then. Yes, I do have my moments of severe pain at ovulation and an occasional bad period. And of course the pain with sex is still there occasionally. But the key word is *occasional*. In addition to which, my pain can now be controlled—or subdued—with Extra Strength Bufferin or Darvocet, not the heavy duty drugs I used to take."

Adhesions can cause havoc particularly with intestinal function. Diana, from Massachusetts, wrote, "I haven't been able to eat right since after my operation and diagnosis after diagnosis of PID, which has been ruled out, [and the] possibility of endo has cropped up again. I am scheduled to have a third laparoscopy . . . with the same doctor, but this time she is having another specialist assist her. I'm scared and frustrated at the same time. Before last year I had upper and lower barium x-rays and a scope in the stomach because I told them my digestive system wasn't right. Well, they told me I had 'spastic colon' and had to live with it also. They also recommended a psychologist, whom I went to." The laparoscopy showed that her large bowel was adhered to her left fallopian tube and ovary. Small adhesions were also formed between her right ovary and the back of her pelvis.

In cases of long-standing endometriosis the adhesions may cause loops of small or large bowel to become entangled, resulting in obstruction and other complications, according to Dr. Ibrahim Ramzy, author of the chapter "Pathology" in Schenken's book. This was apparently the case for Neva, from Indiana. Her story also illustrates the fact that women who have had hysterectomies and removal of the ovaries for endo need to consider adhesions as a possible cause if they have a return of pain (as well as a return of active endo as the cause).

Different courses of action are needed, depending on which is the cause. If it's active endo, for instance, the woman may need to stop estrogen replacement. If it's adhesions, surgery to remove them may be necessary.

Neva had surgery to remove her remaining ovary because of severe pain, loss of bowel function, and adhesions. Neva reports that all was well for six months, until she once again began experiencing severe pain in her lower abdomen, loss of bowel function, partial intestinal blockage, and weight gain. A laparoscopy showed that adhesions had caused her bowel to adhere to the abdominal wall. The adhesions were cut away, but three months later the same problem returned.

She describes the symptoms she experiences when her adhesions begin giving her problems. "I can always tell when my problems start, even the very day. I will experience an extremely large bowel movement and then swelling almost immediately and weight gain. At this time I cannot tolerate regular food and roughage, and I never get better regardless of how I limit my diet. Some foods do not cause as much swelling as others, but all food causes pain. . . .

"In March I went to Nashville, Tennessee, for laser surgery to be performed by way of laparoscopy. During this surgery a video was made of the adhesions and the matting of the intestines. There was no trace of any endo left in the abdominal cavity. All that we were dealing with were adhesions from the endo and all the surgery that I had had over the years.

"The adhesions were in masses, and it was very evident that anyone with this type of adhesions and as many would be in severe pain and have serious problems with bowel function. This was the first time that I had hard-copy evidence that I was not suffering from 'stress' or any other mental condition—the doctors had tried to convince me that 'stress' was the main reason for my colon condition." (Neva also was told she had a spastic colon.)

What causes adhesions? No one knows the exact answer to this question, but a lot of contributing factors are known to play a role. According to Dr. William H. Pfeffer, in an article in *Contemporary Ob/Gyn*,[3] adhesions are caused by operative trauma, temporary loss of blood supply to the tissue, foreign bodies, hemorrhage, raw surfaces, and infection. Pfeffer notes that all these things bring into play other factors leading to adhesions: an inflammatory reaction, release of prostaglandins and histamine, and other elements causing increased permeability of the small blood vessels. Blood seeps through the small blood vessels and collects in the traumatized tissue, clotting factors are activated, and the clot formed provides a matrix for the other cells that give rise to a fibrous adhesion. The disruption of blood flow also leads to inflammation.

Foreign-body reaction might occur from any number of things related to surgery, Pfeffer writes, including suture material, lint, talc,* and fragments from sponge or from cloth or paper drapes. The reaction to any type of foreign body involves lymphocytes, mast cells, macrophages, and other immune cells and immune complexes, all potentially contributing to the development of adhesions.

Pfeffer discusses these contributing factors as they relate to adhesions that form as a result of surgery, but the same factors are involved in adhesions that form because of endometriosis. Inflammation occurs around the misplaced endometrial tissue, internal bleeding occurs as active growths cause cyclic bleeding, and the misplaced tissue may cause a foreign-body reaction.

In addition to the formation of adhesions, smaller amounts of scarring occurs. "Scarring of the peritoneum around endometrial implants is the typical finding," writes Dr. Haney in a chapter of the Wilson book. "In addition to encapsulating an isolated implant, the scar may deform the surrounding peritoneum or result in the development of adhesions between adjacent pelvic viscera" (viscera are abdominal organs). The scarring can also constrict or contract tissues around it, leading to pain and various problems depending on the location.

Women with endometriosis thus can develop scar tissue and adhesions from the endo itself. In addition, of course, surgery brings with it the risk of adhesion formation.

Surgical technique clearly makes a difference as to whether adhesions form postop. Even with good technique, though, adhesions form in some people who seem particularly prone to them. Some physicians believe that if you're a person whose skin heals keloid you may be more prone to developing adhesions. (Keloid is elevated, irregularly shaped scar tissue.)

Pfeffer writes, "Clearly, surgical technique that minimizes trauma, ischemia [loss of blood supply], foreign bodies, hemorrhage, raw surfaces, and infection will best prevent postoperative adhesions formation."

---

*Talc comes from surgical gloves. Careful surgeons will use talc-free gloves or will wash talc-treated gloves before doing surgery to prevent adhesions.

Using certain surgical techniques to reduce the chances of adhesion formation is also discussed by Olive in Schenken's textbook. Olive cautions surgeons to take care not to allow tissue to dry and to prevent loss of blood to tissue as much as possible. Crush injuries and undue tension on peritoneal surfaces should be prevented. Measures should be taken to prevent rather than merely recognize and treat inflammation of the peritoneum. Endometriotic lesions should be removed with minimal tissue trauma. Techniques in which organs (especially the uterus and ovaries) are suspended with sutures away from areas the organs could adhere to are also used at times in an attempt to avoid adhesions.

In addition, many surgeons concerned about preventing adhesions use a variety of solutions or materials put into the pelvis at the time of surgery that may work to prevent adhesion formation. Studies of these materials have been done for many years and reports on them made at research conventions. Some of the most commonly used of these materials (called *adjuvants*) are solutions instilled into the abdomen at the time of surgery (such as dextran and lactated Ringer's); a woven material made of cellulose that forms a gel after it is placed over surfaces at surgery (Interceed); and even small pieces of a plastic material (polytetrafluoroethylene) that is sutured in place and then removed at a later surgery or left (Gore-Tex). The goal of the various materials is to keep raw or cut surfaces separated while healing occurs and, in some cases, to actually inhibit formation of adhesions.

Unfortunately, results from studies of these materials are quite contradictory. Early reports on Interceed, for example, were positive, but later reports were contradictory, and one investigator found the substance may actually cause adhesions. Studies on other substances used for adhesion prevention have also at times been confusing or contradictory. Obviously, more study is needed!

After discussing the importance of surgical technique and the use of various materials in possibly preventing adhesions, you might assume that all surgeons operating on women with endo think about adhesions and make every attempt to prevent them. Unfortunately, this is not the case.

An example from Pfeffer's article shows the problem. A 26-year-old woman attempting to conceive has surgery for ovarian cysts and tubal adhesions. "Her surgeon uses delicate instruments, fine-caliber nonreactive suture, special techniques, and intraperitoneal medications." All this is done to minimize her chances of developing adhesions because the adhesions could contribute to infertility.

A 17-year-old with painful periods also has surgery. She too has ovarian cysts and tubal adhesions. During her surgery the surgeon removes the cysts and adhesions but takes no special measures to prevent adhesions.

Pfeffer questions why women whose chief problem is infertility should receive better surgical care than women who are not yet concerned with their fertility. He points out that later in her life the 17-year-old may also desire children.

But the larger question here is: Why shouldn't surgeons use the best available techniques to reduce adhesion formation for all women with endo, whether they are 17 years old or 44 years old, whether they are trying to become pregnant, trying to resolve pain, or having hysterectomies? Shouldn't prevention of pain, bowel problems, and restricted movement and activities also be priorities? Is the hidden message that the woman herself and her pain don't matter? (Even when a surgery is being done to remove scar tissue and adhesions, many of the techniques used to minimize adhesions are not being used!)

Another surgery issue for women with endo is how should *endo* be removed to prevent adhesions? Few studies have compared the techniques used to remove endometrial growths in relation to adhesion formation. These techniques are excision (cutting them out), fulguration or cauterization (burning the growths to destroy them), and laser (vaporizing or excising them). Unfortunately, the few studies carried out so far have not conclusively shown one technique superior to another.

One positive development in the war against adhesions has been the development of operative laparoscopy (in which laser, electrosurgical, or other tools are used through the laparoscope and a small incision). A number of studies have shown that fewer new adhesions develop with operative laparoscopy compared to laparotomy (surgery involving an incision of several inches and an open abdomen) but that old adhesions still tend to re-form after laparoscopy.

Another development that has helped, especially in women prone to adhesions, is what is called a *second-look laparoscopy*. After a laparoscopic surgery to remove endo and adhesions, a second laparoscopy is carried out a week or so after the first surgery. In the second surgery, adhesions (which form within the first three days after surgery) are cut and removed. (One of the association's advisors, Dr. David Olive of Yale, is doing second-look laparoscopy as an office procedure with a tiny, two-millimeter laparoscope.) With early second-look laparoscopy adhesions are usually quite easy to cut or break up since they have not had sufficient time to form into thick, dense adhesions. Obviously, however, this is yet another surgery for the patient.

The types of stitches used—indeed whether sutures are used at all—also makes a difference in adhesion formation. As noted in a review article on adhesion research, all experimental evidence indicates that peritoneum heals better without sutures and that suturing of peritoneum actually increases the incidence of adhesions.[4] Suturing ovaries has also been reported to result in more adhesions than leaving them unsutured.

So how do you get rid of adhesions once you have them? Unlike endometriosis, adhesions and scar tissue, once in place, do not respond to medical therapy. The usual way to deal with adhesions is through surgery; the catch-22 is that having surgery increases your chances for the formation of more adhesions and re-formation where the old adhesions were.

In removing adhesions in women with endometriosis, Olive notes that care must be taken to excise the entire adhesion rather than simply cut it. The reason is that simple incision may leave tags of tissue that may lead to more adhesion formation. In addition, he notes, active endometrial implants have been found in adhesions.

If scar tissue and adhesions are known problems for you, find the very best surgeon you possibly can and discuss surgical precautions to prevent adhesion re-formation and new adhesions with your chosen surgeon. You need an excellent surgeon also because dense adhesions increase the risk of damaging organs such as the ureter or rectum.

Adhesions can form even when excellent surgical technique is used, but obviously it still makes sense to use the very best techniques possible. Study your operative report(s) from prior surgeries. And if you've had a number of surgeries followed by adhesion formation, consider another surgeon. Not all surgeons are as meticulous as they should be. Of course, as we noted, adhesions can form even when excellent surgical technique is used, but again it makes no sense to take unnecessary risks such as leaving behind blood in the abdomen, allowing tissue to dry out, or being rough with the tissues.

Pain was one of the reasons why Sandy, whose problems with endo began after an IUD lodged in her uterus, consented to a total hysterectomy with removal of her ovaries when she was 26 years old. Seven months after the hysterectomy the severe pain returned: "I was in so much pain that all I did was lie around all curled up. . . . When she [the surgeon] went in, she says that she didn't find any endometriosis but scar tissue. The pains still felt like endometriosis. Two months after surgery the same old pains were back."

The physical and mental distress of dealing with endometriosis put enough stress on her marriage that it ended in divorce. Her third major operation in 16 months also showed that her pain was due not to active endometriosis but to adhesions. Her doctor put her on 800 milligrams of Motrin (ibuprofen) three times a day, which she says helps. However, she continues to have pain in her ribs and lower back.

There may be nonsurgical help for women such as Sandy. One member reported tremendous relief from pain due to adhesions with Rolfing, a deep massage technique intended to help in the realignment of the body by altering the length and tone of myofascial (muscle and connective) tissues. Another member, Shannon, of Ontario, reports the use of ultrasound by a homeopathic doctor, Dr. Lyle Leffler, in relieving the pain caused by adhesions. In an interview Leffler said the ultrasound used for reducing adhesion pain is the type used by physical therapists in treating muscle problems. It works on the same principle as the ultrasound with which most of us are familiar—high-frequency sound waves are emitted by the ultrasound. These sound waves penetrate to the wall of the adhesion and relax it so that its pull on adjacent tissues is reduced.

The ultrasound does not get rid of the adhesion but helps alleviate the pain. Leffler said this type of treatment lessens the chances that a woman will have to undergo a second surgery for pain from adhesions. "I don't think in my years of practice I've had one case that didn't respond favorably to it," he said.

Leffler, who has been in practice for more than 20 years, says it is important to have this done by someone who is knowledgeable in its use. Your gynecologist should be able to refer you to a physical therapist, he said. If your doctor is skeptical about giving you a referral, Leffler suggests you see a chiropractor.

In summary, adhesions can create many problems for women with endo, and although it is not clear what causes adhesions or exactly how to prevent them, it is clear that surgical technique can make a difference. What is encouraging is the recognition by gynecological surgeons that more research is needed on what causes adhesions and what measures can be taken in preventing them.

Notes

1. R. S. Schenken, *Endometriosis: Contemporary Concepts in Clinical Management* (Philadelphia: J. B. Lippincott Company, 1989), 227.
2. E. A. Wilson, *Endometriosis* (New York: Alan R. Liss, 1987).
3. W. H. Pfeffer, "A Surgeon's Guide to Preventing Adhesions," *Contemporary Ob/Gyn* 19 (February 1982).
4. G. diZerega, "Contemporary Adhesion Prevention," *Fertility and Sterility* 61, no. 2 (1994): 219–35.

3

𖦹𖦹

Medical Treatment for Endometriosis: Overview and Alternative Options

By David L. Olive, M.D.

"*My experience has been: (1) Strong suggestion from my M.D. that I take Danocrine. I was unhappy about the cost, but more important, the possible side effects. Being a DES daughter has made me very wary about drugs, and this one carries so many that to me the risk-benefit ratio was not in my favor. . . . (2) Alternate treatment with Ovral birth control pills. I spotted and had erratic mood swings the entire time and also had sensations of pain in the abdominal area. (3) Finally began taking Provera. Had immediate relief from the symptoms I was feeling and continue to feel great. . . .*"

Martha, California

"*All the information I had read on Depo-Provera and even the doctors said that there would be no bleeding while I was on it, just maybe some breakthrough bleeding. Well, I took three shots of it four weeks apart starting in October and ending in December. In November I started spotting every day. By February I was bleeding heavier and every day. I went through every kind of hormone they could use to stop it, and finally I just had a D & C to stop it, which I think it finally did. Also they said the effects of Depo-Provera would last only the four to six weeks between the shots, when actually they can last up to a year. . . .*"

Mary, Delaware

"*I was on Danocrine for nine months about two years ago and felt well while on the drug, but my symptoms recurred shortly after discontinuing the drug. I tried birth control pills but had too much heavy spotting. I get a shot of Depo-Provera every three months (I have been on it nine months), and my symptoms are about 90 percent improved. I had some spotting (light) in the beginning only. . . .*"

"I felt very well physically on the medication. For the first three months I felt fine emotionally also. After that I experienced mild depression and, according to my husband, who is very supportive, I was 'wired.' The least little thing sent me into a rage—the poor children! I am usually a very happy, even-tempered person. I decided to tough it out, hoping that mind over hormones would work. Wrong! Although my feelings were probably not evident to the outside world, I didn't feel really 'normal' mentally until about five months after the shot. . . ."

Elaine, Connecticut

"My endometriosis began shortly after the birth of my only child 21 years ago. I have taken Ortho-Novum for 11 years, have had a laparoscopic examination and surgery, one year on Danocrine, and 30 months on Provera with little or no improvement. (Actually, while on and just after treatment with the Provera my pain and periods were worse. . . .)"

Sally, Indiana

Endometriosis has been the target of countless attempts at therapeutic intervention. At the forefront has been the search for effective medical treatment. Several observations support a role for such an approach. First, endometriosis is encountered in the woman who has had children, but much more often in the woman who has not had children, suggesting a protective effect of the hormonal milieu of pregnancy. Second, endometrium is known to be estrogen-dependent, with ectopic endometrium (that is, endometriosis) presumably behaving in much the same manner. Finally, endometriosis tends to occur nearly exclusively in menstruating, reproductive-age females, again suggesting hormonal dependence.

Although danazol and the GnRH agonists (see the articles on GnRH drugs in this chapter for background) are the only two classes of drugs approved by the Food and Drug Administration for the treatment of endometriosis, numerous other medications have been used both domestically and internationally. Many of these medications have undergone extensive testing in well-designed clinical trials, while for others there is little or no information regarding efficacy. This chapter will provide a comprehensive review of these alternative medical approaches for the treatment of endometriosis.

Assessing Efficacy

The value of a particular medical treatment on endometriosis will vary depending on the therapeutic goal of the intervention. With regard to endometriosis, there are three outcomes that can be assessed to determine drug efficacy: the anatomic manifestations of the disease, pain symptoms, and infertility status.

The anatomic manifestations of endometriosis, implants and adhesions, can be assessed before and after therapy to determine whether the intervention is of value. However, such a simple comparison makes two assumptions. First, it is assumed that endometriosis is an invariably progressive disease, never to regress on its own; this is incorrect, as the disease has in fact been noted to regress in both baboons[1] and humans.[2]

Second, the preceding comparison presupposes that once regression has occurred via medical therapy it is stable. This, too, is not the case, as implant and adhesion regrowth are both time-dependent phenomena (occurring over time, not immediately). Thus, to adequately address the effect of a medical treatment on endometriosis lesions, a proper control group for comparison is needed, with longitudinal follow-up.

A second outcome of interest is the effect on pain. The first requirement of quality pain evaluation is the need for a valid method of assessing pain. While numerous scales have been used in the medical literature, none have been adequately validated specifically for pelvic pain. A second necessity in pain research is the need for longitudinal evaluation, because pain recurrence is a time-dependent phenomenon. Finally, to determine the efficacy of a drug in relieving pain, a placebo effect must be accounted for. [3]

The final outcome of interest is fertility enhancement. It is rare that the woman with endometriosis-associated infertility has absolute infertility due to the disease, as is the case with bilateral tubal blockage or azospermia (absence of sperm). Instead, most women suffering from endometriosis-associated infertility have a relative reduction in their fertility. Thus, they are able to conceive, albeit at a slower rate.[4] To demonstrate improved fertility status after intervention, a comparison group of untreated women is clearly needed. Finally, since fertility is also time-dependent, longitudinal assessment is again critical.

From this discussion it is clear that optimal trials are properly controlled, comparative studies with time-dependent follow-up. Only such studies will be relied on in the subsequent discussion.

Progestogens

Progestogens are a class of compounds that produce progesteronelike effects on endometrial tissue. A large number of progestogens exist, ranging from those chemically derived from progesterone (progestins) such as medroxyprogesterone acetate (MPA) to derivatives of male hormones such as norethindrone and norgestrel. The proposed mechanism of action of these compounds is an inhibition of the estrogen effect on this tissue, resulting in a shrinkage of the endometriosis. This is believed due to a direct effect of progestogens on the estrogen receptors of the endometriosis.

Progestational agents may be administered according to a wide variety of protocols befitting the pharmaceutical diversity of the available drugs. Injectable forms have been utilized, but oral administration is currently felt to be preferable for the patient desiring eventual conception due to the rapid reversibility of the effect. MPA, or Provera, the most commonly used medication in this class, is generally administered in doses of 20 to 100 milligrams daily for three to six months.

Side effects of progestational agents vary greatly, depending on the specific progestogen, the dosage, the interval of treatment, and the route of administration. A common side effect is transient breakthrough bleeding, which occurs in 38 to 47 percent. This is generally well tolerated and, when necessary, can be treated adequately with supplemental estrogen or an increase in the progestogen dose. Other side effects include nausea (0 to 80 percent), breast tenderness (5 percent), fluid retention (50 percent), and depression (6 percent).[5] In published trials few patients have discontinued the medications due to side effects. In contradistinction to danazol, all of the aforementioned adverse effects resolve upon discontinuation of the drugs.

Progestogens may adversely affect serum lipoprotein levels. The 19-nortestosterone derivatives significantly decrease high-density lipoprotein (HDL), a change linked to an increased risk of coronary artery disease.[6] Data on medroxyprogesterone acetate are less clear, with studies demonstrating either no effect[7] or a slight decrease.[8] It is likely that there is a decrease in HDL with all these agents, but the magnitude is related to the specific progestogen and the dose administered. Whether alterations in serum lipoprotein levels for four to six months produce any lasting effects in women is unclear.

Although progestogens clearly affect endometriosis, there is limited information on what the drugs do to the appearance of implants. In the rhesus monkey norgestrel has been shown to decrease lesion size. In the human a single randomized prospective trial demonstrated that 100 milligrams MPA daily for six months produced complete resolution of implants in 50 percent of patients and a partial resolution in 13 percent, whereas corresponding figures for placebos were 12 percent and 6 percent, respectively.[9] The investigators found no difference between MPA and danazol, and both gave greater relief than placebo. Unfortunately, the duration of relief is not well assessed.

Progestogens, like the other medical treatments for endometriosis, have not been shown to be effective in improving fertility. In a nonrandomized trial of women with early-stage disease who were treated with medroxyprogesterone, danazol, or expectant management (observation only), the pregnancy rates over a 30-month period were similar.[10] Another study, including women with all stages of disease, similarly found no difference in pregnancy rates among these three treatments.[11]

In conclusion progestogens appear to be of value in combating the physical manifestations of endometriosis (at least temporarily) as well as the pain associated with the disease (at least temporarily). However, there is no evidence that progestogens can be used to improve fertility rates in women with endometriosis-associated infertility.

Oral Contraceptives
(Combination Estrogen-Progestogen)

The combination of estrogen and progestogen for therapy of endometriosis, the so-called *pseudopregnancy regimen*, has been utilized for 40 years. Like progestational therapy alone, pseudopregnancy is believed to produce shrinkage of endometrial tissue. This has been observed in women[12] but is in direct conflict with data from the rhesus monkey demonstrating larger implants with considerable local growth following the use of these hormones in treating endo.[13]

Pseudopregnancy regimens have been administered both orally and via injection. Combination oral contraceptive pills such as norethynodrel and mestranol, norethindrone acetate and ethanol estradiol, lynestrenol and mestranol, and norgestrel plus ethanol estradiol have all been tried. Injectable combinations have included 17-hydroxyprogesterone or Depo-Provera paired with stilbestrol or Premarin.

Side effects of pseudopregnancy are often quite impressive and include those encountered with progestogens alone, as well as estrogenic- and androgenic-related effects. Estrogens may cause nausea, high blood pressure, blood clots, and enlargement of the uterus. The 19-nortestosterone-derived progestogens may cause androgenic effects such as acne, loss of hair, increased muscle mass, decreased breast size, and deepening of the voice. Noble and Letchworth, in a comparative trial of norethynodrel and mestranol vs. danazol, found that 41 percent of the pseudopregnancy group failed to complete their course of therapy due to side effects of the medication.[14] However, dosages producing significant side effects generally involved more estrogen than found in modern contraceptive preparations. The oral contraceptives commonly prescribed today for combination therapy are more likely to produce a progestogen-dominant picture similar to that of progestogen alone.

Today oral contraceptives are the most commonly prescribed treatment for endometriosis symptoms. Despite this, there are few data regarding efficacy. The effect of these regimens on implants has not been evaluated; only uncontrolled trials assessing pelvic findings via pelvic examination have been reported.

Numerous uncontrolled trials have evaluated pain relief, generally demonstrating improvement in 75 to 89 percent.[5] A recent randomized clinical trial compared cyclic low-dose oral contraceptives to a GnRH agonist and found no substantial difference in the degree of relief afforded these women by the two drugs, except that the GnRH agonist provided greater relief of dysmenorrhea.[15]

Reports of pregnancy rates in women with endometriosis-associated infertility treated with oral contraceptives are sparse and uncontrolled. None provide evidence of improvement of fertility by these medications.

Thus oral contraceptives have been documented to improve endometriosis-related pain symptoms to a degree comparable to other treatments. However, there are no data suggesting a decrease in the size of implants or fertility-enhancing effects.

Gestrinone

Gestrinone (ethylnorgestrienone, R2323) is an antiprogestational steroid used extensively in Europe and South America for the treatment of endometriosis. Its effects include androgenic, antiprogestogenic, and antiestrogenic actions, although the last is not mediated by estrogen receptor binding.

This steroid is believed to act by inducing a progesterone withdrawal effect at the endometrial cellular level, thus enhancing degradation of the cell. There is a rapid decrease in estrogen and progesterone receptors in normal endometrium following administration of gestrinone. Interestingly, these cellular effects did not occur in samples of endometriotic tissue.[16]

Gestrinone may also inhibit production of ovarian hormones. A 50 percent decrease in serum estradiol level is noted after administration,[17] perhaps related to the associated significant decline in sex-hormone-binding globulin concentration (an androgenic or antiprogestogenic effect). No effect on adrenal function or prolactin secretion has been noted.

Gestrinone is administered orally in doses of 2.5 to 10 milligrams weekly, on a daily, twice-weekly, or three-times-weekly schedule. Side effects are androgenic and antiestrogenic. Although most side effects are mild and transient, several, such as voice changes, development of facial hair, and enlargement of the clitoris, are potentially irreversible.

Several randomized trials have assessed the ability of gestrinone to decrease anatomic endometriosis. The drug has been shown to reduce the amount of disease comparably to danazol,[18] and doses as low as 1.25 milligrams twice weekly can accomplish this.[19, 20] Uncontrolled trials suggest pain relief comparable to other medical treatments for endometriosis, and this has been confirmed when compared to danazol.[18] Finally, there is no evidence that gestrinone can enhance fertility in women with endometriosis-associated infertility.[18] Thus gestrinone appears to have clinical efficacy similar to all of the aforementioned medical treatments for endometriosis.

RU486 (Mifepristone)

Apart from its controversial role in pregnancy termination, mifepristone (RU486) may well prove to be of value in a wide variety of gynecologic disorders, including endometriosis. The drug is an antiprogesterone and antiglucocorticoid that can inhibit ovulation and disrupt the normal architecture of the endometrium. Doses of the medication range from 50 to 100 milligrams daily, with side effects ranging from hot flashes to fatigue, nausea, and transient changes in liver function. No effect on lipid profiles or bone mineral density has been reported.

The ability of mifepristone to produce a regression of endometriotic lesions has been variable and apparently dependent on duration of treatment. Trials of two months in rats with surgically induced endometriosis[21] and three months in the human[22] failed to produce regression of disease. However, six months of therapy resulted in less visible disease in women.[23]

Uncontrolled trials suggest possible efficacy for endometriosis-associated pain, although numbers are small.[22] No data have yet been collected regarding fertility enhancement.

Other Medications

A wide variety of additional medical therapies have been attempted in combating endometriosis. Some, such as estrogen and methyltestosterone, have been abandoned due to side effects. Others, such as the antiestrogens tamoxifen and clomiphene, have been tested in only very small, uncontrolled trials. Finally, several medications have appeared promising in the animal model but have yet to undergo testing in human studies; such drugs include pentoxifylline and verapamil.

A promising drug of the latter category is the GnRH *antagonist*. These medications differ from the GnRH *agonists* (Synarel, Lupron, Suprefact or buserelin acetate, Zoladex) in that they produce an immediate inhibition of gonadotropin release. Thus their effect is faster and more direct than the long-acting GnRH agonist. The major problem with human use of this class of pharmaceuticals has been the annoying side effect of histamine release locally at the site of injection, producing an "allergic" response. This has been reduced substantially with the current crop of third-generation antagonists, and it is expected that these drugs will be tested in women within the next six months to one year.

Summary

A wide range of medical interventions is available for endometriosis. Most have been tested inadequately, but a few facts have emerged. It appears that the majority of the medications produce a substantial and roughly equivalent decline in endometriosis implant number, at least temporarily. Furthermore, most seem to generate pain relief, again at least for the short term and to roughly equal degrees. However, there is no evidence that any medical therapy can enhance fertility among women with endometriosis-associated infertility. Given this scenario, it would seem that prudent choices for drug therapy should be based on patient complaints, side effect profiles of the drugs, and cost. It remains to be seen whether the new generation of developing medical therapies can improve on the results with current medications.

Notes

1. T. M. D'Hooghe, C. S. Bambra, M. Isahakia, and P. R. Koninckx, "Evolution of Spontaneous Endometriosis in the Baboon (*Papio anubis, Papio cynocephalus*) over a 12-Month Period," *Fertility and Sterility* 58 (1992): 409.
2. I. D. Cooke and E. J. Thomas, "The Medical Treatment of Mild Endometriosis," *Acta Obstetricia et Gynecologica Scandinavica* 150 (Supplement) (1989): 27.
3. A. Kauppila, J. Puolakka, and O. Ylikorkala, "Prostaglandin Biosynthesis Inhibitors and Endometriosis," *Prostaglandins* 18 (1979): 655.
4. D. L. Olive and A. F. Haney, "Endometriosis Associated Infertility: A Critical Review of Therapeutic Approaches," *Obstetrical and Gynecological Survey* 41 (1986): 538.

5. D. L. Olive, "Medical Treatment: Alternatives to Danazol," *Endometriosis: Contemporary Concepts in Clinical Management*, R. S. Schenken, ed. (Philadelphia: J. B. Lippincott, 1989), 189–211.

6. E. C. Hamblen, "Androgen Treatment of Women," *Southern Medical Journal* 50 (1957): 743.

7. E. Hirvonen, M. Malkonen, and V. Manninen, "Effects of Different Progestogens on Lipoproteins During Postmenopausal Replacement Therapy," *New England Journal of Medicine* 304 (1981): 560.

8. L. Fahraeus, A. Sydsjo, and L. Wallentin, "Lipoprotein Changes During Treatment of Pelvic Endometriosis with Medroxyprogesterone Acetate," *Fertility and Sterility* 45 (1986): 503.

9. S. Telimaa, J. Puolakka, L. Ronnberg, and A. Kauppila, "Placebo-Controlled Comparison of Danazol and High-Dose Medroxyprogesterone Acetate in the Treatment of Endometriosis," *Gynecological Endocrinology* 1 (1987): 13.

10. M. E. Hull, K. S. Moghissi, D. F. Magyar, and M. F. Hayes, "Comparison of Different Treatment Modalities of Endometriosis in Infertile Women," *Fertility and Sterility* 47 (1987): 40.

11. S. Telimaa, "Danazol and Medroxyprogesterone Acetate Inefficacious in the Treatment of Infertility in Endometriosis," *Fertility and Sterility* 50 (1988): 872.

12. M. C. Andrews, W. C. Andrews, and A. F. Strauss, "Effects of Progestin-Induced Pseudopregnancy on Endometriosis; Clinical and Microscopic Studies," *American Journal of Obstetrics and Gynecology* 78 (1959): 776.

13. R. B. Scott and L. R. Wharton, Jr., "The Effect of Estrone and Progesterone on the Growth of Experimental Endometriosis in Rhesus Monkeys," *American Journal of Obstetrics and Gynecology* 74 (1957): 852.

14. A. D. Noble and A. T. Letchworth, "Medical Treatment of Endometriosis: A Comparative Trial," *Postgraduate Medical Journal* (Supplement 5) 55 (1979): 37.

15. P. Vercellini, L. Trespidi, A. Colombo, N. Vendola, M. Marchini, and P. G. Crosignani, "A Gonadotropin-Releasing Hormone Agonist Versus a Low-Dose Oral Contraceptive for Pelvic Pain Associated with Endometriosis," *Fertility and Sterility* 60 (1993): 75.

16. F. J. Cornillie, I. A. Brosens, G. Vasquez, and I. Riphogen, "Histologic and Ultrastructural Changes in Human Endometriotic Implants Treated with the Antiprogesterone Steroid Ethylnorgestrienone (Gestrinone) During 2 Months," *International Journal of Gynecological Pathology* 5 (1986): 95.

17. C. Robyn, J. Delogne-Desnoeck, P. Bourdoux, and G. Copinschi, "Endocrine Effects of Gestrinone," *Medical Management of Endometriosis*, J. P. Raynaud and L. Martini Ojasoot, eds. (New York: Raven Press, 1984), 207.

18. L. Fedele, S. Bianchi, T. Viezzoli, L. Arcaini, and G. B. Cendiani, "Gestrinone vs. Danazol in the Treatment of Endometriosis," *Fertility and Sterility* 51 (1989): 781.

19. M. Worthington, L. M. Irvine, D. Crook, B. Lees, R. W. Shaw, and J. C. Stevenson, "A Randomized Comparative Study of the Metabolic Effects of Two Regimens of Gestrinone in the Treatment of Endometriosis," *Fertility and Sterility* 59 (1993): 522.

20. M. D. Hornstein, R. E. Gleason, and R. L. Barbieri, "A Randomized Double-Blind Prospective Trial of Two Doses of Gestrinone in the Treatment of Endometriosis," *Fertility and Sterility* 53 (1990): 237.

21. B. Tjaden, D. Galetto, J. D. Woodruff, and J. A. Rock, "Time-Related Effects of RU486 Treatment in Experimentally Induced Endometriosis in the Rat," *Fertility and Sterility* 59 (1993): 437.

22. L. M. Kettel, A. A. Murphy, J. F. Mortola, J. H. Liu, A. Ulmann, and S. S. C. Yen, "Endocrine Responses to Long-Term Administration of the Antiprogesterone RU486 in Patients with Pelvic Endometriosis," *Fertility and Sterility* 56 (1991): 402.

23. L. M. Kettel, A. A. Murphy, A. J. Morales, A. Ulmann, E. E. Baulieu, and S. S. C. Yen, "Treatment of Endometriosis with the Antiprogesterone Mifepristone (RU486)," Unpublished data.

■ *David L. Olive, M.D., is associate professor and chief of reproductive endocrinology and infertility, Yale University School of Medicine, and an association advisor.*

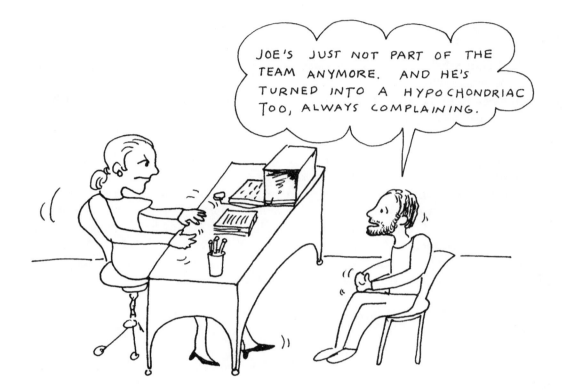

GnRH Update

By Barbara Mains

EDITOR'S NOTE: We have not received many letters from members about their experiences with Zoladex, the GnRH agonist most recently approved in the United States and Canada, because it is newer than Synarel or Lupron. As a long-lasting injectable drug, it is expected to be similar in its effects to Lupron.

"*Through the Endometriosis Association newsletter I read about Synarel. So, I asked my doctor about it and if I could get on it—I had to be persistent, but eventually I got it from him. Right after I started taking the drug I felt no pain: I mean none whatsoever! I have not felt so good for 10 years. I have not had to fill my prescription for Motrin since I started the Synarel. At my last checkup, my doctor said that before the Synarel he could not even move my uterus because the endometriosis had adhered so tightly around it, and now he can move it around. I used to have nodules toward the back of my uterus, and now he cannot find them. Before, when he pressed on my ovaries, I winced every time, and now I don't feel any pain.*

"*I am so thankful for this drug! It has brought me relief worth more than words can say.*"

Sharon, California

"*I am writing to share my experience with the drug Synarel. I was on it for five months. My doctor and I now agree it is no wonder drug. Sure, it helped the pain while I was taking it, but the side effects were terrible, especially when you suffer from migraines to start with. I am living proof that the pain comes back when you stop taking it. I am angry now that I spent over $250 a month for nothing. . . .*"

Tanya, Arizona

"*I have taken Lupron several times. In 1989 and 1990 I got complete relief. But in 1991 I got only minimal relief, and I had three periods while on the Lupron. My estradiol count never went under the desired level. My doctor wanted to try doubling the dosage, but before I agreed I asked him for a bone density test. It showed that I already have osteoporosis, which means I can't take Lupron at all now. I'm in a real catch-22 situation. . . .*"

Nancy, New York

"*My history of endometriosis is long and complicated, but I can tell you that the only time I am symptom-free is when I am taking the Synarel. This includes no relief with two laparo-*

scopies. I do not feel comfortable taking Synarel long-term. I feel the drug is still too new, and they don't have enough long-term information on it. However, I don't see what my other choices are right now."

Elizabeth, New Jersey

"I'd been on Synarel for only one month when my estradiol soared to four times the normal level—and it just wouldn't come down. My doctor told me to double the dose, which meant using the nasal spray four times a day instead of twice a day—but even then my estradiol count just wouldn't budge. Finally I switched to Lupron—and it dropped."

Jill, Washington

"Lupron and Synarel do have some advantages. Being able to go on vacation without getting your period—this always happened to me, even with the best of planning! No more writhing cramps from my waist down; little pelvic pain during the whole month; being able to wear light-colored clothes (my period was so erratic I had to live in dark pants); and no more heavy bleeding. Since I have other medical problems, having endo under control has helped. I am 40 years old and biding my time until either a natural or surgical menopause."

Nancy B., New York

"I'm 33 years old. My last day of six months of GnRH treatment was yesterday. Within a week or two of starting treatment I noticed that I was having trouble remembering really simple things that I had always been sharp about before. Remembering if I left my iron plugged in as I drove to the train station was really bothering me. Another annoying one was that when my alarm went off, I couldn't remember what day of the week it was. Of course, it was a weekday, or my alarm wouldn't have been set. But was it Friday, casual day, or a different day? I found I couldn't remember little things that I had never had a problem with before. I don't feel I'm suffering because of this—my logic hasn't diminished. I'm a computer analyst, and my job hasn't slacked off in any way. . . .

"I'm on continuous birth control pills now (without the usual fourth-week break) because GnRH didn't work for me. I don't know if this will keep my estrogen level high enough that my previously sharp short-term memory will return."

Judith, Illinois

(In an amusing follow-up note, Judith added: "I really get a lot out of the newsletters. Please feel free to use anything from my letter regarding memory loss on GnRH. I'm sure it was profound! Although I don't remember. . . .")

"I feel it is very important to write about my experience with Lupron Depot. I would like anyone considering the drug to realize that once you have that monthly injection, if your body does not tolerate it, you're still stuck with it in your body for 31 days or more.

"I developed an allergic reaction, which erupted as hives and welt patches covering me from head to toe. I went to my physician and later to the emergency room, but their usual treatments were to no avail. I was given epinephrine, Benadryl, and steroids [drugs used to treat severe allergic reactions], but because of the staying power of the drug, there was little that could be done. I was sent to a dermatologist, who put me on large doses of antihistamines and told me I would have to wait it out.

"After one week of watching this drug travel through my body, intense itching, pain, and swelling so bad that I spent two days with my hands in ice packs, I am just starting to get some relief.

"I would like to urge any woman considering the drug maybe to try the daily dose first, to be sure her body can tolerate it. I would hate for anyone else to have to live through the nightmare that I have."

Lisa, Pennsylvania

"As for my side effects on Synarel; I have had hot flashes, dryness, painful intercourse (it was sometimes somewhat painful before going on Synarel but nothing like on Synarel; now it feels as though I have sticker bushes in there and had made love 10 times the night before!), sore joints, and dizziness for about a month, which have gone away, and problems staying asleep, although I had no problem falling asleep. . . ."

Nancy, New York

"Lupron is the best thing that ever happened to me in this whole endo mess. . . . Aside from occasional hot flashes, some headaches that are alleviated with Nuprin or extra-strength acetaminophen, and some diminished sexual desire, I've had no really bad side effects. . . .

"I'm not planning on any more children. . . . However, I do wish to preserve my reproductive organs until I go through natural menopause.

"Soon, more surgery awaits . . . it seems the bowel is involved and Lupron is not doing much in that area.

"My health insurance coverage has paid for 80 percent of all my bills for Lupron, by the way, so that's been a real help. (Why are all these drugs so expensive?) . . ."

A., New York

"I felt so depressed when I was on this medication—side effects included irritability, hot flashes constantly, and I thought everybody was out to get me; the slightest quarrel or problem was such a big thing to me.

"Throughout this I was training to run the New York City Marathon. However, five months into the treatment I woke up one day with severe knee pain (both knees). I had never had problems with my knees. I told my doctor and he said that I had to stop running completely—because my cartilage had dried out. . . . I stopped running—I finished the Lupron in November. It was now January—I still had severe pain in my knees. I told my doctor, and he said that the damage was reversible, but he said it should've been better by now and rec-

ommended that I see an orthopedic specialist. I saw him in January and spent $220 for him to tell me the same thing. He said my cartilage was dried out due to the Lupron, assured me that it is all reversible—however, he said it will take a long time.

"I began running again in March. My knees are much better but far from being the way they used to be. I still wonder if it will ever go back to normal. My doctor did not inform me about joint side effects. Had I known this, I would have opted for laser surgery. . . ."

Anna, New Jersey

EDITOR'S NOTE: Many readers are now familiar with the GnRH family of medications used for managing endometriosis—in North America these are the injectable drugs Lupron (leuprolide acetate) and Zoladex (goserelin acetate) and the nasal sprays Synarel (nafarelin acetate) and Suprefact (buserelin acetate). An inhalation formulation of Lupron is currently under development. Forms more commonly available in Europe, Latin America, and some parts of Asia and Africa include Decapeptyl (tryptorelin acetate) and Supprelin (histrelin acetate). Please see Chapter 3 of *Overcoming Endometriosis* for an introduction to GnRH and GnRH drugs, particularly for background on how the natural hormone and its drug counterparts work.

Gonadotropin-releasing hormone (GnRH) is a hormone produced by a woman's body to regulate her menstrual cycle. GnRH analogs are look-alike drugs, chemically similar to human GnRH but many times more potent than the natural molecule. GnRH analogs can be either agonists (which stimulate, then paradoxically suppress natural hormones) or antagonists (which immediately suppress the natural hormones). Antagonists are being used experimentally at this time, notably in ovulation induction. This article covers GnRH agonists only.

Thank you, Barbara, for your work on this project! We wish to thank not only the author of this article but also the experts who reviewed this chapter: association advisors David Adamson, M.D., Palo Alto, California, and André Lemay, M.D., Ph.D., Québec City, Québec; and the well-known menopause writer Janine O'Leary Cobb, Montreal, Québec.

Introduction

Gonadotropin-releasing hormone (GnRH) agonists were approved for the treatment of endometriosis in the United States in 1990 and in Canada one year later. These drugs have been adopted widely by many gynecologists as first-choice treatment for pain. The pool of potential users for GnRH drugs is growing as researchers in several countries are using these medications to treat many other disorders of women. These include fibroids (noncancerous growths in the uterus), premenstrual syndrome, polycystic ovarian disease, precocious puberty, and heavy menstrual bleeding not related to endometriosis, a condition that becomes more common as women approach menopause.

The gonadotropin-releasing hormones ebb and flow throughout the month in response to the intricate instructions and counterinstructions that travel from a woman's hypothalamus to her ovaries and uterus. GnRH agonists work by overloading and desensitizing the pituitary, a gland in the brain that secretes important hormones under the direction of the hypothalamus. It's a two-step process: During the first phase these drugs actually stimulate the ovaries to produce more estradiol, the most potent form of estrogen. Some women with endometriosis report that their symptoms worsen during this phase. During the second phase, after some 7 to 21 days of constant stimulation, however, the pituitary shuts down production of the "messenger" hormones that control the ovaries. Without direction from the pituitary the ovaries also shut down. Blood tests show estradiol drops sharply and rapidly, sinking in most women to less than 25 picograms per milliliter. Women cease to ovulate or menstruate and enter a state similar to menopause.

Similar but not the same. The menopausal state induced by these and other hormonal drugs may differ from natural menopause in several ways. It's a complicated story, one we're only beginning to understand. Natural menopause is characterized by many changes—some dramatic, others subtle—in the levels and ratios of several hormones. In most women these changes take place over five to seven years. But the suppression of estrogen that follows the administration of GnRH drugs is much more sudden, in some cases plummeting women to castration level within 10 days. Association advisor André Lemay calls this drop in estrogen "an abrupt, deep fall, almost comparable to surgical menopause." The full effects of such a fall are not yet known. Lemay and other writers suggest that some effects of the GnRH drugs may well vary among women of different ages. Women who are very close to natural menopause when they take a GnRH drug may experience the drug somewhat differently from women in their twenties and thirties, whose ovaries would otherwise be producing peak levels of estradiol.

Estrogen plays an important role in endometriosis, which is why women taking GnRH drugs often report significant pain relief. Under the influence of these drugs the lesions of endometriosis tend to shrink in size. But because many other tissues and functions are influenced by the level of estrogen, as well as the ratio of estrogen to other hormones, the suppression of estrogen has many effects, direct as well as indirect. Some researchers are concerned about these effects—especially on bones—as well as other aspects of health, notably pituitary and cognitive function. These mechanisms are still being studied.

How Effective Are the GnRH drugs?

Pain

Randomized comparative trials show that women on the GnRH drugs and women on danazol obtain similar levels of pain relief.[1-4] This seems to be true for several types of pain. Both the GnRH drugs and danazol have been shown to relieve pain with sexual intercourse, especially the pain some women with endometriosis feel with deep thrusting. However, vaginal dryness, which may also cause pain with intercourse, is reported more often with GnRH drugs.

One study compared a GnRH drug to oral contraceptives for managing pain.[5] Two scales were used to measure pain relief. The GnRH drug provided better relief of dyspareunia as measured by one scale but not the other: investigators were unable to explain why the two scales yielded different results. Women who took the GnRH drug did not menstruate, so they were free of dysmenorrhea during treatment. The women who took oral contraceptives continued to menstruate but reported less menstrual pain while taking the oral contraceptives. Interestingly, nonmenstrual pain throughout the month lessened on both scales without differences between treatment.

Not all women obtain pain relief from GnRH drugs or danazol, perhaps because pain may have several causes. Although both medications have been shown to shrink the lesions of endometriosis, neither has been shown to reduce adhesions or scar tissue. Adhesions and/or scar tissue may be responsible for pain in some women. Scar tissue in which disease is deeply embedded may block the action of the medication.

Another reason for the mixed reports on pain relief? The degree of biologic activity of lesions seems to differ widely. Cells from some lesions are richly supplied with hormone receptors, which would make them more responsive to hormone suppression than cells with fewer receptors. "It is not surprising that some of our patients fail to respond to hormone therapy," wrote gynecologist John Rock in 1992.[6] "Patients with low or absent steroid receptors may not be ideal candidates for hormonal therapy."

Recurrence

Reported recurrence rates after GnRH agonist treatment vary, as does the length of follow-up. In the largest sample published to date, the cumulative recurrence rate at five years after treatment was 53.4 percent (among women with severe disease the rate was 74.4 percent).[7] This British study concluded that "patients treated with GnRH-analogues are highly likely to suffer a recurrence of their disease, particularly if their disease is severe at the outset." This and other follow-up studies have also found that pain tends to recur earlier in women with severe disease. Reported recurrence rates after treatment with GnRH drugs appear to be similar to recurrence rates after treatment with other medical therapies.

Infertility

Fertility after medical treatment has been studied in comparative trials (danazol, Provera, or gestrinone, a synthetic testosterone derivative used in Europe, vs. placebo or no treatment; and Provera, gestrinone, or GnRH agonist vs. danazol). Several meta-analyses of controlled trials (statistical summaries that pool together the results from several studies) have been published. These reviews have found no benefit of any medical treatment over no treatment.[8-11] In other words, women who take a GnRH drug are no more likely to get pregnant than women who do not take it.

Table 1. How GnRH Drugs Are Being Used to Treat Women with Endometriosis

• Short term:	1–3 weeks, as preparation for ovulation induction, or 2–3 months before surgery
• Long term:	up to 6 months to relieve pain
• Extended use:	longer than 6 months (experimental or in clinical trials)

Concerns Over Short-Term Use

Treating Infertility in Women with Endometriosis

Many fertility doctors use GnRH agonists in combination with another group of drugs, the gonadotropins (human menopausal gonadotropin and human chorionic gonadotropin), for ovulation induction in in vitro fertilization programs. A small group of women exposed to this or other combinations of drugs appear to be at increased risk for ovarian hyperstimulation syndrome, a rare, serious, and potentially fatal complication of ovulation induction.[12] Use of GnRH agonist in these regimens gives the doctor more control over ovulation but also makes it necessary to expose women to higher doses of gonadotropins to trigger ovulation.[13, 14] Several studies have linked GnRH agonist to the persistent ovarian cysts that develop after ovulation induction in some women.[15] It's not yet known whether the peak levels of estradiol that may follow from this combination of drugs is responsible for the worsening of endo symptoms that some women report after undergoing ovulation induction.

Women taking GnRH drugs are well advised to use a barrier contraceptive to prevent pregnancy while they're on the medication. Although most women on a GnRH drug cease to ovulate or menstruate within the first eight weeks of treatment, a small number of women apparently "escape suppression"—for unknown reasons the drugs fail to suppress estrogen production in these women. Symptoms may include continued bleeding or the absence of hot flashes. (A blood test showing estradiol above 50 picograms per milliliter is further evidence.)

These women may still be fertile. Reports of pregnancies that occurred while women were taking GnRH drugs include a recent case of multiple gestation: a 23-year-old British woman who was undergoing GnRH therapy for endometriosis conceived and miscarried sextuplets.[16] Her doctors suspect that the "flare effect" associated with GnRH treatment in this case resulted in superovulation (ripening of several eggs at the same time). Because exposure to GnRH drugs in baboon pregnancies is associated with a higher incidence of miscarriage, stillbirth, and low birth weight,[17] the development and health of babies from exposed human pregnancies are of concern. Published numbers are small at this point,[18] and full assessment may take decades.

Many readers will remember that the consequences of fetal exposure to diethylstilbestrol (DES) (see Glossary) were not understood until the children resulting from those pregnancies reached sexual maturity and tried to reproduce. The long-term effects of many hormonal medications, including GnRH drugs, danazol, progestins, and fertility drugs on human fetuses and human follicles are not yet known.

GnRH Drugs as Preparation for Surgery

Some surgeons use a GnRH drug before surgery to shrink endometriosis lesions so that they can be removed through the laparoscope. This use is controversial. Surgeons who favor it argue that it simplifies surgery and reduces blood supply to the pelvis,[19, 20] which they believe may result in less blood loss during surgery. Proponents also suggest that reduced blood loss may lower the risk of adhesions. One study has found that GnRH agonist used before surgery did reduce adhesion formation and re-formation in rats.[21]

Opponents say that the GnRH drugs, used before surgery, shrink lesions, so that surgeons have difficulty seeing them.[22] If the purpose of surgery is the removal of disease, anything that makes the disease less visible will make the surgery less effective. Some argue that reduced blood supply may also be associated with delayed healing. The blood supply to postmenopausal tissues has been shown to be somewhat reduced from premenopausal supply, and British surgeon Eric Thomas points out that "all gynaecologists are aware that post-menopausal tissues heal less well than premenopausal tissues."

Some surgeons are taking the middle of the road—using GnRH drugs before surgery in only severe cases, or where other conditions, such as fibroids or adenomyosis, could contribute to blood loss at surgery. In a surgical series reported at the Third World Congress on Endometriosis in Brussels in 1992, GnRH drugs were found to simplify surgery for those cases in which the disease was advanced.[23] But when used in patients with stage I or II disease (as classified by the revised American Society for Reproductive Medicine classification system), the authors added, GnRH drugs "will cause blanching of endometriotic implants and will make the disease more difficult to identify and to treat laparoscopically."

Controversies also surround the use of GnRH drugs after surgery. Doctors who use this approach usually prescribe the medication for several months immediately following surgery. This so-called combination treatment is used most often in severe cases or where removal of disease from delicate areas of the pelvis has proved to be very challenging. It's not yet clear whether combined medical-surgical approaches, in either order, improve recurrence rates. Obviously more study is needed.

Concerns Over Long-Term and Extended Use

Bone Density

EDITOR'S NOTE: See the last article in Chapter 7 of *Overcoming Endometriosis* for a piece on osteoporosis. Also, an association newsletter will look at the factors involved in osteoporosis and whether women with endometriosis run increased risks for this condition. This section covers the bone loss associated with GnRH treatment only.

GnRH treatment is associated with a loss in bone mineral density (a marker for the strength of bones). How much of a loss? Study results vary widely, showing average losses after six months of GnRH treatment that range from 0.2 to 12.8 percent depending on the site and technology of measurement. In his recent literature review, association advisor André Lemay puts the average loss from six months of GnRH treatment at 1 percent per month or 6 percent total, compared with an average loss of 3 percent for the first year of menopause.[24] How meaningful is such a loss over a woman's lifetime? Some researchers describe it as insignificant and point out that women who breast-feed their babies for six months may lose the same amount.[25] But Harvard gynecologist Robert Barbieri points out in the textbook *Modern Approaches to Endometriosis*: "It is conceivable that small losses in trabecular bone density at age 25 have little immediate clinical meaning for that woman. However, when that woman becomes 70 years old, the 4 percent bone loss caused by the GnRH agonist may increase the risk of vertebral fracture."[26]

The rate of loss—and kind of bone lost—may actually be of greater concern than the quantity. This is an "accelerated bone turnover," writes Lemay, "probably much greater than that encountered during progressive estrogen decrease in natural menopause." Data presented at the Fourth World Congress on Endometriosis in Bahia, Brazil (May 1994), indicate there may be "permanent structural changes to bone during GnRH treatment, particularly to strut formation, structure, and strength."[27] Although the study of bone loss has been muddied by debate over the best measurement technique and the sites at which bone density is measured, what's clear is that GnRH drugs trigger changes in bone metabolism. Once initiated, these changes may not be readily reversed in all women.

It's largely for this reason that regulatory agencies in both the United States and Canada have set a limit of six months for the use of GnRH drugs in the treatment of endometriosis. Concerns over bone recovery are the single largest obstacle to extended or repeat courses of these medications. As recently as 1993, the Australian Drug Evaluation Committee (an independent committee that approves or rejects applications for the registration of drugs in Australia) rejected applications to register Synarel and Zoladex, out of concern that the bone loss associated with these drugs would increase the lifetime risk for osteoporosis. (This ruling was later appealed through the efforts of the manufacturers and the Australian patient group, the Victorian Endometriosis Association, and overturned.)

Table 2. Addback Regimens in Pilot Studies or Clinical Trials of GnRH Drugs

GnRH + estrogen

GnRH + oral contraceptives

GnRH + medroxyprogesterone acetate (Provera)

GnRH + medroxyprogesterone acetate + estrogen

GnRH + norethindrone

GnRH + norethindrone + estrogen

GnRH + tibolone (Livial)

As of this writing, doctors who prescribe GnRH drugs for more than six months are operating outside approved limits. Some of these doctors are engaged in research; others are simply trying to help women in persistent pain who have exhausted other treatment options. It is not yet known if this extended use is safe.

Is the Bone Loss Associated with GnRH Treatment Reversible? In many women, apparently it is. But in Lemay's review only three of nine endometriosis studies that evaluated reversibility of bone loss at six months after treatment were able to report complete recovery of the spine. Other investigators, most notably three Japanese teams presenting at the Third World Congress on Endometriosis in 1992,[28–30] found weaker trends toward reversibility. In a recently published multicenter study of nafarelin, investigators followed 183 women for 18 months—but even with this longer period of observation bone mineral density did not return to baseline values. "These findings suggest that the reduction in bone mass after even short-term GnRH agonist treatment may be in part irreversible," concluded the authors.[31] Another study of women who took GnRH drugs for six months to manage fibroids was more worrying still: in this group of women in their forties, bone mineral density of the hip continued to decline a full year after treatment had ended. The author suggests that "the hip bone loss induced by these drugs is not really reversible in the fifth decade of life" (from 40 to 50).[32]

Again, confusion over the best ways to measure bone density may explain some differences, but there may also be a subgroup of women at higher risk for bone loss or who, having once started to lose bone, take much longer to regain it. Product guidelines recommend against use of the GnRH drugs in patients with known risk factors (metabolic bone disease, strong family history of osteoporosis, a history of malabsorption, glucocorticoid use, or a long-standing pattern of irregular periods).

Does Addback Prevent Bone Loss? Addback or give-back regimens are efforts to replace some of the hormones suppressed by GnRH drugs: estrogen and progesterone. In addback studies (see Table 2), women are prescribed estrogen or progesterone or an estrogen/progesterone combination to be taken at the same time as GnRH treatment or shortly after beginning treatment. Do addback regimens prevent bone loss?

Short answer: the jury is still out.

Long answer: each addback regimen has a rationale as well as enthusiasts and detractors. Researchers in the estrogen camp, for instance, are looking for what Robert Barbieri calls an "estrogen window"—a middle ground where estrogen levels will be high enough to prevent both bone loss and hot flashes but low enough to avoid stimulation of endometriosis.[33] Doctors who favor this approach concede that there may not actually be such a window or that the window may not exist for all women. (In some cases even tiny amounts of estrogen appear to stir up disease.)

Two factors have complicated the search for the "estrogen window." One is the varying sensitivity of body tissues to estrogen. Because different body tissues (such as the bones, the breasts, the lining of the vagina) respond to adjustments in estrogen levels in quite different ways, an adjustment that resolves one side effect of treatment may not greatly improve others. Lemay points out that the estrogen sensitivity of abnormal tissues, such as endometriosis and fibroids, may differ from that of normal tissue (endometrium). Again, if some cells in endometriosis growths are well supplied with estrogen receptors, and some are poorly supplied, then estrogen addback may have different effects on different women—and on different cells within the same woman.

The second factor that makes it difficult to calculate the estrogen addback formula is that the bone loss associated with GnRH treatment may not occur in exactly the same way as the bone loss that accompanies natural menopause and may not always respond to the estrogen treatments developed for women in natural menopause. Canadian researcher Akira Sugimoto and co-workers discovered that the standard estrogen dose recommended to prevent bone loss in postmenopausal women (.625 milligram a day) was not sufficient to prevent bone loss in women on GnRH treatment for endometriosis.[34] Higher doses of estrogen, which might be more effective in reducing bone loss, could also have the effect of stimulating the endometriosis.

The problems surrounding estrogen addback have prompted some researchers to look at replacing progesterone instead. (Progesterone is a hormone found in all animals with backbones, and plays an important role in bone formation.) Pilot studies using several forms of progesterone addback have now been published. When medroxyprogesterone acetate (Provera) was prescribed in conjunction with GnRH treatment for endometriosis, hot flashes and bone loss were reduced—but pain scores remained high during treatment.[35] Los Angeles gynecologist Eric Surrey had more success with another progesterone-like drug called *norethindrone*—perhaps because this drug exerts less estrogenic activity. In a prospective, randomized, double-blind trial, norethindrone reduced both hot flashes and bone loss without jeopardizing the low pain scores obtained on GnRH treatment. Unfortunately, the dose of norethindrone necessary to slow down bone turnover was found to trigger adverse changes in lipid ratios (predictors for heart disease).[36]

Proponents of the norethindrone camp are now combining GnRH agonists with low doses of norethindrone and sodium etidronate, a drug used in the treatment of osteoporosis. Calcitonin, another bone-building medication, has also been prescribed in addback trials. Although these bone-building drugs have been studied in postmenopausal women who are simultaneously taking estrogen, their mechanism of action may be different when combined with GnRH treatment for endometriosis. In another recently published study human parathyroid hormone was shown to prevent bone loss in the lumbar spine during GnRH treatment, although small losses from the femoral neck (see glossary) were also recorded.[37]

Other researchers are experimenting with lower levels of suppression (one dose of nasal spray per day instead of two). Some use GnRH drugs in sequence with other drugs (such as Provera for 10 to 12 days) that trigger monthly bleeding. In a paper presented at the Fourth World Congress on Endometriosis in Brazil (May 1994), Belgian researcher Jacques Donnez showed reduced bone loss under combined treatment with tryptorelin (a GnRH drug) and gestrinone (a synthetic testosterone derivative used in Europe and South America).

Addback protocols, some of them quite complicated and many of them expensive, are still experimental. As of this writing, none of the protocols described has been approved for use by either the FDA (Food and Drug Administration, United States) or the HPB (Health Protection Branch, Health Canada). Large clinical trials to investigate the effects of addback treatment are now under way, however, and regulatory agencies in both countries will probably be asked to review the findings from these trials within the next couple of years.

Changes in Lipid Ratios and Markers for Cardiovascular Health

The risk factors for heart disease, a serious public health problem, include changes in lipid patterns. The levels and ratios of certain kinds of lipids are believed to predict coronary disease. Because estrogen has been shown to decrease total cholesterol and LDL cholesterol (the "bad" cholesterol) and to increase HDL cholesterol (the "good" cholesterol), some researchers feared that estrogen suppression during GnRH treatment might raise the risk for cardiovascular disease.

The good news is that GnRH drugs do not appear to exert adverse effects on lipid ratios: the opposite, in fact. Neither total cholesterol nor LDL cholesterol appears to increase over six months of treatment. A small but significant increase in HDL cholesterol, unexpected and not yet explained, has been observed in several studies. In this regard the GnRH drugs appear to hold an advantage over danazol, which has been shown to alter lipid ratios in the other, less favorable direction.

Other studies of cardiovascular health have yielded confusing results. A recent German paper found a reduced risk for thrombosis (a condition that blocks the flow of blood in the arteries or veins) in women on the GnRH drugs.[38] But negative effects on cardiovascular status were shown in another group of women using GnRH drugs, including reduced peak flow velocity through the heart and aorta.[39]

Pituitary Function

Because GnRH agonists appear to work by desensitizing the pituitary gland, some researchers have been concerned about the health of this vital gland in women using GnRH drugs. A California research team found elevated levels of several pituitary hormones during treatment with a GnRH drug but noted a return to normal within one month after treatment.[40]

Changes in pituitary function over a six-month course of treatment with GnRH drugs have not been linked to pituitary health problems. These medications are being used for much longer periods in treating precocious puberty as well as prostate cancer, and studies of pituitary function in these groups of patients may yield useful information for women with endometriosis.

Adverse Effects

Adverse effects were documented carefully in 102 women who took a GnRH drug for six months for fibroids and in a group of women with endometriosis: virtually all experienced one or more adverse effect.[41, 42] Hot flashes were by far the most common side effect. Many women do tolerate GnRH drugs well, but a substantial number of adverse effects have now been reported. (See Table 3.) New reports about several effects are discussed here.

Short-Term Memory Loss

Some mental skills have been shown to deteriorate with age, and there is evidence that both estrogen and progesterone may play a protective role against these age-related losses in women.[43] Although several studies have shown that general mental function in healthy menopausal women does not differ between estrogen users and nonusers, certain specific types of memory function, such as secondary verbal memory (for new verbal material), appear to be influenced by the drop in estrogen that accompanies menopause.[44]

The profound suppression of estrogen in women taking GnRH treatment might explain the short-term memory loss that some women report. A study from London, Ontario, found "mild memory impairment in a substantial proportion of women on GnRH therapy" (40 percent) and "more severe complaints" among 20 percent.[45]

Researcher Andrew Friedman described short-term memory loss and depression as "two of the most disturbing adverse effects" of GnRH treatment.[41] They apparently afflict a minority of women who take the drugs, but they may have very serious consequences for those women. "Although fewer than 10 percent of women experienced these symptoms," wrote Friedman and colleagues of 102 women who took Lupron for fibroids (a somewhat older group closer to menopause than many women with endo), "four women either lost their jobs or had significant disturbances in their personal relationships." These authors

Table 3. Adverse Effects of GnRH Drugs Reported in the Medical Literature, 1987–95 (Sample Sizes Vary)[42]

Very common	Hot flashes
Common	Headaches Insomnia Vaginal dryness
Less common	Decreased sex drive Depression Emotional lability (mood swings) Fatigue
Infrequent	Acne Arthralgia (painful joints) Dizziness Increased sex drive Nausea Short-term memory loss Sweating
Rare	Ascites (accumulation of fluid in the peritoneal cavity) Anaphylaxis (severe allergic reaction) Anxiety Bruising at injection site Diarrhea Hair loss (with treatment or following treatment) Menopause (permanent cessation of periods after treatment) Myalgia (muscle pain) Paresthesia (burning or tingling or numb sensation) Skin rashes Vision changes

recommend that GnRH treatment be terminated if either depression or short-term memory loss develops.

Anaphylaxis, Paresthesia, Vision Problems

A very serious adverse effect from GnRH treatment was reported in 1991, when a 26-year-old woman in Hawaii experienced recurrent anaphylaxis (the most severe form of allergic reaction; see glossary) after an injection of Lupron at twice the dosage approved for endometriosis. Generalized hives and progressive shortness of breath brought her into the emergency room, where she was diagnosed with severe respiratory distress (swelling of tissues in the airway, which can be life-threatening). Prompt intervention saved her life, but the severe allergic reaction persisted over four months and required repeated hospitalizations and aggressive medical and surgical management.[46] This is the only report in the medical literature of such a severe reaction to a GnRH agonist, but several members have written to us to describe serious and persistent allergic reactions, including hives and wheezing that required emergency treatment.

EDITOR'S NOTE: An easy way to avoid long-lasting allergic reactions with GnRH drugs is to use a daily dose of the drug first to determine if you react to it and then continue with that or switch to one of the long-lasting injectables. The unfortunate woman who experienced anaphylaxis had previously developed hives on danazol, a warning that she might be at risk for allergic reactions.

There have been reports of two other uncommon side effects with GnRH drugs. One is paresthesia (sensation of burning, prickling, tingling, or numbness), which was reported after taking Synarel.[47, 48] The other is vision problems, which have also been reported on other hormonal drugs. Vision problems on GnRH drugs reported to the association have included blurring, double vision, and hazing around bright lights. Both these side effects are thought perhaps to occur due to abrupt changes in blood flow patterns on the drugs.

Conclusion

Because the action of the GnRH medications is complex and not yet fully defined, women and doctors who use these drugs find themselves weighing short-term relief of pain against unknown long-term risks. Turning off the estrogen tap interferes with many mechanisms within the body and often seems to disturb some finely tuned internal balance. We will need to know more about how the GnRH drugs act before we'll be able to track their full range of effects, and we'll need more follow-up studies to establish long-term safety.

Trials of the GnRH drugs and the associated addback regimens are yielding new information about the roles of female hormones and hormone

Most manufacturers of the GnRH agonists provide a consumer information hot line. If staff at these numbers are unable to answer your questions, ask for the medical information department.

In the United States

TAP Pharmaceuticals (*Lupron*)	(800) 621-1020
Zeneca Pharmaceuticals (*Zoladex*)	(214) 578-5454

In Canada

Abbott Laboratories, Limited (*Lupron*)	(800) 361-7852
Zeneca Pharma (*Zoladex*)	(800) 268-3992

Note: Syntex, the manufacturer of Synarel, was recently acquired by Hoffmann–La Roche. At time of writing, Hoffmann–La Roche does not provide a consumer hot line in Canada or the United States.

ratios in maintaining bone, blood, and healthy tissues throughout the body. These findings may eventually lead to new treatments or combination treatments that more closely re-create a woman's natural hormonal milieu. Some of the information gleaned from the study of chemical menopause may offer leads for the management of surgical menopause. Because so many women with endometriosis are at risk of losing their ovaries, and because some women cannot take replacement estrogen without stirring up the disease, alternative addback approaches are needed very badly.

Listen to your body while you're on this or any drug—and afterward. Believe in yourself, your awareness of your own body, and your ability to track your symptoms. Listen to the stories of other women. Read about these medications from as many sources as possible. Keep talking to doctors—about this disease, its treatments, and their effects. Ultimately the success of doctors depends on how thoroughly they understand the effects of the treatments they're providing. To do that, they need to hear what we have to say.

Until more is known, women on the GnRH drugs will continue to cope by listening to their bodies, tracking their experiences, and sharing information. We thank the hundreds of members who have shared their experiences on these medications with us and who by so doing have greatly expanded the knowledge base for all of us.

Notes
1. M. R. Henzl, S. L. Corson, K. Moghissi, et al., "Administration of Nasal Nafarelin as Compared with Oral Danazol for Endometriosis: A Multicentre Double-Blind Comparative Clinical Trial," *New England Journal of Medicine* 318 (1988): 485–89.
2. R. Rolland and P. F. M. Van Der Heijden, "Nafarelin vs. Danazol in the Treatment of Endometriosis," *American Journal of Obstetrics and Gynecology* 162 (1990): 586.
3. S. H. Kennedy, I. A. Williams, J. Brodribb, et al., "A Comparison of Nafarelin Acetate and Danazol in the Treatment of Endometriosis," *Fertility and Sterility* 53 (1990): 998–1003.
4. G. D. Adamson, L. Kwei, and R. A. Edgren, "Pain of Endometriosis: Effects of Nafarelin and Danazol Therapy," *International Journal of Fertility* 39, no. 4 (1994): 215–17.
5. P. Vercellini, et al., "A GnRH-Agonist vs. a Low-Dose Oral Contraceptive for Pelvic Pain Associated with Endometriosis," *Fertility and Sterility* 60, no. 1 (1993): 75–79.
6. J. Rock, "Endometriosis: The Present and the Future—An Overview of Treatment Options," *British Journal of Obstetrics and Gynaecology* 99, no. 7 (1992): 1–4.
7. K. Waller and R. Shaw, "Gonadotropin-Releasing Hormone Analogues for the Treatment of Endometriosis: Long-Term Follow-Up," *Fertility and Sterility* 59, no. 3 (1993): 511–15.
8. L. Fedele, S. Bianchi, T. Viezzoli, et al., "Buserelin vs. Danazol in the Treatment of Endometriosis-Associated Infertility," *American Journal of Obstetrics and Gynecology* 161 (1989): 871–76.
9. W. Dmowski, E. Radwanska, Z. Binor, et al., "Ovarian Suppression Induced with Buserelin or Danazol in the Management of Endometriosis: A Randomized, Comparative Study," *Fertility and Sterility* 51 (1989): 395.
10. E. G. Hughes, D. M. Fedorkow, and J. A. Collins, "A Quantitative Overview of Controlled Trials in Endometriosis-Associated Infertility," *Fertility and Sterility* 59, no. 5 (1993): 964–70.

11. G. D. Adamson and D. J. Pasta, "Surgical Treatment of Endometriosis-Associated Infertility: Meta-Analysis Compared with Survival Analysis," *American Journal of Obstetrics and Gynecology* 171, no. 6 (December 1994): 1488–1505.

12. J. Yeh, R. L. Barbieri, et al., "Ovarian Hyperstimulation Syndrome Associated with Leuprolide Suppression: A Case Report," *Journal of In Vitro Fertilization and Embryo Transfer* 6 (1989): 261.

13. A. Leader, "Ovarian Hyperstimulation Syndrome," *Journal of Society of Obstetrics and Gynaecologists of Canada* 16 (1994): 1895–1901.

14. S. Van der Meer, "OHSS: Use of GnRH Agonist to Trigger Ovulation Does Not Prevent This Syndrome," Poster O-008. Conjoint annual meetings of the American Fertility Society and the Canadian Fertility & Andrology Society. (Montreal, October 1993.)

15. I. S. Tummon, I. Henig, E. Radwanska, Z. Binor, R. Rawlins, and W. P. Dmowski, "Persistent Ovarian Cysts Following Administration of Human Menopausal and Chorionic Gonadotropins: An Attenuated Form of Ovarian Hyperstimulation Syndrome," *Fertility and Sterility* 49 (1988): 244–48.

16. A. Pickersgill, C. Kingland, A. S. Garden, and R. G. Farquharson, "Multiple Gestation Following Gonadotropin-Releasing Hormone Therapy for the Treatment of Minimal Endometriosis," *British Journal of Obstetrics and Gynaecology* 101 (1994): 260–62.

17. I. S. Kang, T. J. Kuehl, and T. M. Siler-Khodr, "Effect of Treatment with Gonadotropin-Releasing Hormone Analogues on Pregnancy Outcome in the Baboon," *Fertility and Sterility* 52 (1989): 846–53.

18. J. Har-Toov, S. Brenner, and A. Jaffa, "Pregnancy During Long-Term Gonadotropin-Releasing Hormone Agonist Therapy Associated with Clinical Pseudomenopause," *Fertility and Sterility* 59, no. 2 (1993): 446–47.

19. J. Donnez, M. Nisolle, P. Grandjean, et al., "The Place of GnRH Agonists in the Treatment of Endometriosis and Fibroids by Advanced Endoscopic Techniques," *British Journal of Obstetrics and Gynaecology* 99, no. 7 (1992): 31–33.

20. R. M. Miller and R. A. Frank, "Zoladex (Goserelin) in the Treatment of Benign Gynecological Disorders: An Overview of Safety and Efficacy," *British Journal of Obstetrics and Gynaecology* 99, no. 7 (1992): 37–41.

21. J. A. Wright and K. L. Sharpe-Timms, "Gonadotropin-Releasing Hormone Agonist Therapy Reduces Postoperative Adhesion Formation and Reformation After Adhesiolysis in Rat Models for Adhesion Formation and Endometriosis," *Fertility and Sterility* 63, no. 5 (May 1995): 1094–1100.

22. E. J. Thomas, "Combining Medical and Surgical Treatment for Endometriosis: The Best of Both Worlds?" *British Journal of Obstetrics and Gynaecology* 99, no. 7 (1992): 5–8.

23. H. A. Goldfarb, "The Pre-Operative Use of GnRH Agonists in Operative Laser Laparoscopy for Advanced Endometriosis," Abstract P-17. Third World Congress on Endometriosis. (Brussels, June 1992.)

24. A. Lemay, et al., "Extending the Use of GnRH Agonists: The Emerging Role of Steroidal and Nonsteroidal Agents," *Fertility and Sterility* 61, no. 1 (1994): 21–34.

25. L. M. Kent, et al., "Human Lactation: Forearm Trabecular Bone Loss, Increased Bone Turnover, and Renal Conservation of Calcium and Inorganic Phosphate with Recovery of Bone Mass Following Weaning," *Journal of Bone and Mineral Research* 5 (1990): 361–69.

26. R. L. Barbieri, "Danazol as a Treatment of Endometriosis," *Modern Approaches to Endometriosis,* E. Thomas and J. Rock, eds. (Lancaster: Kluwer Academic Publishers, 1991), 252–53.

27. "Skeletal Effects of GnRH Agonist Treatment in Women with Endometriosis," Abstract PA-VIII. Fourth World Congress on Endometriosis. (Bahia, Brazil, May 1994.)

28. H. Tanaka, T. Kawai, and M. Kiguchi, "Trabecular Bone Mineral Density Loss Following Hormonal Therapy in Endometriosis and Factors Concerning the Loss," Abstract P-51. Third World Congress on Endometriosis. (Brussels, June 1992.)

29. T. Hamamoto, J. Deguchi, T. Maruoka, and R. Nishimura, "Quantitative Computed Tomography (QCT) Reveals Decreased Trabecular Bone Mineral Density After Treatment with Gonadotropin-Releasing Hormone Agonist, Buserelin, Compared with Danazol in Japanese Patients with Endometriosis," Abstract P-53. Third World Congress on Endometriosis. (Brussels, June 1992.)

30. M. Fukushima, M. Shindo, and K. Sato, "Effects of GnRH Agonist and Danazol Treatments in Endometriosis on Bone Mass," Abstract P-62. Third World Congress on Endometriosis. (Brussels, June 1992.)

31. E. S. Orwoll, A. A. Yuzpe, K. A. Burry, L. Heinrichs, V. C. Buttram, and M. D. Hornstein, "Nafarelin Therapy in Endometriosis: Long-Term Effects on Bone Mineral Density," *American Journal of Obstetrics and Gynecology* 171 (1994): 1221–25.

32. L. Fedele, et al., "Is Bone Loss Induced by Gonadotropin-Releasing Hormone (GnRH) Agonist Treatment Really Reversible?" Abstract 0-146. Conjoint annual meetings of the American Fertility Society and the Canadian Fertility & Andrology Society. (Montreal, October 1993.)

33. R. L. Barbieri, "Hormone Treatment of Endometriosis: The Estrogen Threshold Hypothesis," *American Journal of Obstetrics and Gynecology* 166, no. 2 (1992): 740–45.

34. A. K. Sugimoto, A. B. Hodsman, and J. A. Nisker, "Long-Term Gonadotropin-Releasing Hormone Agonist with Standard Postmenopausal Estrogen Replacement Failed to Prevent Vertebral Bone Loss in Premenopausal Women," *Fertility and Sterility* 60, no. 4 (1993): 672–74.

35. M. Cedars, et al., "Treatment of Endometriosis with Gonadotropin-Releasing Hormone Agonists (GnRH-a) and Medroxyprogesterone Acetate," *Obstetrics and Gynecology* 75 (1990): 641–45.

36. E. S. Surrey and H. L. Judd, "Reduction of Vasomotor Symptoms and Bone Mineral Density Loss with Combined Norethindrone and Long-Acting Gonadotropin-Releasing Hormone Agonist Therapy of Symptomatic Endometriosis: A Prospective Randomized Trial," *Obstetrics and Gynecology* 75 (1992): 641–45.

37. J. S. Finkelstein, A. Klibanski, E. H. Schaefer, M. D. Hornstein, I. Schiff, and R. M. Neer, "Parathyroid Hormone for the Prevention of Bone Loss Induced by Estrogen Deficiency," *New England Journal of Medicine* 331 (1994): 1618–23.

38. U. H. Winkler, "Medical Therapy of Endometriosis: Effects on Coagulation and Fibrinolysis," Abstract 0-61. Third World Congress on Endometriosis. (Brussels, June 1992.)

39. N. Eckstein, A. Pines, Z. Fisman, et al., "The Effect of the Hypoestrogenic State Induced by Gonadotropin-Releasing Hormone Agonist on Doppler-Derived Parameters of Aortic Flow," *Journal of Clinical Endocrinology and Metabolism* 77 (1993): 910–12.

40. M. I. Cedars, K. A. Steingold, and J. H. L. Lu, "Pituitary Function Before, During, and After Chronic Gonadotropin-Releasing Hormone Agonist Therapy," *Fertility and Sterility* 58, no. 6 (1992): 1104–7.

41. A. J. Friedman, M. Juneau-Norcross, and M. S. Rein, "Adverse Effects of Leuprolide Acetate Depot Treatment," *Fertility and Sterility* 59, no. 2 (1993): 448–50.

42. R. W. Shaw, "The Role of GnRH Analogues in the Treatment of Endometriosis," *British Journal of Obstetrics and Gynaecology* 99, Supplement 7 (February 1992): 9–12.

43. E. Barret-Connor and D. Kritz-Silverstein, "Estrogen Replacement Therapy and Cognitive Function in Older Women," *Journal of the American Medical Association* 269 (1993): 2637–41.

44. D. L. Kampen and B. S. Sherwin, "Estrogen Use and Verbal Memory in Healthy Postmenopausal Women," *Obstetrics and Gynecology* 83, no. 6 (1994): 979–83.

45. C. R. Newton, A. A. Yuzpe, I. S. Tummon, and M. D. Slota, "Memory Complaints: A Side Effect of Continued Exposure to Gonadotropin-Releasing Hormone Agonists (GnRHa)," Abstract 0–137. Conjoint annual meetings of the American Fertility Society and the Canadian Fertility & Andrology Society. (Montreal, October 1993.)

46. G. S. Letterie, D. Stevenson, and A. Shah, "Recurrent Anaphylaxis to a Depot Form of GnRH Analogue," *Obstetrics and Gynecology* 78 (5), no. 2 (1991): 943–46.

47. J. Ashkenazi, D. Feldberg, J. A. Goldman, et al., "Adverse Neurological Symptoms After Gonadotropin-Releasing Hormone Analog Therapy for In Vitro Fertilization Cycles." *Fertility and Sterility* 53 (1990): 738–40.
48. A. S. Penzias, J. N. Gutmann, D. B. Seifer, and A. H. DeCherney, "Facial and Neck Paresthesia Associated with Nafarelin Administration," *Fertility and Sterility* 56 (1991): 357–58.

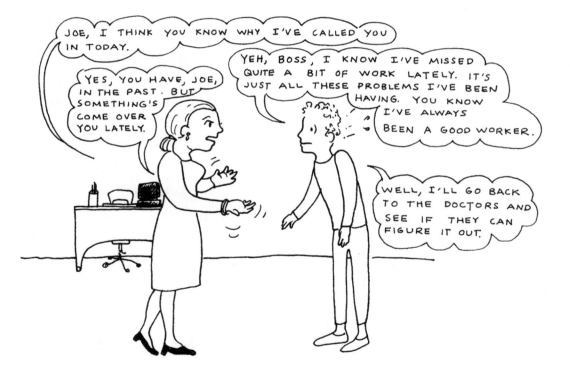

Tips for Coping with GnRH Drug Side Effects

By Nancy Fletcher

In response to the many members who have written to us regarding their experiences with GnRH drugs (in particular the menopauselike side effects), we have put together a list of coping strategies from a variety of sources, most directed at naturally occurring menopause. These sources include *Earl Mindell's New & Revised Vitamin Bible*, Earl Mindell (New York: Warner Books, 1989); *Menopause: A Positive Approach*, Rosetta Reitz (New York: Viking Penguin, 1979); *The Medical Self Care Book of Women's Health*, Sadja Greenwood, M.D., et al. (New York: Doubleday & Company Inc., 1987); *No More Hot Flashes and Other Good News*, Penny Wise Budoff, M.D. (New York: G. P. Putnam's Sons, 1983); *Coping with a Hysterectomy*, Susanne Morgan, Ph.D. (New York: New American Library, 1986); *The Doctor's Book of Home Remedies*, Rodale Press (Pennsylvania: Rodale Press, 1990); *Hysterectomy: Before & After*, Winnifred B. Cutler, Ph.D. (New York: HarperCollins, 1988); *Women and the Crisis in Sex Hormones*, Barbara Seaman & Gideon Seaman, M.D. (New York: Bantam Books, 1977); *Ourselves Growing Older*, Paula Brown Doress, et al. (New York: Simon & Schuster, 1994), in cooperation with the Boston Women's Health Book Collective.

Checking with knowledgeable health care practitioners before starting any vitamin, herbal, or exercise therapy is always recommended. As always, thorough education regarding any therapy, whether it be homeopathic, natural, traditional, or medical, is essential before deciding if it is appropriate for any individual.

Hot Flashes

According to *Ourselves Growing Older*, during a hot flash internal body temperature decreases while skin temperature increases, which is why many women may feel chilled afterward. Layers of clothing, including vests, sweaters, and blazers or jackets, can provide you with the opportunity to add or subtract clothing as needed. Loose clothing and clothes made of natural fibers such as wool and cotton can aid in transferring heat and perspiration from the body. Other tips: loosen anything tight, such as collars, belts, and headbands; fan yourself; rinse or towel off if possible, turn down the heat, open a window, and take off your shoes.

The Medical Self Care Book of Women's Health states that the body's temperature regulation is impacted by norepinephrine, a chemical involved in the transmission of nerve impulses, and that strong emotions and certain foods such as caffeine and alcohol may stimulate production of norepinephrine, which in turn may trigger hot flashes. Hot foods and liquids may also cause them. Eating many small meals during the day rather than three larger meals may help, and drinking lots of water is important.

All sources suggest vitamin therapy as an aid in dealing with menopausal side effects, particularly hot flashes. They do not all agree, however, on dosage. Typically vitamin E is suggested, with the dose ranging from 30 IU (international units) all the way up to 1,200 IU. *Earl Mindell's New & Revised Vitamin Bible* suggests 400 IU (mixed tocopherols) one to three times a day to relieve hot flashes. Mindell also says a 600-milligram stress B complex twice a day helps. Individuals with rheumatic heart disease, high blood pressure, or diabetes need to be aware that they should use vitamin E very conservatively (no more than 100 to 150 IU according to one source; we would suggest consulting your health care practitioner before using vitamin E if you have any of these conditions). Vitamin E is more effective when taken in conjunction with selenium. In fact numerous reports from the British Endometriosis Society tell us that vitamin E taken with selenium and vitamins C and A (most safely taken in its precursor form, beta-carotene) has improved endo symptoms. Readers need to be aware, however, that vitamin E affects hormone levels—follicle- stimulating hormone and luteinizing hormone levels according to *Women and the Crisis in Sex Hormones*.

All sources consistently touted vitamin C with bioflavonoids, vitamin A, calcium (from dolomite, which also contains magnesium), and vitamin D as aiding in the reduction of menopausal symptoms.

The herb ginseng is often mentioned as beneficial to women with menopausal symptoms. Earl Mindell reports that it does, however, contain estriol (estrogen) and therefore may not be appropriate for women on GnRH drugs. *Ourselves Growing Older* states that black cohosh, another herb often suggested for hot flashes, also contains natural estrogen. Possibly these substances could serve as natural addbacks, but they have not been studied.

Getting a good night's sleep may be a problem for some. If hot flashes or night sweats are a problem, sticking a leg or foot out from under the covers instead of throwing the covers off completely may be less disruptive and help ease you back into sleep after the episode passes. If you're sleeping with a partner, using separate covers may help in regulating your own space. Other types of sleep disturbances may be alleviated by avoiding caffeine. Chamomile tea also has soothing qualities.

The amino acid L-tryptophan is often cited as having sedative qualities and therefore being a potential sleeping aid, but its manufactured form has been taken off the market due to the presence of toxins produced by improper processing. Homeopathic and herbal alternatives available on health food shelves may be worth investigating.

If possible, a good workout during the day can contribute to a good night's sleep as well as to your total well-being. Aerobic exercise such as bicycle riding, walking, jogging, running, and swimming is especially beneficial. As mentioned previously, many members have reported joint pain and therefore may not be able to perform jarring exercise. (Swimming may be an option for these people.) One member found relief from her joint pain by taking aspirin and keeping her joints warm. If muscle cramps are a problem, calcium in combination with magnesium may help.

Medications used to alleviate hot flashes described by members and others include Bellergal-S and clonidine. According to the *Physicians' Desk Reference*, Bellergal-S contains the barbiturate sedative phenobarbital (which may be habit-forming), ergotamine tartrate, and Bellafoline (derived from belladonna). It acts on the nervous system and shouldn't be taken by those with peripheral vascular disease, coronary heart disease, high blood pressure, liver or kidney problems, sepsis (a serious blood infection), or glaucoma. Bellergal-S also contains FD&C yellow #5 (dye), which some individuals are allergic to (apparently those who cannot tolerate aspirin are more likely to react to this dye). Among possible side effects of this drug are tingling, blurred vision, palpitations, dry mouth, decreased sweating, decreased gastrointestinal mobility, urinary retention, tachycardia (accelerated heartbeat), flushing, and drowsiness.

Clonidine is typically prescribed for high blood pressure. It acts by causing dilation (increasing the diameter) of certain blood vessels. According to Penny Wise Budoff, M.D., in *No More Hot Flashes and Other Good News*, in small doses (.05 milligram twice a day) the drug has been shown to reduce the frequency, duration, and severity of hot flashes. Possible side effects include dry mouth, drowsiness, sedation, constipation, dizziness, headache, and fatigue. Other less frequent side effects may include loss of appetite, hives, thinning or loss of scalp hair, difficulty urinating, and dryness and burning of the eyes.

Vaginal Dryness

Products on the market to ease the discomfort of intercourse while on GnRH drugs include K-Y Jelly (or any non-petroleum-based products), Creme de la Femme (from Especially Products), Replens (Columbia Labs), Gyne-Moistrin, Astroglide, and Lubrin. Any water-soluble unscented lubricant or vegetable oil could be used, as could vitamin E oil.

Winnifred Cutler, in *Hysterectomy: Before & After*, suggests that regular vaginal massage (by intercourse, sexual play, or self-stimulation) helps to thicken vaginal walls that have thinned due to lack of estrogen and therefore may alleviate painful intercourse over time (in other words, regular sexual stimulation may keep painful intercourse to a minimum).

Ourselves Growing Older suggests that adding moisture to the air in your living/working space and drinking eight cups of fluid a day will help keep skin and other tissues from drying out (it also suggests that this may help women who experience dry eyes).

Susanne Morgan, in *Coping with a Hysterectomy*, states that during menopause vaginal pH may become less acidic, causing the vagina to be irritated easily, making intercourse painful. She suggests that douching with yogurt can help restore the pH balance. (See the caution on this in Chapter 5.)

Other suggestions regarding sexual behavior during this difficult time include investigating less traditional lovemaking techniques such as oral sex, various sexual positions that you may find more comfortable, and nonpenetrating methods of achieving orgasm such as clitoral stimulation (stroking the penis, or masturbation, is a nonpenetrating way of achieving orgasm for your male partner). More touching, hugging, cuddling, kissing, massaging, and talking are wonderful ways of loving each other. Rent an erotic film and explore all the sensual areas of your bodies!

Headaches

Rosetta Reitz, in *Menopause: A Positive Approach*, suggests that menopause-related headaches may occur as a result of premenstrual tension symptoms (specifically water retention) that may continue even after menstruation stops. Blurred vision may also result. She explains that many women produce aldosterone (a hormone that regulates the sodium and potassium balance in the blood) prior to menstruation, which causes fluid retention. She suggests that increased fluid may also occur in the brain, which could cause headaches. Limiting salt and avoiding monosodium glutamate (MSG) and red wine may help, since they contain tyramine, an amino acid that stimulates the release of epinephrine and norepinephrine, adrenal hormones that cause blood vessels to contract. Products made with yeast, alcohol, aged cheeses, and meats are other foods that contain tyramine. Many headaches are caused by constriction of blood vessels.

Mood Changes

Talking helps. If there is an Endometriosis Association support group or chapter in your area, consider attending the meetings and talking to other women who know what you're going through. Sharing feelings is good therapy. (If there is no group in your area, order an association contact list for your area—members who've given permission for their name and phone number to be given to other members—and share via the phone. Or join one of the computer endo support networks. Contact the association—see "Additional Resources"—for information.)

Take care of yourself, eat well, and listen to your body. If fatigued, rest. Exercise, if you're able to do it, is a wonderful way of working off stress and inducing physical and emotional well-being.

Winnifred Cutler discusses the possible correlation between estrogen and tryptophan deficiency, which may cause depression. As previously discussed, tryptophan is an amino acid that, according to Earl Mindell, is found in the brain and used to produce serotonin (a neurotransmitter that aids in sleep). Tryptophan can be found in cottage cheese, milk, meat, fish, turkey, bananas, dried dates, and protein-rich foods.

■ *Nancy Fletcher became a volunteer for the association in 1984, assisting with development of its library and computer systems. She served on the association's board as vice president of research from 1986 to 1988 and then joined the association staff as support program/development coordinator, a position she held for 3½ years, followed by a stint as education/development assistant.*

Danazol Revisited: Does an "Old" Drug Have "New" Tricks?

By Mona Trempe Norcum, Ph.D.

"*In my late 20s and early 30s I had two D & Cs, two laser laparoscopies, a term on Lupron with no improvement, and Danocrine. I continue to use Danocrine as my main treatment, but only on 200 milligrams a day, which has kept me pain-free.*"

Caroline, Colorado

"*The pain came back and got worse, and I just did not know what to do. Finally I saw another gynecologist, who told me about the Endometriosis Association. He did a laparoscopy and found a cyst the size of a small orange on one of my ovaries, and afterward he put me on danazol. I did not feel any better, but I kept hoping. . . .*"

Sharon, California

"*I followed my doctor's recommendation and went on danazol. However, I had tried that course in 1982 and was literally knocked flat by the side effects. I asked my doctor if a smaller dose than 800 milligrams a day was better for someone of my size. I'm five feet tall and weigh less than 90 pounds. He wasn't sure but was willing to try it. After one episode of breakthrough bleeding after two weeks on the danazol at 400 milligrams, my periods were stopped for nine months. The side effects were minimal. This may be of interest to teens and others who are small or may have had side effect problems.*"

Susan, Wisconsin

"*The doctor then placed me on 400 milligrams a day of Danocrine. This dosage wasn't high enough, so . . . he increased the dosage to 800 milligrams a day. By February I was feeling much better. I had a calm, peaceful feeling in my abdomen. . . .*"

Linda, Ohio

"*I was on danazol for almost 11 months. . . . When I first started taking it, my side effects included nausea, lack of appetite, fatigue (extreme), and hot flashes. I would wake up completely soaked almost every night. Immediately after taking a pill I would feel a head rush for a couple of hours. I also suffered from vaginal dryness, slight hair loss (my frontal hairline receded), and weight gain. . . . By far the most severe side effect I had was depression. . . . I have never felt so utterly worthless in my entire life. I'd had low self-esteem practically from day one of my treatment. . . .*"

Anne, Québec

Preface

When beginning the research for this article, I must admit that I held a preconceived bias against this drug. This was due primarily to its side effects and the temporary nature of its benefits. Also, when I was diagnosed in the late eighties as having endo, the treatment trends were toward newer drugs and laparoscopic surgery. Indeed my gynecologist never even discussed danazol as an option, and now danazol is no longer considered a first-line therapy by many. However, as I describe in this article, it appears to be time for another look at an "old" drug that may have important "new" benefits.

History and Pharmacology

Danazol is a synthetic testosterone derivative marketed under the trade names Danocrine and Cyclomen. It was the first drug approved by the U.S. Food and Drug Administration specifically for treatment of endometriosis and has been used widely since the late seventies. It is now one of several medical therapies available.

In the United States danazol is typically given orally in a 400- to 800-milligrams-a-day dose,[1] although some physicians prescribe lower doses. Treatment is usually for six months at a cost of up to $1,200. Danazol is rapidly absorbed by the gastrointestinal tract. It is then converted in the liver to a large number of compounds, most of which are considered metabolically inactive. Over half of each dose is processed within only four to five hours, so danazol is taken two or three times a day.

Because of its structural similarity to natural steroids, danazol has a variety of biological effects.[1] The best-documented of these that are relevant to treatment of endometriosis are:

1. suppression of normal pituitary-ovarian signaling, which decreases estrogen production
2. inhibition of enzymes in estrogen production pathways in both the adrenal glands and the ovaries
3. binding to androgen and progesterone receptors on endometriosis implants
4. displacement of testosterone from sex hormone–binding globulin
5. reduction of the circulating levels of sex hormone–binding globulin

There is still no *consistent* evidence that danazol directly affects endometrial lesions. Thus it is likely much of danazol's effect in reducing symptoms is due to the overall low-estrogen/high-androgen state it induces. However, the mechanisms for this are as yet unknown. Some of the effects of danazol may come from its influence on the immune system. For example, it lowers autoantibody levels,[2] which are common in women with endometriosis. It also decreases the inflammatory response to pelvic endometrial cells that may play a role in development of the disease.[3] (These are discussed in more detail later.)

From the combination of hormonelike effects and modulation of immune responses, it is clear that the overall physiological effect of danazol is extremely complex. This has led the Canadian Consensus Conference on Endometriosis[4] to recommend that, as for the GnRH drugs, danazol be used only after a *confirmed* diagnosis of endometriosis by surgery or biopsy. However, *because* of this variety of effects, danazol is also used in treatment of several other endocrine, blood, and autoimmune disorders. For example, it decreases breast pain in fibrocystic disease by suppressing estrogen levels, restores normal platelet counts, increases clotting factors, and restores normal enzyme levels in the complement cascade (a key immune process) in several diseases, and decreases autoantibodies in systemic lupus erythematosus.

How Effective Is Danazol?

The goals of medical treatment of endometriosis are pain relief and reduction of lesions.[4] The effectiveness of a particular therapy is clinically assessed on the basis of one or more of the following criteria:[5]
1. decrease in laparoscopic score (meaning reduction in the stage of disease based on the American Society for Reproductive Medicine classification system)
2. alleviation of pain
3. restoration of fertility in the approximately one-third of endo patients who are also infertile

Because danazol was the first medication specifically for endometriosis, it has been used as the standard against which the newer therapies have been measured. A review of the multicenter, randomized controlled trials from 1988 through 1992[5] comparing danazol to the other types of medical treatment show that all are comparable in effectiveness. The findings of more recent trials (through 1995) are consistent with this conclusion.

Extent of Disease
A six-month course of danazol therapy typically decreases disease scores (revised American Society for Reproductive Medicine system) from 30 to 50 percent as determined by second-look laparoscopy. This translates into a decrease of one to two stages; for example, from severe (stage III) to moderate (stage II) or mild (stage I) disease. When described in terms of percentage disappearance of visible lesions (which we now know may not be all that are there), there is complete remission in about 25 percent of patients, partial remission in 60 percent, no change in 5 to 10 percent, and progression of disease in 5 to 10 percent.[5]

The primary effect is on the number and size of endometrial implants, with little, if any, effect on the extent of adhesions. Moreover, no authors report any reduction in size of cysts larger than three centimeters, and it is unlikely that even ones as small as one centimeter will be affected significantly. Thus the greatest regression of lesions is seen in initially moderate or mild disease. But overall, danazol (as well as other available drug therapies) induces some level of remission in 70 to 100 percent of women.

Pain

Danazol is also highly effective in reducing pain associated with endometriosis. By both objective and subjective assessment, over 80 percent of women report pain relief, often within the first month of therapy. Because the standard doses of danazol prevent normal menstruation, painful periods are abolished during treatment. Also, the periodic activation of endometrial implants is interrupted, so the associated pelvic and back pain are reduced markedly. Significant decreases in pain with sex and painful bowel movements are also observed. However, in cases where distortion of pelvic anatomy due to adhesions is causing the pain experienced with menstruation, intercourse, or intestinal function, danazol therapy is ineffective.

Recurrence

The excellent success rate of danazol in pain relief and reduction of lesions is unfortunately temporary in most cases. As is typical for all types of medical treatments of endometriosis, 30 to 60 percent of women will have experienced a gradual return of pain within one year after ending danazol treatment.[1, 5] For some women the level of pain has been reported to be less than before treatment,[6] but for about 20 percent the severity of symptoms will require further therapy. This is often another course of danazol, other medical therapy, and/or surgical intervention. Unlike the GnRH drugs, danazol has not been limited by regulatory authorities to one course of treatment. (This may change with addback therapies for GnRH therapy—see the preceding articles.) However, there is still no medical option that cures endometriosis.

Infertility

Over the years many physicians were of the opinion that pregnancy rates for women with endometriosis were significantly improved after danazol therapy. Indeed, even in the absence of symptoms, some recommended that infertile women with mild endometriosis receive medical therapies to prevent disease progression and so increase chances of pregnancy.[7] It is now clear that the available drugs suppress endometriosis only temporarily. Moreover, combined analysis of controlled trials from 1977 to 1992[8] indicates that none of these studies has shown any benefit of medical therapies on pregnancy rates in women with endometriosis. Extension of this analysis by inclusion of studies through 1993[9] emphasizes that medical treatment alone, or in addition to surgical therapies, did *not* produce higher pregnancy rates than no treatment at all.

Although still highly controversial, current opinion is turning toward the view "that suppressive hormone therapy has no place in the treatment of infertility associated with endometriosis."[10] However, as discussed later, there may still be a role for danazol because of its ability to affect immunological factors that have been implicated in endometriosis and related infertility.

Use Before and After Surgery

Another controversial aspect of the effectiveness of danazol concerns its use before and/or after surgical treatment of endometriosis. With regard to preoperative treatment, most issues are similar for all medical therapies (see the earlier GnRH drug articles). For example, some physicians want to reduce the extent of endometriosis prior to surgery, while others fear that such reduction will cause them to miss some active lesions. However, an argument in favor of danazol is the observation that a preoperative course of danazol reduces pelvic inflammation,[11] which is likely due to its effect on immune system cells. This in turn could reduce formation of adhesions resulting from surgery.

Conflicting opinions also exist on postoperative use of medical treatment. One controlled trial showed that patients receiving danazol or Provera after surgical removal of endometriosis had significantly less pain and other "inconveniences" for at least six months.[10] However, others feel that postoperative medical treatment should be reserved for those patients who have continuing symptoms or residual lesions inaccessible at surgery.[5] This view is based on the unsuitability of current medical treatments for long-term use because of their significant side effects. However, if a decision is made to use medical treatment before or after surgery, danazol is as effective as the other types in use.

Adverse Effects of Danazol

With what is known of the multiple biological effects of danazol, it is not surprising that it is associated with many adverse effects. Quantifying the occurrence of these side effects is difficult because each study reports widely varied numbers and not every study reports each side effect. Also, not every person taking danazol will experience all of the effects, although almost everyone will have some.

Common Side Effects

Combining data from a variety of studies,[12–15] Table 1 is a representative listing of the most common side effects of danazol. Those reported most often are related directly to the altered steroid hormone state induced by danazol. For example, hot flushes, decreased sex drive, and vaginal irritation are all attributable to low estrogen levels. Weight gain and acne are due to the anabolic effects of this steroid. All of these effects are readily reversible when treatment is stopped. In contrast, some effects of the high-testosterone environment, such as loss of frontal head hair and deepening of the voice, may be irreversible. Enlargement of the clitoris is also possible, although rare. Many women (and physicians) find these side effects to be intolerable (or undesirable) and so opt not to use danazol despite its effectiveness in reducing the lesions and the pain of endometriosis.

Table 1. Adverse Effects Associated with Danazol Therapy

Common (30–55 percent)	Acne
	Decreased sex drive
	Headache
	Hot flushes
	Oily skin and hair
	Reduction in breast size
	Weight gain (usually up to 10 pounds)
Less common (15–25 percent)	Abnormal facial and body hair growth
	Emotional instability, depression, nervousness
	Fatigue
	Fluid retention
	Muscle aches and cramps
	Vaginal dryness and irritation
Infrequent (<10 percent)	Breast pain
	Deepening of the voice
	Insomnia
	Nausea
	Rash
	Visual disturbances

Values are averages of reported incidences.[12–15] Sample sizes vary, and not all effects were reported in each study.

Effects on General Metabolism

More recently additional reservations regarding the use of danazol have been described based on the changes it causes in several types of biological processes (see Table 2). A review of several studies[16] clearly documents alteration of lipid metabolism during danazol therapy. Overall HDL cholesterol (the "good" cholesterol) falls while LDL cholesterol (the "bad" cholesterol) increases. Although the exact mechanisms are not known, the net effect mimics the usual postmenopausal changes that increase the risk of arterial blockages and heart disease. Therefore, for women with other risk factors for cardiovascular disease (high cholesterol levels, high blood pressure, smoking, or a family history of heart disease), lipid profiles should be monitored closely during danazol treatment or an alternate therapy used.

Danazol can also affect the function of the liver, the organ that processes it. The rate of production of several proteins is changed, leading to decreases in some and increases in others. This in turn can lead to a variety of other changes. For example, danazol causes

Table 2. Metabolic Changes During Danazol Therapy

Changes in lipid metabolism:
Decrease in HDL cholesterol
Increase in LDL cholesterol

Changes in liver function:
Increase or decrease in circulating levels of several proteins

Changes in carbohydrate metabolism:
Prolonged insulin and glucagon presence

less hormone-binding proteins to be made, so higher levels of free (biologically active) testosterone and thyroid hormone are found in the blood. Although a number of other proteins are affected, changes in them are usually mild.[13, 17] However, periodic tests are suggested while on danazol to monitor for possible liver toxicity. Women with decreased liver function should not take danazol.

Danazol also alters the level of hormones involved in controlling blood glucose levels. Both insulin and glucagon remain elevated in the blood longer than normal.[18] This does not appear to affect overall glucose metabolism but could produce erroneous results when measuring the two hormones or in glucose tolerance tests (which are important in diagnosing hypoglycemia or diabetes). In addition, there may be changes in insulin requirements of diabetic women during danazol treatment.

Neither the short-term nor the long-term overall biological effects of these metabolic changes are well understood. However, all of the indicators mentioned return quickly to normal levels when danazol is stopped.

Additional Precautions and Warnings (Table 3)

Danazol has at least two documented adverse drug interactions.[19] Patients taking warfarin to inhibit blood clot formation should be aware that danazol may further increase clotting time. This has the potential of causing episodes of uncontrolled bleeding. Also, concurrent danazol can induce carbamazepine toxicity by inhibiting its normal metabolism. Carbamazepine is commonly used for control of epileptic seizures and as an analgesic for pain associated with certain nerve disorders.

Certain rare diseases are associated with danazol use. Several cases of increased pressure within the skull and brain swelling known as *pseudotumor cerebri* have been documented.[20] This can result in strokes and vision problems. Also, there has been a recent report of acute pancreatitis associated with danazol taken for endometriosis.[21]

TABLE 3. Precautions and Warnings for Danazol

Adverse drug interactions	Warfarin
	Carbamazepine
Rare diseases	Blood clots
	Pseudotumor cerebri
	Pancreatitis
	Liver abnormalities
Birth defects	Masculinization of female fetus

The *Physicians' Desk Reference* warns of cases of blood clots resulting from danazol treatment.[19] It also cautions that long-term use may cause physical changes in the liver that usually remain hidden until a potentially life-threatening abdominal hemorrhage occurs. *The primary warning is against danazol use during pregnancy.* This is because danazol is a potent teratogen; it produces deformities in developing fetuses. The most common are androgenic effects seen as masculinization of females. Therefore, women taking danazol *must* use barrier contraception!

Positive Aspects

Despite its undesirable physical and metabolic effects, danazol treatment does have certain positive aspects.

Bone Metabolism
A recent review of studies examining the effect of medical therapies on bone mass[22] shows that danazol does not cause bone loss typical of a hypoestrogenic state. In complete contrast to the persistent bone mass loss seen after treatment with the GnRH drugs, women taking danazol have either no change or a net *gain* in bone. For example, an increase of 2 to 17 percent in spinal bone has been reported after three to six months of treatment with 800 milligrams a day of danazol. A bone surplus of approximately 8 percent remained in some patients at one year posttreatment. Thus danazol may be the preferred medical treatment for women with low bone mass or several known high-risk factors for osteoporosis (low calcium intake, smoking, high caffeine or alcohol intake, thin individuals).

Immune Function
Within the last decade several investigators have observed significant alterations in the immune system of women with endometriosis. Changes in both the local pelvic cell–mediated inflammatory response and the general systemic responses are seen. Briefly, peritoneal

macrophages are overactivated, producing high levels of cellular growth factors, prosta-glandins, and other enzymes. Paradoxically, the cytotoxic ability of these cells is decreased, as is that of other types of cells that "clean up" foreign, diseased, or dead cells. In addition, immature macrophages (known as *peripheral blood monocytes*), especially from women with severe endometriosis, stimulate the growth of endometrial cells grown in the laboratory. The overall effect favors the growth and possibly the implantation of the misplaced endometrial cells. This clearly increases pelvic inflammation, which in turn promotes adhesion formation.[3]

In addition, high levels of a variety of autoantibodies have been measured in the blood of women with endometriosis.[2] Some of these "antiself" antibodies react specifically with endometrial cells, but most are directed against general cellular structures, such as membrane phospholipids. The presence of these general types of autoantibodies is also common in women with unexplained infertility.[23] Moreover, a recent study shows that for women with endometriosis and autoantibodies, successful pregnancies following in vitro fertilization occur at only half the rate of that for women with endometriosis that do not have autoantibodies.[27]

Based on these immunologic abnormalities, there is an emerging view that endometriosis is actually an autoimmune disease. However, it is not yet clear whether altered immune function is a cause or result of endometriosis. Danazol has potential in helping to answer this question and in determining the cellular mechanisms involved.

For example, already known is that, even though danazol does not affect endometrial cell growth directly, it decreases the ability of peripheral blood monocytes to stimulate endometrial cell growth. This seems to be due to a reduction in growth factor secretion by monocytes, as well as a decreased response of endometrial cells to the factors.[24] Overall, an activation signal is removed. This may be part of the explanation for decreased pelvic inflammation after danazol treatment. Similarly, danazol significantly decreases the auto-antibody levels in women with endometriosis.[2] This is apparently a unique property of danazol—the GnRH drugs do not do so.

New Directions

If endometriosis really is a systemic disease that is mediated by abnormal immune function, then neither localized surgery nor hormonal suppression can be expected to completely prevent or eradicate it. Indeed the high recurrence (or relapse) rate of endometriosis documents that current treatments are not adequate. In light of the current research focus on the immunological factors associated with endometriosis, it is likely that the next therapeutic approach will be aimed at modulation of the immune response. A logical starting point in development of immunosuppressive drugs for endometriosis might be danazol (or danazollike molecules) because of the already existing data showing that it can reduce the function of several types of lymphocytes. Meanwhile, danazol is involved in some new twists in the standard treatment regimens.

Lower Doses

There has been a recent reassessment of the amount of danazol needed to treat endometriosis-associated pain. For example, a review of studies involving doses of 100, 200, 400, or 600 milligrams a day for six months concluded that there was no significant difference in the amount of pain relief provided, even though most women taking the lowest dose continued to menstruate.[25] The authors also performed a pilot study of a very-low-dose regimen of 50 milligrams a day for nine months. Average pain scores were effectively decreased, while the incidence and severity of the usual side effects were much less. A novel biphasic treatment of three months of Lupron followed by six months of very-low-dose danazol gave similar results.

In addition the frequency and occurrence of all types of adverse effects attributed to danazol are dose-dependent (the more drug, the more side effects), so, a logical approach is to use the lowest dose necessary to control symptoms of endometriosis to reduce these unwanted effects. The *Physicians' Desk Reference*[19] still recommends a starting dose of a total of 800 milligrams a day but does remind physicians that they should consider lowering the dose when periods have stopped.

Increasing numbers of published reports directed at physicians advocate lower initial doses, such as 200 to 400 milligrams a day, that are already common practice in many countries other than the United States. However, at these levels many patients may still have breakthrough bleeding or spotting. More important, higher doses are often needed to completely suppress ovulation. This means that at these intermediate doses there is a significant chance of pregnancy (see earlier warning)!

Shorter Length of Treatment

There are also new trends in the length of medical therapy. The full effect of medical therapy reduction of endometrial lesions is usually achieved in two to three months.[26, 28] Thus there is little evidence that the high-dose regimens (and the associated side effects) need to be tolerated for the standard six months. However, knowing the temporary nature of improvement after taking danazol, shorter duration of treatment implies shorter time free of symptoms. Long-term treatment at high doses has always been discouraged because of the multiple adverse effects of danazol (not to mention the high cost).

Perhaps additional studies on the effectiveness and safety of lower doses of danazol will encourage treatment aimed at long-term partial suppression of lesions sufficient to relieve symptoms instead of short-term, profound suppression. This could provide longer periods of remission with manageable side effects and cost.

Other Approaches

Continuing attempts are being made to increase the effectiveness of medical therapy and of conservative surgery by combining them.[26] For example, a three-step technique used a three-month medical therapy between laparoscopic destruction of lesions and excision of large cysts.

In addition, alternative delivery systems may be beneficial. One team[10] used a vaginal ring and an intrauterine device to slowly release up to 3.5 grams of danazol. Both intravaginal and intrauterine administration reduced pelvic lesions and pain. Of interest is that ovulation was not suppressed. This suggests that the mechanism of action of danazol (and perhaps the level of adverse effects) may vary with route of delivery. Unfortunately, the newer delivery methods used for other hormonal drugs, such as creams, transdermal patches, and slow-release implants, have not yet been evaluated for endometriosis.

Epilogue

Classic high-dose danazol (600 to 800 milligrams a day) *is* highly effective in reducing endometriotic lesions and pain. Unfortunately, as with other drugs for endometriosis, its use is compromised by multiple adverse side effects, and treatment provides only a temporary suppression of disease. However, in light of recent information on bone sparing and immunological effects, danazol perhaps should be considered carefully when medical therapy is chosen. In particular, intermediate (200 to 400 milligrams a day) or even lower-dose regimens should be strongly encouraged, with the awareness that extra care must be taken so as *not* to become pregnant while taking danazol.

Notes
1. W. P. Dmowski, "Danazol: A Synthetic Steroid with Diverse Biologic Effects," *Journal of Reproductive Medicine* 35 (1990): 69–75.
2. A. El-Roiey, W. P. Dmowski, N. Gleicher, E. Radwanska, L. Harlow, Z. Binor, I. Tummon, and R. G. Rawlins, "Danazol But Not Gonadotropin-Releasing Hormone Agonists Suppresses Autoantibodies in Endometriosis," *Fertility and Sterility* 50 (1988): 864–71.
3. W. P. Dmowski, H. M. Gebel, and D. P. Braun, "The Role of Cell-Mediated Immunity in Pathogenesis of Endometriosis," *Acta Obstetricia et Gynecologica Scandinavica* 159 (1994): 7–14.
4. The Canadian Consensus Conference on Endometriosis, "How Should Endometriosis Be Treated Medically?" *Journal of the Society of Obstetricians and Gynaecologists* Special supplement 15 (1993): 23–31.
5. M. Wingfield and D. L. Healy, "Endometriosis: Medical Therapy," *Baillières Clinical Obstetrics and Gynaecology* 7 (1993): 813–38.
6. S. Telimaa, J. Puolakka, L. Ronnberg, and A. Kauppila, "Placebo-Controlled Comparison of Danazol and High-Dose Medroxyprogesterone Acetate in the Treatment of Endometriosis," *Gynecological Endocrinology* 1 (1987): 13–23.
7. E. J. Thomas and I. D. Cooke, "Impact of Gestrinone on the Course of Asymptomatic Endometriosis," *British Medical Journal* 294 (1987): 272–74.
8. E. G. Hughes, D. M. Fedorkow, and J. A. Collins, "A Quantitative Overview of Controlled Trials in Endometriosis-Associated Infertility," *Fertility and Sterility* 59 (1993): 963–70.
9. G. D. Adamson and D. J. Pasta, "Surgical Treatment of Endometriosis-Associated Infertility: Meta-Analysis Compared with Survival Analysis," *American Journal of Obstetrics and Gynecology* 171 (1994): 1488–1505.
10. A. Kauppila, "Changing Concepts of Medical Treatment of Endometriosis," *Acta Obstetricia et Gynecologica Scandinavica* 72 (1993): 324–36.

11. V. C. Buttram, "Use of Danazol in Conservative Surgery," *Journal of Reproductive Medicine* 35 (1990): 82–86.

12. R. W. Shaw, "Treatment of Endometriosis," *Lancet* 340 (1992): 1267–71.

13. J. M. Wheeler, J. D. Knittle, and J. D. Miller, "Depot Leuprolide Acetate Versus Danazol in the Treatment of Women with Symptomatic Endometriosis: A Multicenter, Double-Blind Randomized Clinical Trial," *American Journal of Obstetrics and Gynecology* 169 (1993): 26–33.

14. J. A. Rock, J. A. Truglia, and R. J. Caplan, "Zoladex (Goserelin Acetate Implant) in the Treatment of Endometriosis: A Randomized Comparison with Danazol," *Obstetrics and Gynecology* 82 (1993): 198–205.

15. B. S. Hurst and W. D. Schlaff, "Treatment Options for Endometriosis—Medical Therapies," *Infertility and Reproductive Medicine Clinics of North America: Endometriosis* 3: 3 (1992): 645–55.

16. C. J. Packard and J. Shepherd, "Action of Danazol on Plasma Lipids and Lipoprotein Metabolism," *Acta Obstetricia et Gynecologica Scandinavica* supplement 159 (1994): 35–40.

17. M. Y. Dawood, "Considerations in Selecting Appropriate Medical Therapy for Endometriosis," *International Journal of Gynecology and Obstetrics* 40 supplement (1993): S29–42.

18. R. Bruce, I. Godsland, J. Stevenson, M. Devenport, F. Borth, D. Crook, M. Ghatei, M. Whitehead, and V. Wynn, "Danazol Induces Resistance to Both Insulin and Glucagon in Young Women," *Clinical Science* 82 (1992): 211–17.

19. *Physicians' Desk Reference* (Montvale, NJ: Medical Economics Data Production Co, 1994), 2092–93.

20. L. M. Hamed, J. S. Glaser, N. J. Schatz, and T. H. Perez, "Pseudotumor Cerebri Induced by Danazol," *Journal of Ophthamology* 107 (1989): 105–10.

21. J. Balasch, S. Martinez-Roman, J. Carreras, and J. A. Vanrell, "Acute Pancreatitis Associated with Danazol Treatment for Endometriosis," *Human Reproduction* 9 (1994): 1163–65.

22. M. Y. Dawood, "Impact of Medical Treatment of Endometriosis on Bone Mass," *American Journal of Obstetrics and Gynecology* 168 (1993): 674–84.

23. N. Gleicher and D. Pratt, "Abnormal (Auto)Immunity and Endometriosis," *International Journal of Gynecology and Obstetrics* 40 supplement (1993): S21–27.

24. D. P. Braun, H. Gebel, and W. P. Dmowski, "Effect of Danazol In Vitro and In Vivo on Monocyte-Mediated Enhancement of Endometrial Cell Proliferation in Women with Endometriosis," *Fertility and Sterility* 62 (1994): 89–95.

25. P. Vercellini, T. Bramante, L. Trespidi, F. Mauro, S. Panazza, and P. G. Crosignani, "Very Low Dose Danazol for Relief of Endometriosis-Associated Pelvic Pain: A Pilot Study," *Fertility and Sterility* 62 (1994): 1136–42.

26. I. A. Brosens, "New Principles in the Management of Endometriosis," *Acta Obstetricia et Gynecologica Scandinavica* supplement 159 (1994): 18–21.

27. W. P. Dmowski, N. Rana, J. Michalowska, J. Friberg, C. Papiernak, and A. El-Roiey, "The Effect of Endometriosis, Its Stage and Activity, and of Autoantibodies on In Vitro Fertilization and Embryo Transfer Success Rates," *Fertility and Sterility* 63 (1995): 555–62.

28. S. Wright, C. T. Valdes, R. C. Dunn, and R. R. Franklin, "Short-Term Lupron or Danazol Therapy for Pelvic Endometriosis, *Fertility and Sterility* 63 (1995): 504–07.

■ **Mona Trempe Norcum** *earned a B.S. in chemistry at the University of Vermont and a Ph.D. in biological chemistry at UCLA. She is currently an associate professor of biochemistry at the University of Mississippi Medical Center in Jackson.*

4

❦❦

Endometriosis and the Intestines

By Mary Lou Ballweg

"*I want to express my sincere appreciation. After numerous tests and surgeries, I was thoroughly frustrated, aggravated, and sick! I was having tremendous pelvic pain, severe constipation, and flulike symptoms while my gynecologist and gastroenterologist both felt I had two separate unrelated problems—even though it was coinciding with my monthly cycle. I called the association and simply said, 'I have a feeling they are very related and somehow my intestinal problems are related to my endometriosis.' I asked if any other women had complained of similar problems. The person I spoke with was very helpful and said numerous women had these problems.* [EDITOR'S NOTE:* The letter writer then describes how, through the help of association members, she was able to find a physician who was able to help.]

"*I called Dr. B. in New Orleans, and without hesitation he felt my problem was very related. . . . I had major laser microsurgery with Dr. B.*

"*I have been able to return to work and feel absolutely wonderful. My endometriosis was in stage IV in numerous locations, especially in the small bowel, appendix, and several other locations.*

"*Thanks again for your assistance, and I hope this letter will help other women with similar problems.*"

Linda, Texas

"*For over a year I have gone from doctor to doctor trying to find out what was wrong with me. I had excessive bleeding, passing out, severe pain, and finally a year ago the diarrhea started. I went to one ob-gyn, and he said some people bled heavier than others—try to live with it.*

"*I went to a gastrointestinal specialist, and he did every test there is on bowels, intestines, and stomach, and he found nothing. So, I still didn't know what was wrong with me.*

"I went to a third ob-gyn in town. He agreed to do a 'lap-scope' to see if I had endo. He didn't think so, saying it was very rare for it to affect the bowel.* Even he suggested it was probably stress, as had all the other doctors. Well, it was endo. He found my uterus is badly tipped, lying right on the bowel, and covered with implants."

Mary, New York

"When I was 12, I began having menstrual periods with excruciating cramps. Each month I suffered about 24 hours of vomiting and diarrhea with the cramps. When I was 18, I also began having colon problems. Every day I would strain for 45 minutes trying to have a bowel movement and then finally have diarrhea. I was 5'8" and weighed 100 pounds. I went to several doctors, but they dismissed the menstrual cramps as irrelevant, psychosomatic symptoms and said I had a spastic colon. I suffered with this for 10 years. By the time I was 28 I was crippled with pain. Blood was in my urine, and pain shot down my right leg.

"I finally found a doctor who believed me when I said I was overwhelmed with pain. He performed a hysterectomy and discovered endometriosis on my colon, bladder, and sciatic nerve. He cauterized the lesions, and I immediately had the first relief from pain I had known in years. A week after surgery I had normal bowel movements, without pain, and my poor colon has functioned normally for years now."

Janice, Colorado

"Before a laparoscopy was performed, I had been to numerous doctors who had mentioned spastic colon as the problem I was experiencing. Ever since the onset of my endometriosis I have experienced bad gas pains, a bloated stomach, frequent nausea, and chronic constipation. . . . I had never experienced any of these symptoms other than constipation before the onset of endometriosis. . . ."

Katherine, Virginia

"I am home recuperating from my third surgery for endo. During my first surgery, eight inches of my sigmoid colon were removed. There was quite a large mass of endo, and it would bleed whenever I had a period. I had immense discomfort whenever I moved my bowels, and the rectal bleeding was awful, and digestion was also affected.

"Four years later not much has happened to improve my lot. I am taking Bentyl and Donnatal to help with the spasms in my colon. I also need Tylenol with codeine to help me endure the pain. During this last operation the doctors discovered endo under my rectum. This is especially uncomfortable. I find it difficult to sit down during my period, and I am always making sure that I eat properly to assure less painful bowel movements."

Ethel, Louisiana

---

*Endo affecting the bowel is certainly not rare, as is clear from the statistics given in this chapter.

"I am one of the endometriosis sufferers who put up with regular nausea; dizziness; non-cyclic diarrhea; extreme headaches; abdominal pain; bloating; numerous allergies, etc., even intermittent extreme and sudden, totally disabling, grabbing abdominal cramps when I would stand up or lean over that would leave me in agony and unable to move. I finally got to the point where I could not bend at the waist or lean down. Over about a seven-year period I was diagnosed as irritable bowel syndrome, spastic colon, colitis, peptic ulcers, nervous duodenal, hypochondriac, mentally unbalanced, seeking attention, pelvic inflammatory disease, and just plain fat. I was treated with everything from whirlpool baths to antidepressants, antibiotics, aspirin, Darvocets, Valium, etc. The ninth doctor I saw finally recognized that I really had a problem and sent me to a gynecologist with experience in endometriosis. Needless to say, it was endometriosis with a nearly solid block attached to the bowels and intestines behind the uterus."

Nancy, Illinois

"I have constant bowel problems and notice that after surgery these problems leave for a while but return within a few months. . . . It was determined I had many food allergies. The elimination of these foods helped quite a bit; however, there still remains much bowel and intestinal discomfort. . . ."

Diane, New York

Since the early days of the association we've been aware of the many intestinal symptoms experienced by women with endo. In our first data registry results published in May 1983, 68 percent of a group of 365 women with endo reported "diarrhea, painful bowel movements, and intestinal upset" at the time of their periods.[1] In a later series of 3,020 women with endo 79 percent reported these symptoms. In fact intestinal symptoms are the most frequently reported symptoms in women with endo, along with dysmenorrhea and fatigue/exhaustion. The only symptom more common in our survey was pain with menstruation—96 percent of the women in the survey reported it.

It has been difficult to sort out what is happening with endo and intestinal symptoms. Typically the gynecology textbooks don't address these symptoms unless there is evidence of endo invading the bowel walls or endometriosis directly on the intestinal tract. Yet many women with endo who experience intestinal symptoms have neither. If the woman goes to see a gastrointestinal specialist about the bowel symptoms, chances are the specialist will see the symptoms as unrelated to the endometriosis. Work-ups often include bowel x-rays, barium enema, sigmoidoscopy, and even colonoscopy. Then, more often than not, the bowel tests come back negative and the woman is told there is no problem or, even worse, the problem is stress or a psychological problem.

So what is going on? We decided it was time to do an exploratory article on the subject. We expect that by pulling together what we have learned thus far and presenting it here, we'll get the ball rolling for our readers, doctors, and others interested in endo to start comparing notes on endo and intestinal problems. Let us hear from you—we'll keep building our understanding, and when new insights or treatment approaches emerge in the future, we'll share them in the association newsletter.

Endo in or on the Bowels

Four groups of intestinal problems seem to occur in women with endo. First and most straightforward are problems possible with direct involvement of endometriosis in or on the intestines. Endometriosis on the intestines, most often the portion of the large intestine at the end of the gastrointestinal system (the sigmoid colon, rectovaginal septum, and rectum) can cause painful bowel movements, a sense of rectal pressure and urgency to move the bowels, bloody stools, and, at its worst, partial or complete bowel obstruction. The last is rare.

According to the medical text *Endometriosis*, edited by Dr. Emery Wilson, 10 to 15 percent of women with endo will have significant gastrointestinal disease (meaning endo is found in or on the intestines). Another source says as many as 37 percent of women with endo have gastrointestinal involvement.

It's possible the frequency is actually higher because gynecologists are attuned primarily to the reproductive organs. Endometriosis specialists would, of course, check the bowel closely, especially at the end of the large intestines. Even if they are on the lookout for intestinal endo, however, the length of the intestines makes it easy to miss. The large intestine, where most endo occurs, is about 5 feet long, the small intestine about 20 feet long.

The same treatments are used for intestinal endo as for other endo. Hormonally, GnRH drugs, danazol, progestins, and birth control pills are used.

Surgically, the best endo experts recommend removal of intestinal endo. Most lesions of the bowel, according to Drs. Malinak and Wheeler in Dr. Wilson's text on endometriosis, "are superficial and may be destroyed by electrocautery/laser or sharply excised. Nodules invading the bowel wall must be excised." (*Superficial* means on the surface of the bowels and not invading the bowel wall. Even when the growths or nodules invade the bowel walls, it is generally only into the outside layers, not all the way through, although the latter is possible and, of course, much more serious.)

These and other experts go on to explain that women with severe endo and gastrointestinal involvement should have their bowels prepared before major surgery for endo so a resection (removal of the damaged part of the intestines) can be done if endo is found to have invaded the bowel deeply. (Bowel preparation usually involves clearing the intestines with solutions and enemas.) "It is always preferable to prep a patient who does not require bowel surgery than to run the risk of not prepping a patient who does," say two other experts, Drs. Grunert and Franklin, in the Wilson book. They also note that if the need for bowel surgery is expected (based on bowel studies prior to the surgery), a general surgeon or surgeon specializing in colon surgery should be involved. Drs. Grunert and Franklin note they have become more aggressive in surgically treating endo of the bowel as they've had more experience with it.

And Drs. Barbieri and Kistner in the book *Gynecology: Principles and Practice* also note that "small endometrial implants on the intestines should be excised." However, they write that when there is more involvement, "since bilateral oophorectomy [removal of both ovaries] will bring about permanent arrest of the disease, this procedure should be performed in preference to extensive bowel resection." (It's possible that without immediate hormone replacement after removal of the ovaries, the endo remaining on the bowel would die out, but unfortunately numerous reports to the association show the disease often continues after removal of the ovaries when the endo was severe. This would seem particularly likely if the amount of endo was great enough to warrant extensive bowel resection. See the hysterectomy articles in Chapter 2 for more information.) Innovative endo specialists have now pioneered new resection techniques, and the trend is to attempt to remove the diseased portion of the bowel.

A gynecologist trained only in traditional surgical techniques and electrocautery is at a disadvantage in treating endo of the bowels because of general skittishness related to surgery near or on organs not part of the reproductive tract and because of the inability to control precisely the depth of tissue destroyed via electrocautery. This inability is particularly important for the bowel, since a cut or burn that goes too deep could cause leakage of bowel contents into the abdomen. The bacteria and other microorganisms of the bowel, as well as fecal matter, can lead to peritonitis, a serious and potentially life-threatening inflammation of the peritoneum, the tissue lining the abdomen. The use of laser and sharp excision may be better surgical approaches for removing endo on the bowels. (For an in-depth discussion of surgical techniques for endo, see Chapter 2.) Drs. Malinak and Wheeler, in the gynecology textbook *Endometriosis*, note: "Cautery—in particular unipolar—should be avoided in areas near bowel, bladder, ureter, and broad ligaments as control of depth of tissue destruction is much less than that with carbon dioxide laser." They go on to cite the "precise incision of tissues with a very shallow depth of tissue destruction" of the carbon dioxide laser as the reason for its use in infertility surgery. The same need for minimal tissue destruction and precise control exists for surgery for endo of the bowels.

Despite the recommendation of experts, "the failure to completely resect cul-de-sac or rectosigmoid implants is common," write Drs. Grunert and Franklin. Reasons they cite for failure to remove all the endometriosis seen in surgery are inadequate evaluation of the patient before surgery, inadequate preparation of the patient, "an injudiciously timid approach to surgery, a lack of appreciation for the natural history of the disease, and the feeling that medical therapy will somehow take care of lesions that are difficult to remove. . . ."

"Endometriosis of the bowel is often left untouched, and pain can continue even if other measures were taken to alleviate it," according to Dr. Dean Sharpe, a general surgeon who has worked on endo of the bowel with Dr. David Redwine of Bend, Oregon. Among the reasons he cites are that endo of the bowel is difficult to detect before surgery, most patients are not prepared for possible bowel resection, and a surgeon who could do a resection is usually not involved in the surgery. (Most gynecologists are not trained to do surgery on the bowels.) Finally, when endo on the bowel is addressed, Dr. Sharpe notes, "Full-thickness resection is the norm even when the endo has not penetrated deeply."

In other words, disease on the bowel is not being treated surgically even when it could be handled by simple removal without a complete cut through the bowel wall by some surgeons. By others the disease on the bowel is simply being ignored or treated hormonally, regardless of the nature of the particular growths. Dr. Sharpe argues that "by liberally preparing patients for bowel resection, combining the skills of both gynecologic and general surgeons, and following the philosophy that all disease (rather than organs, such as ovaries) should be removed for optimum pain relief, I feel we have developed a positive new approach to treating endometriosis of the bowel."

Bowel Problems Due to Adhesions

A second group of intestinal problems seems to occur in women with endo related to adhesions. Bowel symptoms can result from adhesions pulling on the bowel even if there is no active endometriosis on the bowel, write Drs. Grunert and Franklin in the gynecology textbook *Endometriosis*. Adhesions can result from the disease itself or from surgery for the disease. They and other specialists recommend great care in endo surgery to reduce the chance of adhesions.

Symptoms due to adhesions are similar to symptoms due to active endo. Adhesions often seem to cause pain after activities that can stretch them, such as exercise, intercourse, or pelvic and rectal exams. If the adhesions pull on the bowels, the same activities can then cause bowel symptoms. (See the article on adhesions in Chapter 2 for more information.)

Gastrointestinal Symptoms and Prostaglandins

The presence of gastrointestinal symptoms does not necessarily indicate endometriosis in or on the bowel, however, or even that there are adhesions on the intestines. Our third group of symptoms seems to occur in many women with endo who have no evidence of endo on the bowel, as well as in those who do. These gastrointestinal symptoms are usually at their worst at the time of the period. They include diarrhea, nausea and vomiting, and general intestinal discomfort (sometimes described as an unpleasant jumpiness in the intestines). These are well-known symptoms of primary dysmenorrhea. Primary dysmenorrhea is painful periods, diarrhea, intestinal upset during periods, sometimes nausea and vomiting, dizziness and fainting, hot/cold flashes, headache, and other discomforts due to an imbalance in prostaglandins.

Prostaglandins are substances that control the smooth muscle tissue of the body, the nonvoluntary muscles. These muscles cause contractions of the uterus, change blood vessel diameter, and regulate intestinal activity. Prostaglandins are produced by the lining of the uterus, by endometriosis lesions, and by macrophages. The same prostaglandin imbalance at work in primary dysmenorrhea has been documented in the peritoneal fluid of women with endometriosis. (The cause of the imbalance is unknown, although many factors are potentially involved—imbalance in the modern food supply of the essential fatty acids from which our body produces prostaglandins; overactivation or malfunction of macrophages caused by toxins, allergies, viruses; or other triggers such as *Candida albicans*.) A major study reported in the *Journal of the American Medical Association* found primary dysmenorrhea to be a risk factor for endometriosis—meaning women with primary dysmenorrhea were more likely to develop endo.

Indeed, primary dysmenorrhea and endometriosis seem to be part of the same continuum, with mild primary dysmenorrhea on one end and full-blown endometriosis on the other. This is a concept the Endometriosis Association has remarked on since 1983, but women and doctors still often ignore primary dysmenorrhea as unimportant or "normal."

Dr. Penny Budoff describes the effects of this imbalance in her book, *No More Menstrual Cramps and Other Good News*:

The uterine lining [and, we add, endometriosis] produces two prostaglandins, prostaglandin E and prostaglandin F (eight groups have been identified so far, dubbed A through I). Their levels increase as the time of menstruation approaches. The highest levels occur at the onset of flow. Prostaglandin F probably causes a greater increase in muscle tone and contraction of the uterus than prostaglandin E. When prostaglandins are produced in excess amounts or F is in excess of E, the uterus is overactive and contracts too much, causing cramps and pain. The uterus squeezes so hard that it compresses the uterine blood vessels and cuts off the blood supply. This situation is very much like what occurs in the heart when its blood supply is cut off by a clot or blood vessel spasm during a heart attack. The heart also is a muscle, and when it suffers a decrease in its blood supply the pain (angina) is excruciating. The result is the same in both instances: pain occurs when a muscle does not have sufficient oxygen because the blood flow has been cut off. The pain of dysmenorrhea is analogous to the pain experienced during a heart attack.

Some of the excess prostaglandin escapes from the uterus and into the blood-stream, where it may affect other smooth muscles in the body before it is destroyed. The smooth muscle of the gut is stimulated and contracts too rapidly and propels food along too quickly, causing diarrhea. The smooth muscle in blood vessels may cause blood vessels to constrict and dilate. That's why some women feel cold and hot flashes. And some women will faint because a sudden dilation of the blood vessels causes a pooling of blood in their legs and feet, depriving the brain of blood and oxygen.

For more on prostaglandins and endometriosis, see Chapter 16 in the association's first book, *Overcoming Endometriosis*.

Gastrointestinal Symptoms and Candidiasis

There's another group of intestinal problems experienced frequently by women with endo that is possibly related to the prostaglandin group. These include chronic or episodic constipation and diarrhea, abdominal pain, gas and bloating, rectal itching, and irritable bowel syndrome (also called *spastic colon* and *mucous colitis*). These symptoms all occur with candidiasis, a condition of sensitivity to a fungus (*Candida albicans*) or an overgrowth of the fungus. *Candida albicans* lives in great numbers in the colon and can cause many colon symptoms if not kept in check. People with candidiasis typically develop numerous allergies, including food allergies, which can cause gastrointestinal and other symptoms.[2] We have covered this problem so common in women with endo in our first book, so will not go into detail here except to note that women with endo have found relief from gastrointestinal symptoms with proper treatment for candidiasis.

Proper diagnosis and treatment for candidiasis can be hard to obtain because it is relatively new and somewhat controversial. However, we continue to hear so many reports of improvement in women with endo who follow the candidiasis treatment programs that we would be remiss not to continue to bring this to readers' attention.

Why, despite some good research, is the information related to candidiasis controversial? The best answer is plain resistance to change, to new information that contradicts what was taught in medical school (that *Candida albicans* is harmless, for instance, although no one understands its role in the body). James S. Goodwin, M.D., of the Department of Medicine and Jean M. Goodwin, M.D., M.P.H., of the Department of Psychiatry at the University of New Mexico School of Medicine call this "the tomato effect." Their paper, "The Tomato Effect . . . Rejection of Highly Efficacious Therapies," was published in the *Journal of the American Medical Assocation* in 1984. It describes how tomatoes were rejected as a food by North Americans almost until the 20th century because "everyone knew they were poisonous." In fact, part of the debunking of this myth involved public demonstrations of tomato eating by "brave" individuals proving they could eat tomatoes and not die on the spot:

> The tomato effect occurs in medicine when an efficacious treatment for a certain disease is ignored or rejected because it does not 'make sense' in the light of accepted theories of disease mechanism and drug action. . . . The tomato effect has retarded the use of effective therapies, including the use of gold, colchicine, and aspirin for the treatment of various types of arthritic joint dysfunction.
>
> Modern medicine is particularly vulnerable to the tomato effect. What gets lost are the only three issues that matter in picking a therapy: Does it work? How toxic is it? How much does it cost? We are at risk for rejecting a safe, inexpensive therapy in favor of an alternative treatment perhaps less efficacious and more toxic. . . . Before we accept a treatment we should ask, "Is this a placebo?" and before we reject a treatment we should ask, "Is this a tomato?"

Resistance to change is a common human trait and afflicts doctors and scientists as well as all other humans. It's a dangerous trait for endometriosis, though, since endometriosis is a disease without answers. The answers as to the cause, cure, prevention, and better treatment of the disease can come only from new information or a new way of looking at information we already have.

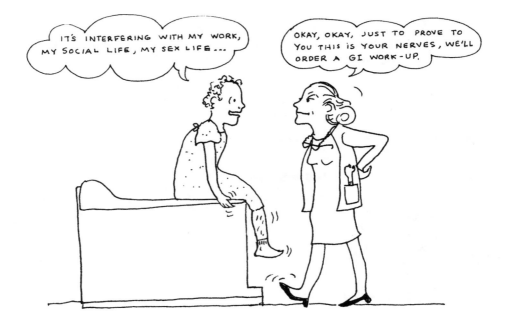

Irritable Bowel Syndrome and Endo

As is clear from the four groups of intestinal problems and symptoms presented here, women with endo suffer from many gastrointestinal ailments. It is not impossible, of course, to have a bowel disease along with the endo, but more often than not the standard bowel tests are negative.

Women with endo are sometimes told they have irritable bowel syndrome, a catch-all nondiagnosis used to describe bowel problems when no other diagnosis is found. Among 3,020 women with endo whose case histories are included in our data research registry, 85 (2.8 percent) were told they have irritable bowel syndrome, colitis, or spastic colon.[3]

Irritable bowel syndrome, colitis, and spastic colon are all names for the same thing—a condition in which the muscular contractions of the bowel become uncoordinated, causing abdominal cramping and pain, constipation and/or diarrhea, nausea, bloating, rectal urgency, and excessive gas. When the stool contains a lot of mucus, it may be called *mucous colitis*, a noninflammatory condition. (Be aware there are other types of colitis, which are true colitis—meaning an inflammation of the bowel. The other types are amebic, granulomatous, regional or segmental, transmural, and ulcerative.) Irritable bowel syndrome (*IBS* for short) is twice as common in women as in men and begins most often in early adult life, according to *The AMA Family Medical Guide* (1987). The cause of the syndrome is not understood; not surprisingly, IBS is often thought to be due to psychological problems, the standard explanation for puzzling problems not yet explained by science (especially if they affect primarily women).

We think *uncoordinated contractions of the intestines* sounds a lot like the work of the prostaglandins. As a diagnosis, irritable bowel syndrome is singularly unhelpful. Reading

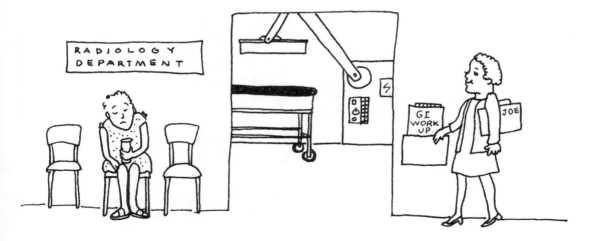

the recommendations for it sounds much like the literature from before 1980 on what to do about painful menstruation. The advice is nebulous, sometimes contradictory (one group of drugs used can cause constipation, one of the symptoms of IBS, for example); references are made to things like "hypochondriasis, hysteria, and depression"; inevitably the suggestion is made that the patient be referred for psychological counseling; and it's clear physicians don't like to deal with it. ("This particularly distressing disorder is as frustrating for the patient as it is for the physician," notes one source. Shouldn't that be in reverse order?!) Finally, in echoes nearly every woman with endo will recognize, patients with IBS are told, "Eventually you will need to learn to live with and control your own symptoms."

In Summary—What to Do About Gastrointestinal Symptoms

So in summary, what can you do about gastrointestinal symptoms and endometriosis other than learn to live with them? We suggest women with endo with bowel symptoms do the following:

1. Treat the endo—as noted in the letters from women with endo and gastrointestinal symptoms that accompany this story, treating the endo frequently brought relief of the gastrointestinal symptoms.

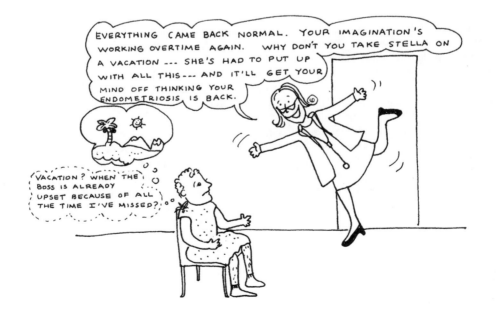

2. Work with the very best doctor you can find. Ask questions about how your doctor intends to handle endo on or near the bowel if found in surgery. To find that special doctor, an endometriosis specialist, attend meetings of your local association chapter or group and/or call other members in your area. Get in touch with headquarters for contact information (see "Additional Resources").

3. If you have a lot of intestinal upset at the time of your period and have never tried antiprostaglandins, give them a try. They may not work for the intense pain of endo (although they do help some women), but they might help lessen the sickening intestinal symptoms, nausea/vomiting, and hot/cold flashes so many women with endo experience with their periods.

4. Eat as healthy a diet as possible. Consider eliminating or cutting down on things that might irritate your intestines, including coffee, teas, and colas containing caffeine; and soft drinks and gums containing artificial sweeteners (some of these have been found to be irritating to the intestines and contribute to diarrhea). Consider an allergy to milk or milk products if you haven't considered it in the past. Adequate fiber (as in vegetables, fruits, etc.) is also generally suggested to improve bowel health.

5. If you suspect candidiasis, food allergies, or other allergies as contributing factors, seek competent medical help. Treating these problems has brought gastrointestinal health for some women with endo who did not have endometriosis right on or in the bowels but rather were suffering from prostaglandin effects or candidiasis problems. Remember, the healthier you can get overall, the better you'll feel in spite of the endo.

Notes

1. The association's data registry was begun in 1980 and consists of computerized data from more than 3,000 case histories of women with endo. It was the first registry in the world for ongoing information gathering and research on endometriosis.

2. The association was the first to document multiple allergic manifestations in women with endo. The findings were reported in the *American Journal of Preventive Medicine* 2, no. 6 ("Endometriosis: A Comparison of Associated Disease Histories"), and *Annals of Allergy* 59, no. 11 ("The Association of Atopic Diseases with Endometriosis").

3. Because the questionnaire used for our data registry does not specifically ask about irritable bowel syndrome but rather is an open-ended question asking if the woman has any other health problems, the numbers here are likely to be on the low side. Informal observation by the author over the years indicates more than 2.8 percent of women with endo are told they have IBS. In any case, the symptoms of IBS clearly parallel the gastrointestinal symptoms reported by women with endo and candidiasis.

Endometriosis, Irritable Bowel Syndrome, and Me

By Sandy Nemeroff

EDITOR'S NOTE: Member Sandy Nemeroff's story about struggling with bowel problems that were actually endometriosis is like so many others we've heard through the years. We urge readers with bowel problems to consider treatment of endo as a possible step in resolving them. For more on lasers, see Chapter 2.

Since 1975 I have been suffering from bowel symptoms that have become progressively worse through the years. I have submitted myself to the usual testing procedures (including GI series, barium enema, gallbladder sonography, sigmoidoscopy, colonoscopy, etc.), all of which were negative. I pursued every avenue of medical help of which I was aware, generally to no avail. Symptomatically, I was experiencing many bowel movements throughout each day. These episodes generally left me weak and nauseated.

The acute attacks that seemed to "come out of the blue" were, however, the worst aspect of the condition. These were characterized by (1) occurring one-half to one hour following the ingestion of food and (2) a peculiar abdominal sensation that inevitably resulted in an urgent visit to the bathroom. The bowel movement generally deteriorated to diarrhea, which was accompanied, at its worst, by excruciating pain. This situation usually required pharmacological remediation (Lomotil, paregoric) and sent me to bed physically depleted, anxious for the pain to subside, and frightened by the thought of subsequent attacks.

My life was a nightmare that resulted in my fearing my body's abnormal reactions. As a last resort I underwent psychotherapy—this, too, to no avail. In the ninth year of my illness (which, as I mentioned earlier, became increasingly more debilitating) I came under the care of a physician who sent me to a psychiatrist who had done some pioneer work with tricyclic antidepressants. One of the side effects of certain members of this family of drugs is that they slow down gastrointestinal motility. This, they thought, was the only hope of getting my intestines to perform more normally on a daily basis.

While under the psychiatrist's care, the facts that (1) I had extremely painful menstrual periods and (2) my "colitis" became worse during my menstrual period were discussed. He insisted that I return to my gynecologist and emphasize these facts to him. Interestingly enough I had complained to my gynecologist for years about my GI problems. His response had been that my uterus was retroverted and therefore I would experience increased "discomfort" during my menstrual period as the uterus became engorged and added pressure to the colon. The psychiatrist found the gynecologist's rationale for my symptoms unacceptable.

I returned to the gynecologist for the visit that ultimately led to my first laparoscopy. Endometriosis was diagnosed, and I was put on Danocrine for seven months, during which time I did not experience one acute "colitis" attack. My condition was generally improved, but I have to admit that I still didn't feel "great." With the return of my menstrual period (two months after discontinuing drug therapy), I experienced my first acute colitis attack in nine months. My gynecologist felt that this was a psychosomatic phenomenon and insisted that the endo had to have disappeared after seven months of Danocrine.

I stopped the Danocrine and underwent surgery in Atlanta, Georgia, with Dr. Camran Nezhat. Endo was again found [and removed with the laser], and my acute attacks of "colitis" came to an end. I would like to add that my local gynecologist refused upon several requests to view the videotape of my surgery and, even after having read the hospital report, denies that the endo still existed at the time of surgery by Dr. Nezhat.

■ *Sandy Nemeroff, Northport, New York, is a member of the Endometriosis Association.*

5

⊘⊘

Endometriosis and the Urinary Tract

By Andrea Lea Yap

"*Four years ago I began to have problems with pain in my bladder. My general practitioner found no reason for this. I went next to a urologist. By this time I was actually getting bladder infections, but the pain continued after the infection was cured. The urologist believed my symptoms were due to stress. He said, 'Many of our career gals experience this.'*

"*Next I went to a gynecologist, who said nothing was wrong. . . . Finally I read about the disease endometriosis in Time. I went to a highly respected doctor. He thought I had endo but warned that the bladder problems were not part of the problem—after all, the urologist had viewed the bladder and ruled this out.*

"*I took the medication danazol for three months, and the bladder problems gradually improved. I then had the laparoscopy, which showed endo on the ovary but none on the bladder. The endo was vaporized with the laser; I stopped the danazol and felt completely better for the next two years! Although none of the doctors agree, I am absolutely convinced that the bladder problems were due to endo.*"

Kathleen, Pennsylvania

"*I have had three laparoscopies and two laparotomies, including hysterectomy and removal of the ovaries, in the last three years. It wasn't until the third laparoscopy that a few small endometrial lesions were seen on my bladder, but symptoms were present both before and after diagnosis and treatment, whether or not lesions were seen on the bladder.*

"*I am sometimes awakened at night with severe back pain that ends after urination. This usually occurs if I drink liquids after 6:00 P.M. and fail to completely empty my bladder before bed. I also cannot tolerate having a full bladder, as it is extremely painful, as is urination. I have seen urologists both near home and at Mayo Clinic, and no one seems to have an answer. I did not have a urinary tract problem before the endo symptoms began.*

"*I continue to have the problem even though I am in 'remission' and am feeling well otherwise.*

"At the time of my last surgery, adhesions were found and removed from my ureters, but the pain continues. Perhaps the adhesions have regrown already. Apparently my physicians do not doubt my continued bladder pain since I consistently have blood in my urine that is found each time I have a urinalysis. Two cystoscopies have not revealed the source of the problem.

"Since I have also had three IVPs (intravenous pyelography) to x-ray the entire urinary tract, I don't know what other investigations can be done.

"I've taken birth control pills, danazol, Lupron injections, and had more tests and surgeries than an otherwise healthy person can imagine. At this time I have resigned myself just to dealing with the problem as best I can without further medical tests."

Martha, Illinois

"My bladder symptoms started about one year ago. Like magic, overnight I woke up with bad cystitis symptoms—frequency, urgency (the feeling that you must empty your bladder immediately), pain, etc. . . . When the GP examined my abdomen, it was very tender, and that didn't seem to go along with cystitis. The urine culture came back negative.

"In the next couple months I had several cultures that were all negative. Anyway, finally one of the gynecologists in my group thought I might have endo because I also had pelvic and back pains. Diagnosis was confirmed at the same time I was having the laser surgery."

Cristine, Georgia

"I would like to suggest a book that helped me overcome my problem of chronic bladder inflammation. The book is You Don't Have to Live with Cystitis *by Dr. Larrian Gillespie (Avon Books, 1986). It was recommended by my urologist.*

"By following the diet in the book, I immediately became more comfortable and ceased to have any symptoms within four weeks; after six months I was able to go back to my regular diet, although I continue to go easy on acidic foods. I should mention that I am not a food faddist and that observing strict rules about what I ate was an unusual step for me. But it worked, and I am delighted that I can recommend something that will help.

"Here are some of the rules in the book that I found helpful; this is not a complete list, just enough to put you in enough comfort to run out and buy the book:

"1. If you have pain in the bladder, drink ¼ teaspoon of baking soda in a glass of water. This will alkalinize your urine and prevent the acids in the urine from interacting with sore or damaged tissue. The action is rapid.

"2. A few hours later, take four Tums or another form of calcium carbonate. Repeat the dose 12 hours later.

"3. Drink lots of clear fluids. Don't drink abnormal amounts, though; drinking a quart at a time will distend the bladder and add to your discomfort.

"4. Do not eat or drink anything on the following list, cooked or uncooked: acidic juices, fruit, caffeine (coffee, tea, chocolate), alcoholic beverages, tomato sauce, chilies/spicy

foods, vinegar, carbonated drinks, aged cheese, brewer's yeast, chicken livers, onions, nuts, raisins and prunes, soy sauce, fava beans and lima beans, mayonnaise, NutraSweet, avocados, yogurt, corned beef, rye bread, and sour cream.

"Be aware that what you eat can irritate your bladder just as it can irritate your bowel. Although the list above is relatively short, the diet is hard to follow. You will find yourself eating a lot of cooked vegetables and basic foods like Mother used to make (e.g., tapioca pudding), because this is a bland diet and avoids salad dressings and fruit. Try to plan one day at a time and make a list before you go to the store. After a couple of weeks you will get used to the diet and it will be no problem."

Judith, Massachusetts

EDITOR'S NOTE: Another book that may be helpful is *Conquering Cystitis, A Self-Help Guide to Understanding and Controlling Cystitis*, by Dr. Patrick Kingsley (London: Ebury Press, 1987), which describes the links between cystitis and food allergies and sometimes *Candida* yeast.

"I have had bladder problems as a result of endometriosis damaging my bladder. I had endo in and on the bladder. I had a total hysterectomy four years ago. This freed me from constant chronic disabling pain, bowel pain and problems, and lower abdominal pain in the bladder area. This is a blessing because I have a life today, and before hysterectomy I did not.

"The bladder problems are diminished but did not leave entirely. I take propantheline as needed when bladder spasms are a problem, which they are from time to time. The bladder spasms are sometimes quite painful, and I find this is aggravated by stress. I also urinate frequently, but after hysterectomy I am able to sleep through the night, except for getting up once about midway through. . . . P.S. I've found Kegel exercises help some."

Althea, Louisiana

EDITOR'S NOTE: Kegel exercises involve tightening and relaxing the muscles in the pelvic floor to keep them firm. You can locate the right muscles by experimenting until you can stop your urine in midstream and restart it at will.

"My gut feeling at this point is that the endo and the IC [interstitial cystitis] are both manifestations of a general problem with my immune system—that both are autoimmune diseases caused by one genetic defect. What is it? I don't know. It's got to be related to hormones, monthly cycles, ability to fight off infections (I also wage war on chronic vaginal yeast), and other factors I don't understand.

"Choose urologists with care. They tend to be far more interested in men's prostate problems than women's complaints of nonspecific pain. They also have an amazing ability to make women with chronic bladder pain feel frantic and hysterical, and they have been known to suggest psychiatric help as an alternative to any concrete physical protocol.

I'm not knocking psychiatrists (mine has been very helpful), but I caution you not to let anyone tell you that your bladder pain is a manifestation of psychological disease. If anything, the process works in reverse. Who wouldn't start to lose it with all the pain and so little relief?"

Cathy, Connecticut

In February 1990 I was urinating up to 60 times a day. Desperate, I requested contact in the association newsletter from other members with bladder problems. It was a spontaneous act, and I thought I'd receive three or four letters. At this writing I am still astounded that I have been contacted by almost 50 members with bladder problems.

Members also have reported bladder difficulties to the association headquarters, which responded by establishing the Bladder Correspondence Network, an informal correspondence network of members with bladder problems. (To join, write to association headquarters; see "Additional Resources.")

The exact number of women with endo who have urinary tract difficulties is unknown. The first reported case of bladder endo occurred in 1921. Most researchers cite the incidence of urinary involvement at 1 to 2 percent of all cases but admit that underdiagnosis is a problem. In a May 1988 *Journal of Reproductive Medicine* study, the incidence was quoted at 1 percent, "but most physicians have seen bladder involvement."[1] In one large study of patients 16 percent had urinary involvement. Most had endo implants on the bladder. Only 1.5 percent had involvement of the ureters.[2] (The urinary tract includes the kidneys, two ureters, the bladder, and the urethra; see diagram.)

We wonder if the incidence of urinary involvement with endometriosis is much higher than 1 or 2 percent. In the association's Data Research Registry, 24.9 percent of the 3,020 registry participants reported that their doctors had told them endometrial implants were located on the bladder.

Australian gynecologist Daniel T. O'Connor reported that in a study of 717 endo patients 108 (15 percent) had bladder involvement and two had involvement of the ureter. This is a higher percentage than reported on the uterine surface, fallopian tubes, bowel, appendix, vagina, or cervix in his study. The most common site reported was the cul-de-sac, followed by the uterosacral ligaments, peritoneum, left ovary, and right ovary, respectively.[3]

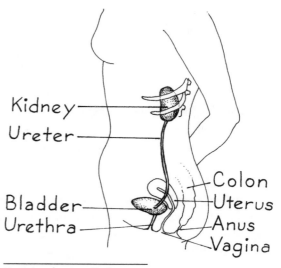

Drawing by Jan Kruk.

Symptoms

A review of endometriosis research yielded a variety of symptoms found when endometriosis involves the urinary tract. By far the most common complaint was abdominal pain, either related to the menstrual cycle or constant. Also common were dysmenorrhea, urinary frequency, low-back pain, difficult urination (dysuria), and pain in the flank (the fleshy part of the side of the torso, between the ribs and hip). Less commonly patients mentioned blood in the urine (hematuria), suprapubic pain (pain above the pubic bone), painful intercourse, rectal pain and pressure, fatigue and high blood pressure, urinary urgency, fluid retention, and incontinence.

Blood in the urine can also be a sign of bladder cancer. The authors of an *American Journal of Obstetrics and Gynecology* article claim that only 25 percent of bladder endo cases involve hematuria.[4] According to *Overcoming Bladder Disorders*, "If blood is discovered in your urine, it does *not* necessarily mean that you have cancer."[5] Bladder cancer doesn't usually affect people under age 50, and men are at least three times more likely to develop this type of cancer than women.

Urinary urgency is probably best described as "When I have to go, I have to go *now*." It is the urgent demand by your bladder for relief. The two types of incontinence described in the research are stress incontinence and urge incontinence. Stress incontinence is a leakage of urine in response to a cough, sneeze, laugh, or sudden movement. Urge incontinence is a leakage of urine when you feel the urge to urinate but may not have enough warning to get to the bathroom in time.

Medical textbooks, including *Endometriosis: Contemporary Concepts in Clinical Management* edited by Robert S. Schenken, M.D., list the most common complaints associated with bladder endo as difficult urination, frequency, and suprapubic pain or pressure. Endometriosis obstructing the ureters also tends to cause difficult urination, plus urgency, frequency, blood in the urine, flank pain, fever, and, rarely, vomiting.

An article in a newer medical textbook, *Modern Approaches to Endometriosis*, states: "Presenting symptoms of vesical [bladder-related] endometriosis frequently include dysuria, urgency and frequency, while ureteral and kidney endometriosis are more commonly present with hematuria and abdominal flank pain."[6]

In 75 percent of cases of bladder endo the patients have a history of "symptoms usually suggestive of cystitis," according to the article in the *American Journal of Obstetrics and Gynecology*.[7]

Roberta, an East Coast member, had several of these symptoms a few years ago: "I started having bladder problems—frequent and painful urination aggravated by alcohol or caffeine, agony if I had to go but must wait, and feeling like I have to go when I don't have to. As for whether I have endo on my bladder or not, I'm not really sure. . . ."

As with endo in other locations, bladder symptoms also can occur when adhesions pull on the bladder or scar tissue involves the ureters. Adhesions are bands of scar tissue that stretch between areas of the pelvis or abdomen. Adhesions and scar tissue can result from the endo itself or from surgery and can cause problems even when no active endo is present. (For more on adhesions and endo, see the article on adhesions in Chapter 2.)

Diagnosis

An article in *Endometriosis: Contemporary Concepts in Clinical Management* says cystoscopy is required to make the diagnosis of bladder endo. During a cystoscopy a urologist looks inside the bladder by inserting an instrument called the *cystoscope* through the urethra. "Cystography [x-ray of the bladder after it has been filled with a substance to show contrast] and pelvic ultrasonography may show a mass in the pelvis close to the bladder, but these tests are not diagnostic . . . cystoscopic diagnosis is optimal during menstruation; however, biopsy is necessary to make a definitive diagnosis."[8]

Interestingly, six cases of endo of the urinary tract reported by researchers had no urinary symptoms at all. This may contribute to the problem of underdiagnosis that plagues endometriosis patients. When urinary tract endo goes undetected, the result can be life-threatening damage to the kidneys. In the previously mentioned article the author states: "The prognosis is serious; in one series of 62 patients, loss of kidney function occurred in 46 percent, mostly because of delay in diagnosis."[9]

Bladder endo can easily be confused with urinary tract infections (UTIs for short). Jane from Oklahoma has expressed the frustration that misdiagnosis can cause: "I hate to go running to the doctor's office every time I'm in pain. The 'what if' questions go through my head: What if I don't have a bladder infection? What if I do have a bladder infection? What if something serious is wrong and I don't go in? What if nothing is wrong?"

Jane has had many UTIs, but eventually she began getting the symptoms without the bacteria showing up in her urine: "Before being diagnosed as having endo, I thought I had urinary tract infections, etc. (I have a history of bladder infections way back when I was six years old.) I went to my urologist three different times with my bladder. My symptom was low-back pain. I drank lots and lots of water and still had pain. My urine never showed infection. In December of 1989, I found out it was not my bladder; it was endo."

Interestingly, about half of all women with urinary tract endo have had previous pelvic surgery. A 1985 *Journal of Urology* article reports that as many as 50 percent of the patients have a history of pelvic surgery. "Diagnosis often is delayed, with a reported average of 54 months between the onset of symptoms and diagnosis."[10] A 1982 *American Journal of Obstetrics and Gynecology* article stated: "The patient's history frequently reveals that she had had several pelvic operations before signs and symptoms of urinary tract involvement developed. This suggests that long-standing disease or an aggressive process is found when the urinary tract is involved."[11]

Swedish researchers in 1980 reported a study of 17 women with endo on the bladder over a period of years from 1953 to 1967.[12] In all cases the endometriosis had followed vaginal hysterotomy—incision of the uterus—for legal abortion. This procedure was used commonly in Sweden in the late 1940s for legal abortion after the twelfth week of pregnancy. Modern techniques have now replaced hysterotomy for abortion. "Up to ten years after the abortion, however, endometriosis often appeared at the site of the scar. . . ."

EDITOR'S NOTE: Endometriosis also has been detected in scars from other surgeries, including cesarean sections, and episiotomies.

The *American Journal of Obstetrics and Gynecology* in December 1985 detailed a case of bladder endometriosis in a woman whose bladder had been injured during surgery.[13] Two years earlier she had had a total vaginal hysterectomy, during which the left posterior wall of the bladder was injured and repaired transvaginally. The endometriosis was found in the same area as the old injury. She complained of difficult urination, frequency, and urgency. She also had blood in the urine for five days each month.

Treatment of Urinary Tract Endo

Generally urinary tract endometriosis is treated the same as other forms of the disease—with surgery and/or hormonal therapy. Treatment choices depend on the location of the disease, severity of symptoms, patient's age, and childbearing desires. In the September 1984 issue of the journal *Urology*, a group of physicians in Brazil states: "There are a variety of management modalities in vesical [bladder] endometriosis, the choice depending on the patient's age, marital status, desire for progeny, extent of the vesical lesion, severity of urinary symptoms or menstrual disorders, and associated pelvic pathology."[14]

A review of three medical textbooks on endometriosis showed two recommending hormonal therapy and/or surgery and one recommending surgery only. In the textbook *Endometriosis,* edited by Emery A. Wilson, M.D., authors Rock and Markham conclude: "Therapy . . . would depend on the extent of the disease, but should include local excision and/or hormonal suppression. Occasionally, castration [removal of the ovaries] is indicated in such patients, and then only when fertility is no longer desired."[15]

The textbook *Endometriosis: Contemporary Concepts in Clinical Management* explains:

Treatment depends upon the status of the patient and her reproductive desires. Castration ordinarily results in resolution of lesions and relieves symptoms. Occasionally, this is not successful and segmental resection of the bladder may become necessary. [**EDITOR'S NOTE:** Unfortunately, as found in an association study reported in the article "Does Hysterectomy and Removal of the Ovaries Offer a Cure for Endometriosis?" continuation of endometriosis is all too often the result when endo involves the bowel and/or bladder and the disease is left behind.] Treatment with progestogens and danazol is reported to be temporarily successful in a few cases, but accurate data are not available, and long-term administration of these agents is unwarranted. Recurrence of the disease is likely when treatment is discontinued. For this reason medical therapy is limited to a few selected cases.[16]

One reason hormonal therapy sometimes fails is that scar tissue, which does not respond to hormones, is often present. A March 1985 article in *Obstetrics and Gynecology* mentioned this:[17]

Gardner and Whitaker reported success in relieving ureteral obstruction in one patient using danazol as an adjunct after right salpingo-oophorectomy [removal of the right fallopian tube and ovary] failed to relieve the patient's pain. Other authors state that hormonal relief should not be expected in patients with obstructive uropathy [blocked ureters] due to endometriosis because of the presence of dense scarring by hormonally unresponsive tissue.

Surgically, endometriosis of the bladder can be excised or lasered. In a case report, Dr. Camran Nezhat, endometriosis specialist and association advisor, describes a surgery he performed on an endometriosis patient along with Drs. Farr Nezhat and urologist Bruce Green at the Center for Special Pelvic Surgery and Fertility and Endoscopy Center, Endometriosis Clinic in Atlanta. The surgeons carried out a laparoscopic partial bladder resection and repair to treat bladder wall endometriosis. The article states that laparoscopic partial bladder resection and repair has not previously been reported—in the past these procedures have been done through laparotomy, major open abdominal surgery.

The 39-year-old woman had a history of pelvic pain and hematuria during menstruation. She had already had a cystoscopy with coagulation of endometriosis, but the hematuria continued. Treatment with danazol and a GnRH drug stopped the bleeding, but it recurred when the medications were stopped.

If endometriosis has deeply penetrated the bladder, a partial cystectomy (removal of part of the bladder) may be required. A study published in the *Scandinavian Journal of Urologic Nephrology* in 1980 examined the effects of partial cystectomy more than 10 years afterward in four women. These women had most or all of the trigone of the bladder—a triangular area at the base of the bladder—removed. The researchers wanted to determine how this affected the function of the urethra and the bladder. The four women were found to have "normal" bladders: "Knowledge that the trigone can be extirpated [cut out by surgery] without disturbance to bladder function is also valuable. In endometriosis of the urinary bladder, radical extirpation of the affected area can therefore be regarded as appropriate treatment, particularly as no recurrence appeared during the period of observation."[18]

The textbooks touch on treatments for urinary tract endo only briefly. There is little discussion of how patients fare after partial cystectomy or of recurrence rates.

Another study, published in March 1990, did show both subjective and objective improvement from danazol and surgery. (*Subjective* means the patient felt better; *objective* means there's evidence that the disease is diminishing.) The *Mount Sinai Journal of Medicine* contained a case report of a woman who had urinary frequency, nocturia (frequency at night), urgency, and urge incontinence.[19] The patient had a laparotomy with removal of fibroid tumors and endometriosis from the surface of the bladder. She then took danazol for three months. The nocturia, frequency, urgency, and urge incontinence all improved. The capacity of the bladder was measured and had also improved from 100 cubic centimeters to 450 cubic centimeters. The stability of her bladder and the urine flow rate were also measured and had improved. She was still without symptoms a year later.

As is the case with all forms of endometriosis, some researchers maintain that the only cure for urinary tract endo is removal of the uterus, tubes, and ovaries. Sadly, sometimes even radical surgery fails to curb this insidious disease. Several cases are reported in the research literature. Most cases seem to be the result of estrogen replacement therapy activating endo of the urinary tract that was not eradicated at surgery. Endo can also be activated if all ovarian tissue is not removed. One article on the subject states: "Although Langmade and Gantt et al. stated that estrogen replacement usually does not cause reactivation of endometriosis, it is our impression that it is a factor in recurrence. However, when endometriosis recurs during estrogen replacement, it can also be due to incomplete removal of ovarian tissue."[20]

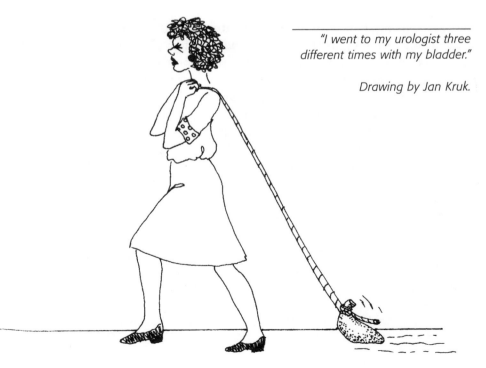

"I went to my urologist three different times with my bladder."

Drawing by Jan Kruk.

However, there is at least one report of a 68-year-old woman who did not take estrogen therapy and still experienced recurrence of endometriosis: "Our case is unusual in that the patient had not received any exogenous estrogens and the hormone study showed low estrogen levels found normally after menopause or castration. The severe inflammatory and granulomatous changes in our patient were thought to be due to previous endometriosis that had degenerated after menopause."[21] (*Exogenous* means coming from outside the body, not made by the body. *Granulomatous* means nodular, masslike tissue.)

They also claim their patient is the oldest patient on record to have bladder endo. This patient was treated with partial cystectomy, which is what the authors recommend for postmenopausal women with bladder endo. The authors conclude, "Vesical endometriosis should be considered as a cause of pyuria [pus in the urine] or a lesion of the bladder, even if the patient is postmenopausal and has received no exogenous estrogen therapy."

Another case of bladder endo in a 64-year-old woman was reported in the journal *Urology* in 1983. This woman had not taken estrogen either; and the same treatment was used—partial cystectomy.[22]

Endometriosis of the Ureters

Treatment is usually more aggressive when endometriosis is obstructing one or both ureters because of the risk of kidney failure. An article in the *British Journal of Urology* warns: "One has to bear in mind that treating ureteric obstruction with hormonal manipulation alone involves the risk of recurrence and loss of renal [kidney] function."[23] The article reported on a 23-year-old with both ureters obstructed.

Where endo involves the ureters, a urologist should be involved in the surgery according to one text. Unfortunately, just as has been the case with bowel endo in the past (and is now fortunately changing), rarely is a urologist trained in endo surgery available or on standby. Hopefully, this will change as pioneers such as Drs. Camran and Farr Nezhat involve urologists in complicated cases.

Drs. Nezhat, in addition to treating bladder endo through laparoscopy, have treated endo of the ureters in this manner. With urologist Dr. Bruce Green, they detailed a case report of a patient with an obstructed ureter due to endometriosis.

The patient was a 36-year-old with a history of long-standing endometriosis and pelvic pain. She had one previous laparoscopy but had declined other treatments since then. The surgeons used the CO_2 laser to excise the three- to four-centimeter section of the ureter involved with endometriosis and reconnected the ends through the scope. The patient left the hospital the following day and 15 months later was still well, without symptoms.[24]

The textbook *Endometriosis* says in most cases of obstruction of the ureters, surgical therapy, and total abdominal hysterectomy are recommended.[25] The textbook *Endometriosis: Contemporary Concepts in Clinical Management* concurs:

> Reversal of ureteral obstruction has been reported with progestogen and danazol therapy, but in several cases there has been recurrence after discontinuance of treatment. Preoperative and postoperative use of medical therapy, either to facilitate surgery or prevent postoperative recurrence, has been attempted, with discouraging results. It is unwise to persist with medical treatment unless early return of normal kidney function is noted by repetitive radiologic [x-ray] evaluation, and long-term follow-up is instituted.[26]

For ureteral obstruction by endometriosis, the blocked portion of the ureters is usually resected, or cut and removed. The ureter is then reimplanted into the bladder.

Sometimes a ureter will not be reimplanted if kidney function is minimal or nonexistent. The *British Journal of Urology* article notes that 25 percent of kidneys with ureteral obstruction because of endo are not functioning at the time of diagnosis.[27] This was the case with several women studied in an article reported in the *American Journal of Obstetrics and Gynecology*. The authors concluded that earlier diagnosis might have prevented this. They report the average time for diagnosis for eight patients in Ottawa, Ontario, hospitals was 24 months. After treatment for endometriosis some patients still had chronic kidney failure; others improved but still had some damage. Endometriosis was not diagnosed before surgery to treat the ureteral destruction in half of these patients.

> The conclusion reached after study of this small but important population is that physicians should have a heightened awareness of this uncommon but serious manifestation of the disease. Earlier diagnosis might be achieved on the basis of a high index of suspicion and careful physical and pelvic examination. The liberal use of intravenous pyelography [IVP] even in cases of minimal endometriosis is urged.[28]

IVP is an x-ray of the kidneys and urinary tract done by injecting a dye into the veins that is concentrated by the kidneys and outlines the kidneys, ureters, and bladder. The dye contains iodine, so if you are allergic to it, you should have an ultrasound instead. The authors also state that when the ovaries are left in, 27 percent of patients need further surgery for urinary tract endo.

Another consequence of ureteral obstruction can be hypertension—high blood pressure. This complication has been reported rarely, but a case was reported in May 1988 in the *Journal of Reproductive Medicine*. The patient had a hysterectomy but kept her ovaries. The endometriosis recurred, and she developed high blood pressure. When the blocked ureter was cut and reimplanted, her blood pressure fell quickly. Again, it is noted that "medical therapy is usually unsuccessful because the obstruction typically results from scarring caused by hormonally unresponsive tissue." The authors, Davis and Schiff, conclude:

> Our case illustrates the importance of a thorough workup for patients with new-onset hypertension, particularly if they are known to have endometriosis. Further, it underscores one possible risk of ovarian conservation at the time of definitive surgery for endometriosis, even in the apparent absence of residual disease.[29]

Practical Applications

Now, how do you assimilate the information about urinary tract endo into something you can practically apply to your life? Sometimes a lot of information can make you feel overwhelmed and confused. In the long run, however, taking time to sift through information should help you learn more about your body and how to improve your health. It is our responsibility to educate ourselves, because many of us have discovered we can't expect health care practitioners to do the job.

Try to see the best doctors you can find in your area. This can be very difficult if you are limited financially or belong to an HMO. If you must work with doctors who are not very knowledgeable, maybe you can get them to read more on endometriosis. If you are financially restricted, teaching hospitals are often more flexible with billing than private physicians. They usually have access to modern equipment and ideas, and you have several doctors working together instead of just one. If you notice any new symptoms, such as urinary frequency or high blood pressure, report them to your doctor immediately.

If you are already being treated for endometriosis and develop urinary symptoms, consider seeking a urologist, but choose cautiously. Association headquarters has heard "horror stories" from a number of members about how urologists have treated them. I also have heard many complaints about insensitive or unknowledgeable urologists from members.

However, in the last 10 years a new medical specialty has emerged that may benefit women with urinary tract endo—urogynecology. The authors of the book *Overcoming Bladder Disorders* describe the new American Urogynecological Society (see "Additional Resources" at the back of the book) as "urologists or gynecologists who have a special interest in and, hopefully, a special sensitivity to women's urological problems." Ideally, the number of female urologists will also increase—currently there are about 100 in the United States.

I went through two urologists before I found one I'm happy with—and I have to drive 3½ hours to see him. The time is worth it. One of the urologists I saw did a cystoscopy on me and said my problems were from stress, even though my bladder had some abnormalities. He gave me one medication to try, but when it failed he said I would have to "live with it." That's when I decided to find another doctor.

I was diagnosed with interstitial cystitis in December 1991. I no longer urinate 60 times a day—the number varies from about 15 to 30 times a day. If I don't drink much fluid, I will go 15 times, but I usually drink *at least* eight glasses of water a day. If I don't drink enough water, I have more pain and burning, and given the choice I'd rather urinate more often. I have had to give up caffeinated beverages and drinks with NutraSweet, since they both irritate my bladder, but I can drink flavored seltzer or soda with sugar. I am in the process of evaluating my diet, trying to determine exactly which foods bother me. So far I know that very spicy foods such as chili peppers will set my bladder off.

I am on several medications for IC right now. One is a narcotic painkiller—I have to be careful I don't become addicted. I never had any relief from anti-inflammatories, and they rile my gastrointestinal tract. I also take a drug for bladder spasms twice a day, and the bladder analgesic Pyridium as needed. They all help me quite a bit. I will be trying a smooth muscle relaxer for my bladder, and if that doesn't work there are other alternatives.

One thing that has helped me considerably is setting my alarm clock for the middle of the night to get up to urinate. Sometimes I am very tired and will not wake up before the pain in my bladder becomes unbearable from the need to urinate. I never hold my urine during the day, because it always causes excruciating pain throughout my entire pelvis. When I set the clock, I go very quickly and am able to fall asleep immediately after I empty my bladder.

When the pain is very bad, I often will try ice packs or a heating pad. When I am trying to fall asleep at night, I have a favorite visualization trick that helps me relax. It may sound strange, but it helps! I simply imagine that I am a large sponge and that the pain, instead of something bad, is merely a neutral force—it is the water the sponge absorbs. Then I imagine the sponge being squeezed, and the pain flows through me and away.

Although I have been diagnosed with IC, I firmly believe that endo was causing some of my bladder problems. Perhaps it still is—it's hard to say when we know so little about the disease. Endo was found on my bladder in February 1991, when I had a laparoscopy with an endo specialist, as well as in a few other spots. I also had ovarian cysts and repeated pelvic infections, plus some mild adhesions, complicating things. The specialist cut the endo off the surface of my bladder. Unfortunately, I continued to have severe pain and fevers, etc., from all my problems. I had tried many medications for endo and had three laparoscopies, so I decided to have a hysterectomy in June 1991. The number of times I was urinating each day immediately dropped by half after the hysterectomy, which is why I believe endo played a part in my problems.

Another helpful exercise is to try thinking of your doctor as a partner, not a superior. Partners work together, complementing each other, while superiors sometimes simply dictate. Your doctor may have some knowledge that you lack and skills you need such as surgical techniques. But *you* are the only one who really knows how your body feels. You are the one that lives in it every day, not your doctor. All too often we allow ourselves to be intimidated by doctors who tell us it's in our heads.

No matter what is causing your bladder symptoms, it can't hurt to try to maintain your overall health by drinking at least eight glasses of water (preferably purified) a day and trying to eat the best diet you can. The water will flush and soothe your bladder no matter what ails it. Also try to get enough sleep, which we know of course is difficult if you're forever running to the bathroom.

Exercise should help you sleep better and keep your spirits up, but don't let anyone tell you how much or what kind is right for you—only you know. Some of us know from experience that overdoing exercise can bring a backlash of pain.

If you are experiencing urinary frequency and voiding small amounts of urine, you can help your doctor if you keep track on paper of what you drink, how much, how many times you urinate, and how much. You can buy a device to put in your toilet to measure your urine in cubic centimeters and ounces. You may have seen one—they are used in hospitals after you have surgery to measure your urine output. They are white plastic, and some people describe them as looking like the shape of a nurse's cap. The part that holds the urine is round, but there is an edge that goes between the toilet seat and bowl to hold it in place. I bought two at a medical supply store—one for the upstairs bathroom and one for the downstairs bathroom. Each one cost only $1.83. If you don't do this and you see a urologist, he or she may ask you to do it anyway.

Last, try to have a sense of humor and be creative. The authors of *Overcoming Bladder Disorders*[30] interviewed a woman who did just that—every week, she took the crossword puzzle to the copy store to have it enlarged and laminated. Then she put it up on the bathroom wall to pass the time enjoyably! I keep good reading material in my bathrooms and have upgraded the scenery with candles, potpourri, etc. I'm amazed at all the reading I get done while I'm in the bathroom.

I sincerely hope that someday soon there will be cures for endo, IC, and many other puzzling diseases that affect women. But until that time I am focusing on trying to achieve balance in my life, which isn't easy. I have to accept some limitations but at the same time not be passive and give up trying to improve my health. If I do too many activities, I get into trouble, but if I don't do enough, I get depressed. Exactly the kind of balance that women with endo struggle to achieve with every other aspect of the disease is what's needed in urinary tract endo. And, as is true for other aspects of the disease, *together* we will learn how to overcome bladder endometriosis.

Notes

1. O. K. Davis and I. Schiff, "Endometriosis with Ureteral Obstruction and Hypertension," *Journal of Reproductive Medicine* 3 no. 5 (May 1988): 470–72.
2. T. J. Williams and J. H. Pratt, "Endometriosis in 1,000 Consecutive Celiotomies: Incidence and Management," *American Journal of Obstetrics and Gynecology* 129 (1977): 245.
3. D. T. O'Connor, "Endometriosis," *Current Reviews in Obstetrics and Gynecology,* A. Singer and J. Jordan, series eds. (Edinburgh/New York: Churchill Livingstone, 1987), 45.
4. M. Vermesh et al., "Vesical Endometriosis Following Bladder Injury," *American Journal of Obstetrics and Gynecology* 153 (December 1985): 894–95.
5. R. Chalker and K. Whitmore, *Overcoming Bladder Disorders* (New York: Harper & Row, 1990).

6. S. M. Markham, "Extrapelvic Endometriosis," *Modern Approaches to Endometriosis,* E. J. Thomas and J. A. Rock, eds. (Dordrecht/Boston/London: Kluwer Academic Publishers, 1991), 151–82.

7. M. Vermesh et al., 894–95.

8. G. W. Mitchell, "Extrapelvic Endometriosis: Urinary Endometriosis," *Endometriosis: Contemporary Concepts in Clinical Management,* Robert S. Schenken, ed. (Philadelphia: Lippincott, 1989), 314–16.

9. G. W. Mitchell, 314–16.

10. K. W. Aldridge, J. R. Burns, and B. Singh, "Vesical Endometriosis: A Review and 2 Case Reports," *Journal of Urology* 134 (September 1985): 539–41.

11. T. L. Ball and M. A. Platt, "Urologic Complications of Endometriosis," *American Journal of Obstetrics and Gynecology* 84, no. 11, part 1 (December 1982): 1516–20.

12. S. Fianu et al., "Surgical Treatment of Post Abortum Endometriosis of the Bladder and Postoperative Bladder Function," *Scandinavian Journal of Urology and Nephrology* 14 (1980): 151–55.

13. M. Vermesh et al., 894–95.

14. W. Arap Neto et al., "Vesical Endometriosis," *Urology* 24, no. 3 (September 1984): 271–74.

15. J. A. Rock and S. M. Markham, "Extrapelvic Endometriosis," *Endometriosis,* E. A. Wilson, ed. (New York: Alan R. Liss, 1987), 185–206.

16. G. W. Mitchell, 314–16.

17. D. W. Laube, G. W. Calderwood, and J. A. Bend, "Endometriosis Causing Ureteral Obstruction," *Obstetrics and Gynecology* 65, no. 3 (March 1985): 69S–71S.

18. S. Fianu et al., 151–55.

19. M. S. Goldstein and M. L. Brodman, "Cystometric Evaluation of Vesical Endometriosis Before and After Hormonal or Surgical Treatment," *Mount Sinai Journal of Medicine* 57, no. 2 (March 1990): 109–11.

20. C. Kane and P. Drouin, "Obstructive Uropathy Associated with Endometriosis," *American Journal of Obstetrics and Gynecology* 151 (January 1985): 207–11.

21. T. Habuci et al., "Endometriosis of Bladder After Menopause," *The Journal of Urology* 145 (February 1991): 361–63.

22. B. Vorstman et al., "Postmenopausal Vesical Endometriosis," *Urology* 22, no. 5 (November 1983): 540–42.

23. T. Esen et al., "Bilateral Ureteric Obstruction Secondary to Endometriosis," *British Journal of Urology* 66 (July 1990): 98–99.

24. C. Nezhat, F. Nezhat, and B. Green, "Laparoscopic Treatment of Obstructed Ureter Due to Endometriosis: Resection by Ureteroureterostomy," *Journal of Urology* 148 (September 1992): 865–68.

25. J. A. Rock and S. M. Markham, 194.

26. G. W. Mitchell, 315.

27. T. Esen et al., 98–99.

28. C. Kane and P. Drouin, 207.

29. O. K. Davis and I. Schiff, 472.

30. R. Chalker and K. Whitmore, *Overcoming Bladder Disorders* (New York: Harper & Row, 1990).

■ ***Andrea Lea Yap*** *lives in Shiprock, New Mexico, on the Navajo Reservation. She's a teacher. Her endometriosis seems to be gone since her hysterectomy/oophorectomy in 1991, but she is battling another chronic illness—interstitial cystitis.*

Conditions That Can Mimic
Urinary Tract Endometriosis

By Andrea Lea Yap

EDITOR'S NOTE: We are grateful to Rebecca Chalker and Kristene Whitmore, M.D., for their enormously helpful book *Overcoming Bladder Disorders* (New York: Harper & Row, 1990). Readers with the bladder conditions described here may want to obtain it based on recommendations of a number of members.

Myriad conditions can mimic urinary tract endometriosis, making diagnosis difficult. These conditions include an overgrowth of the yeast *Candida*, interstitial cystitis, urinary tract infections, urethral syndrome, estrogen deprivation, and even kidney stones.

Kidney stones come in various forms, but most are made of calcium oxalate, a hard salt compound.[1] They can be caused by repeated kidney infections, not drinking enough water, or eating high-oxalate foods such as chocolate, colas, tea, peanuts, and spinach. The symptoms of kidney stones are severe pain that may begin in the lower back and move to the side or groin, nausea, fever, bloody urine, or burning on urination. Middle-aged men are three times more likely to get kidney stones than women of the same age.

A case of endometriosis originally diagnosed as kidney stones was reported in the May 1990 issue of *Prevention* magazine. The woman had low-back pain, nausea, flulike symptoms, and overall body stiffness. However, treatment for the stones did not improve her symptoms. She then realized that her attacks were coming at regular monthly intervals. She had had a hysterectomy years earlier for endo and was taking hormones. The attacks had begun just after her doctor had changed the dosage schedule of her estrogen. When she began taking progesterone daily, the attacks stopped and tests showed her ureter was no longer blocked.

Urinary Tract Infections (UTIs)

In contrast to kidney stones, women are about 30 times more likely to develop UTIs than males until after age 60, when "the score evens out somewhat"[2] according to the authors of *Overcoming Bladder Disorders*.

Urinary tract infection means an infection anywhere in the urinary system—kidneys, ureters, bladder, or urethra. *Cystitis* means infection of the bladder only. Cystitis has classic symptoms, according to Chalker and Whitmore: burning or stinging during urination, urgent need to urinate, frequent urination, voiding small amounts of urine, and frequent waking at night to urinate. One reason women seem to be more susceptible to UTIs may be "partly due to the fact that the urine of women has a higher, or less acidic, pH reading. In fact, one study found that the urinary pH of infection-prone women was even more alkaline than that of women who did not have infections." (For more on the pH of urine and the vagina, see the discussion under "Bladder Problems Due to *Candida Albicans*" later in this article.)

Some doctors will prescribe antibiotics over the phone for a woman even if no bacteria is found in a urine culture. However, Chalker and Whitmore say "a urinalysis (or at least a urine dipstick test at home) should always be done to make sure that bacteria are present." You can test your own urine with chemically treated dipsticks. They do not test for bacteria but show the presence of white blood cells and nitrites. The white blood cells indicate the body is fighting infection, and nitrites are by-products of bacterial attack. You can obtain dipsticks in most pharmacies or order them by mail.

One problem with taking antibiotics is they can cause overgrowth of the yeast *Candida albicans*. Women with *Candida* problems often complain of urgent or frequent urination. If you take antibiotics only when you have a proven infection, it should help, but many women with endo are so susceptible to *Candida* that even limited antibiotic use causes trouble. For more information on *Candida*-related problems in women with endo, see the section in this article and Chapter 11 in the association's first book, *Overcoming Endometriosis*.

Susan, an association member from Missouri, has had numerous UTIs. She was diagnosed with bladder endo at her last surgery. To make matters even more complex, one time last year a doctor told her her bladder flare-up was caused by yeast: "The last time my bladder was acting up and there was no sign of infection, a doctor told me to go buy something over-the-counter for yeast infection. He hadn't even seen me. I didn't do it, and eventually the problem went away by itself. I tried to get some of those strips that they use to check urine so I could test it myself and not have to run to the doctor's office unless I was sure I had a UTI. The doctor acted like that was a silly idea. She said, 'You'll know if you have an infection.'" Before the endo was removed from her bladder, Susan didn't get UTIs. "I never had any urinary tract infections before I had bladder surgery. I keep wondering if there is any connection," she wrote in another letter.

Chalker and Whitmore also recommend you start looking for the cause of your cystitis if you have more than three episodes annually. For example, diaphragm use has been connected to cystitis, as has sexual intercourse. Nuns have a very low incidence of cystitis according to the authors of *Overcoming Bladder Disorders*. You can help prevent infections by drinking a large amount of liquid, especially water. Do not hold your urine.

Many women also swear by drinking cranberry juice to help the bladder, even though theoretically you'd have to drink huge amounts to reap any benefit. Drinking large amounts of the juice *will* flush the bladder, possibly getting rid of bacteria. Cranberry juice breaks down in the body into hippuric acid, which has antibacterial properties. Nitrofurantoin, a drug often used for UTIs, is made more effective by the acidity of the juice. However, cranberry juice hinders the function of the antibiotic erythromycin.

Other preventive methods include avoiding or only moderately consuming bladder irritants such as alcohol and caffeinated beverages. You can avoid vigorous sexual activity that puts direct pressure on the urethra; wear loose clothing and cotton underwear; wipe from front to back; and try to reduce stress. Often it is recommended that you try increasing the amount of lactobacillus in your vagina. "Lactobacillus is a 'friendly' bacteria that lives in both the bowel and the vagina," according to *Overcoming Bladder Disorders*. "Its presence appears to inhibit the growth of yeast and to interfere with the proliferation of *E. coli* (a common bowel bacteria) as well as with its adherence to the bladder wall." The authors say the method of administering lactobacillus is not important. You can douche with yogurt containing live lactobacillus acidophilus; use a plastic speculum to pour an ounce in and hold it for three to four minutes; or insert a few acidophilus gelatin capsules into the vagina. The best way to get a live culture is the liquid or crystal forms in the refrigerator at health food stores.

Although it is often recommended that women with vaginal yeast infections increase the lactobacillus in their vagina, one authority on the subject, Marjorie Crandall, Ph.D., author of the booklet *How to Prevent Yeast Infections*, states that you should *not* insert yogurt or lactobacillus into the vagina. She states that these products contain live bacteria and can cause a vaginal infection due to bacteria. Perhaps the best way to take in lactobacillus is through *eating* good-quality yogurt or taking capsules orally with lactobacillus.

If you do get an infection, several antibiotics are used to treat bladder infections. Some women find they do better with large single doses taken just after sex to nip bacteria in the bud. Others find a short course for three days or so works just as well as a 10- to 14-day course.

It might be worthwhile to have your sexual partner(s) treated as well. Chalker and Whitmore mention this in their discussion of urethritis—infection of the urethra: "Because the organisms that cause urethritis are almost always sexually transmitted, diagnosing and treating your sexual partners at the same time is another extremely important measure. . . . REMEMBER: Using condoms in *all* non-monogamous situations could prevent most cases of urethritis."

Interstitial Cystitis (IC)

IC is a chronic inflammation of the bladder wall in the absence of bacteria. The cause of IC is unknown, and there is no cure. According to Chalker and Whitmore, the most common symptoms of IC are: frequency of urination; urgency of urination; waking at night to urinate; pain in the bladder, urethra, or vagina; pain relieved by voiding; painful intercourse; difficulty emptying the bladder; and difficulty starting the flow.

The association has heard from some members who have been diagnosed with IC. The disease has another common denominator with endometriosis: it is difficult to diagnose. Chalker and Whitmore discovered in their research that IC sufferers see an average of two to five doctors over a period of more than four years before obtaining a correct diagnosis. Diagnosis is usually made by looking inside the bladder with a cystoscope. Cystoscopy usually reveals tiny pinpoint hemorrhages in the bladder—the bladder cracks or bleeds when it is filled with water during the procedure. Many IC patients also have decreased bladder capacity, and some have actual ulcers in the bladder.

If a woman has urinary symptoms but no other complaints, a cystoscopy will probably be done. The drawback of this procedure is that it views only the *inside* of the bladder. The urologist is unable to see the outside of the bladder, the ureters, and the pelvic organs. So if a woman has endo on the outside of the bladder, it will likely go undetected. Or if she has an endometrioma (cyst) on her ovary that is pressing on the bladder, it will not be seen at cystoscopy.

Laparoscopy, on the other hand, does not offer a view of the inside of the bladder. It also does not allow for bladder biopsy, which is often done to help diagnose IC and bladder cancer.

If a woman has both gynecologic and urinary symptoms, the two procedures can be done one after the other while the patient is under general anesthesia. A cystoscopy can be done in the doctor's office under local anesthesia, but many urologists prefer to use general anesthesia because the procedure can be painful since the bladder is overdistended with water to check its capacity. (The pinpoint hemorrhages characteristic of IC will often not be noticeable in the office procedure.) A cystoscopy does not require an incision, but there is a risk of infection. The length of time for a cystoscopy varies from a few minutes to about half an hour. Both of mine were about half an hour.

While a cystoscopy under local anesthesia is more painful, it has a couple of advantages. For example, my doctor was able to learn more about my case than possible with general anesthesia. My first cystoscopy was done under general and was easier than my laparoscopies were. My doctor at the time did see some pinpoint hemorrhages, but he told me he decided it was not IC because my capacity was normal. He had filled my bladder with 600 cubic centimeters of water easily, he said. When I changed urologists, my new doctor said that under local anesthesia I would be able to tell him when I first felt the urge to urinate and when it became unbearable. Obviously, when you're asleep you can't do that. So I agreed to the procedure, because after measuring my urine for several weeks I *knew* I couldn't stand 600 cubic centimeters while I was awake. I was right. After the cystoscopy my doctor said that I first needed to urinate at 150 cubic centimeters and was in agony at around 350 cubic centimeters. Based on that and the hemorrhages, he diagnosed IC.

In their research Chalker and Whitmore uncovered a long list of 30 familiar labels IC patients have been stuck with. The list of diagnoses includes endometriosis, adhesions from surgery, yeast overgrowth, and "suffering from not having a baby." In fact the journal *Urology* in October 1988 reported a case of bladder endometriosis that had been mistaken for IC. The researchers concluded:

> The symptoms of bladder endometriosis can be similar to those of interstitial cystitis. Some premenopausal patients with interstitial cystitis experience worsening of their symptoms peri-menstrually [around the time of menstruation]. This is similar to the cyclical symptomatology present in patients with bladder muscle endometriosis. . . . The possibility of bladder endometriosis should be considered in patients with symptoms of interstitial cystitis because "menstrual dysuria" [difficult urination menstrually] occurs in both conditions. Endometriosis is more likely to be present in patients who have had prior pelvic or gynecologic surgery. Bimanual examination and cystoscopy should be scheduled during or near a menstrual period to allow for the best chance of diagnosis.[3]

Another fascinating similarity is the theory that IC, like endo, is possibly the result of some immune system abnormality. Chalker and Whitmore explain:

> Although it is a singular disease in many respects, interstitial cystitis has some striking similarities with certain other diseases in which inflammatory processes predominate: lupus erythematosus, rheumatoid arthritis, asthma, irritable bowel syndrome, allergic rhinitis, and polyarteritis (inflammation of the smaller arteries). While many IC patients have no other major diseases, it is not uncommon for people with IC to have a constellation of these conditions.

In addition to the autoimmune disorder theory, the authors list nine other theories on the cause of IC, "but so far there is little evidence to support any of them." They are a history of UTIs; a bacteria, virus, or fungus; antibiotics; a deficiency in the bladder lining; abnormal metabolism of serotonin and/or tryptophan; toxic substances in the urine; pelvic surgery; hormonal factors; and abnormal number of mast cells, commonly found in connective tissues, which release histamine. Histamine is a substance released during allergic reactions.

If you have IC, help is available from the Interstitial Cystitis Association. The group describes itself as "a not-for-profit health organization working to find a cure for interstitial cystitis." (See "Additional Resources.")

Bladder Problems Due to *Candida Albicans*

Candida is present in all humans, especially in the intestines and vagina. Normally the yeast is kept in check by the immune system and various "good" bacteria that also live within us. However, when factors conspire to change the pH to one more favorable to yeast, *Candida* grows rapidly. The pH scale measures the acidity on a scale of 1 to 14. One is extremely acidic, 7 is neutral, and 14 is extremely alkaline. According to *Womancare* by Lynda Madaras and Jane Patterson, M.D.,[4] the average pH of the vagina is 4.5 to 5.0. "Monilia [*Candida*], the organisms responsible for yeast infections, prefer a pH of about 5.4," the authors state. The pH of the vagina can be changed unfavorably by antibiotics, excessive douching, and hormonal fluctuations.

The normal pH of urine is about 5, according to *Overcoming Bladder Disorders*. The urine pH can fluctuate as well, depending on your diet. Some foods that are acidic are broken down into alkaline substances and vice versa. Orange juice, for example, appears in the urine as alkaline, the book says. "There doesn't seem to be a rule about what will come out acid and what will come out alkaline." You can test your own urine with litmus paper or nitrazine paper, available in most pharmacies.

In their book *The Yeast Syndrome*, John Parks Trowbridge, M.D., and Morton Walker, D.P.M., state: "Vaginitis—inflammation of the vagina—often manifests itself with irritation, increased vaginal discharge and pain on passing urine (cystitis symptoms)."[5] The authors also give case examples of women who had numerous health problems, including urinary tract symptoms due to *Candida albicans*. They all resolved their urinary problems when they undertook an antiyeast diet and medication.

At least three of the women who answered my request for contact from others with bladder problems highly recommended an antiyeast diet, as well as taking acidophilus supplements. *Lactobacillus acidophilus* is a "good" bacteria that helps to keep *Candida* in check.

Wanda, an association member from Alabama, wrote about her problem with candidiasis—which is both an infection/overgrowth of *Candida* and an allergy to it. When her bladder problems recurred after surgery, Wanda decided to reread the chapters on yeast in the EA's first book, *Overcoming Endometriosis*. As a result Wanda "began to follow the recommendations in the article, especially the one about taking acidophilus tablets to combat excess yeast in the body, and taking B vitamins. . . . I had cut out drinking anything but water and cranberry juice and had limited the amount of spicy food I ate. But nothing helped until I began taking the acidophilus and the B vitamins."

It's also very helpful to see a physician who can test for *Candida* sensitivities as well as other sensitivities, including food allergies, and help you with all the related problems. The Candida and Dysbiosis Information Foundation, listed in "Additional Resources" at the back of this book, can help you find a knowledgeable practitioner.

Patti, an EA member from Pennsylvania, experienced a significant improvement in her bladder symptoms when she implemented an antiyeast diet. In a letter to me she described her symptoms and her efforts to alleviate them: "I have had great bladder problems, including bladder pain, frequent urination, and bladder pressure. For a long time (before endo was diagnosed) I was repeatedly treated for urinary tract infections. The bladder problems were secondary only to the pelvic pain as far as my needing to get treatment for endometriosis. I can't give you any ideas as far as medical treatment that has been effective for relief—I can't even get adequate medical treatment for the more familiar symptoms of endo. Something I have done on my own is to do extensive reading (just to survive). I have found that I do appear to have many yeast-related problems. In working with the yeast, I have had *dramatic* relief of my bladder problems. I also have started to really watch my fluid intake to assure I drink at least eight glasses of water daily. I have read several books on yeast-related problems and, through trial and error, have found many things to help me. The yeast diet has helped me. I also have learned that the chronic vaginal irritation I have is also yeast-related, so I constantly battle it with home remedies. I also have found an allergist who works with yeast problems and have started therapy."

The last time I heard from Patti, almost a year ago, she was doing pretty well. She was trying to get into aerobics again since it had helped her in the past. The ironic thing about Patti's inability to get "adequate" medical care is that she herself is a nurse!

Urethral Syndrome

If your symptoms include problems with the urethra, you may be told you have "urethral syndrome." This poorly defined label is applied only to women. The symptoms include prickly, tingling, or burning sensations around the urethra and/or vulva and occasional episodes of urinary frequency, urgency, and dysuria. According to Chalker and Whitmore, this term is often used when a woman's symptoms are present but are not specific enough to be called interstitial cystitis. The only way to be sure is to have a cystoscopy. "The condition is very ill-defined, and since it is neither life-threatening nor very dramatic, it has not been of much interest to researchers. What causes this condition, and which treatments are appropriate for it, constitute one of the most obscure controversies in urology."

Urethral syndrome sufferers, like IC sufferers, are often told they have other problems, according to *Overcoming Bladder Disorders*: "Many doctors are baffled by these symptoms and may not be much help to you. If you are lucky, they will tell you that they don't know what is causing your problem and treat it empirically, that is, with basically anything that experience tells them might work. . . ." So even if you are told you have the syndrome, your doctor might not know what to do, and he or she will not have a cure for the syndrome, since there is no cure.

It is estimated that up to three million women have symptoms that would be classified as urethral syndrome. Information on the condition is sketchy at best, and diagnosis is not precise. The syndrome is diagnosed by excluding other conditions such as UTIs. Because the urethral syndrome is enshrouded in vagueness, it seems likely that some women who actually have endo or other problems are told they have urethral syndrome.

Like the proposed possible causes of endo and IC, the proposed possible causes of urethral syndrome are intriguing. They include urinary tract infections; dysfunction of the urethral nerves; pelvic surgery, especially hysterectomy; estrogen deficiency; allergies; chronic inflammation due to infection, trauma, autoimmune reactions, or other causes; and stress. Infections include the sexually transmitted virus chlamydia and other organisms.

Several EA members have been told they have urethras that are "too small," possibly a euphemism for the urethral syndrome. *Overcoming Bladder Disorders* mentions this: "Many women are simply told . . . they have a small bladder or a small, damaged or fibrotic urethra. In many cases, the functional capacity of the bladder may be diminished, but unless the bladder is distended under anesthesia, it is not possible to tell what its *true* capacity is. And when a urethra is 'too small' has yet to be defined. It may be that swelling from inflammation causes a diminished urinary flow and prevents the bladder from emptying completely—making the urethra *seem* smaller. Or it may be that in response to irritation or inflammation, urinary frequency develops, causing the bladder's *functional capacity* to decrease—so you feel as if you need to urinate more frequently."

Some association members with bladder or urethral symptoms have had their urethras dilated with graduated metal rods. Janet from Oklahoma had this done and briefly mentioned her bad experience in a letter to the EA: "I was sent to another gynecologist . . . he led me to believe I had pelvic inflammatory disease and sent me home for four more weeks with antibiotics—also sent me to a urologist for my bladder spasms. The urologist proceeded to stretch my urethra tube, which was very painful and caused me to have a mechanically induced bladder infection, and sent me home with more antispasm medicine and antibiotics."

According to *Overcoming Bladder Disorders*, "This practice is now generally frowned upon, but it has been shown to be helpful in some cases. Occasional dilations, or two or three at spaced intervals, will probably not harm the urethra, but over-use of dilation, referred to by some urologists as 'the rape of the urethra,' may cause scarring or even incontinence."

The authors go on to say that some urologists also do a meatotomy, cutting the urethral opening to enlarge it, or a urethrotomy, a lengthwise cut in the urethra, to enlarge it permanently. "These procedures are considered very dangerous by most urologists and are strongly discouraged. At present, no studies have been done to show that dilation, meatotomy, or urethrotomy has any medical value," say Chalker and Whitmore.

The speculation that the urethral syndrome is the product of inflammation is fascinating. If so, what is causing the inflammation? Some fingers are pointing at prostaglandins. Prostaglandins are naturally occurring hormonelike substances that are thought to affect many functions, including lowering blood pressure and controlling inflammation. In the study mentioned previously about a case of bladder endo masquerading as IC, the authors speculate "the symptoms in both conditions may be attributable to prostaglandin release."[6]

More questions arise when one considers our limited knowledge of endometriosis—and that some women with endo receive some pain relief from anti-inflammatory drugs that suppress some prostaglandins. Also, in the textbook *Endometriosis*, authors Wild and Wilson state that prostaglandins may sensitize nerve endings to pain stimuli. For more information on these substances, see Chapter 16 in the EA's first book, *Overcoming Endometriosis*.

Estrogen Deficiency and Bladder Symptoms

One cause of urinary tract symptoms that *is* well documented is estrogen deficiency. Because women with endometriosis often take measures to decrease estrogen levels, they are obviously at risk of developing this problem. EA member Rosa experienced this. She wrote: "I went on Lupron a couple months prior to my videolaseroscopy. Within a short period of time I experienced a burning sensation in the bladder area. About a month after the surgery I was losing bladder control and the bladder pain was so great I collapsed at work. I saw a urologist on an emergency basis. He found that I had urethral stenosis, which he thought was caused by the lack of estrogen from the Lupron."

In her book *Hysterectomy: Before and After*, Winnifred Cutler discusses the role estrogen plays in urinary tract health: "The sex hormones play a critical role in maintaining the structural integrity of various parts of the urinary system. The lower urinary tract and the vagina are composed of very similar tissue; both depend on estrogen to maintain their full health. Estrogen depletion produces atrophy [shrinking in size and function] and when atrophy occurs, incontinence follows. Particularly sensitive to estrogen are mucous membranes, the connective tissue, the blood vessels, and the muscles of the urethra. If you are estrogen-deficient, these tissues deteriorate, and estrogen is needed to restore them."[7]

Danforth's *Obstetrics and Gynecology* explains that estrogen and progesterone receptors are present in the lower urogenital tract. These receptors do not decrease in number after menopause: "In postmenopausal women, it is clear that estrogen deficiency is a cause of irritative voiding symptoms. Many women become increasingly symptomatic as their estrogen levels decrease during the peri-menopausal years. Urgency often is associated with urge incontinence. Endoscopically, an estrogen-deficient urethra appears pale and somewhat friable. The trigone may share that appearance. It is well-documented that estrogen replacement therapy may have a beneficial effect on the female lower urinary tract."

Estrogen replacement therapy is very effective in treating urinary problems due to estrogen deficiency. But when a woman is forced to forgo her estrogen or doesn't want to take estrogen, medications that may help the symptoms are available: drugs that soothe the inside of the bladder, such as Pyridium; drugs that relax the bladder muscle and stop spasms, such as Ditropan and Levsinex; antidepressants such as Doxepin and Elavil; anti-inflammatories, antihistamines, etc. These drugs are also commonly prescribed for IC.

Remember that all medications have side effects—you can research them in the *Physicians' Desk Reference* and ask your pharmacist for the informational package insert. You can also try drinking lots of water and avoiding bladder irritants such as caffeine and alcohol or just using them in moderation. Experimenting with hot and cold compresses on your lower abdomen over the bladder area also may be useful.

Practical Applications

The more you know about your own body and about what can go wrong with it, the better you will be able to help yourself. Knowledge is power! Keep a journal tracking your symptoms—just a short description each day or month about how you feel in what part of your cycle. This helps me be more objective about whether I'm actually improving, maintaining the status quo, or worsening.

Talk to other association members who have had bladder problems and join the Bladder Correspondence Network—it's free with your membership in the EA. You are not alone! Sometimes we become embarrassed to discuss subjects such as urinary difficulties. Sometimes you might feel embarrassed when you have to run to the bathroom in the middle of something important such as a business meeting, but perhaps knowing many other women go through this will make it easier.

Notes
1. Krames Communications, "Understanding Kidney Stones" (1988), 5.
2. R. Chalker and K. Whitmore, *Overcoming Bladder Disorders* (New York: Harper & Row, 1990).
3. S. I. Sircus, G. R. Sant, and A. A. Ucci, Jr., "Bladder Detrusor Endometriosis Mimicking Interstitial Cystitis," *Urology* 32, no. 4 (October 1988): 342.
4. L. Madaras and J. Patterson, *Womancare* (New York: Avon, 1981): 272–75.
5. J. P. Trowbridge and M. Walker, *The Yeast Syndrome* (Toronto: Bantam Books, 1986).
6. S. I. Sircus et al., 342.
7. W. Cutler, *Hysterectomy: Before and After* (New York: Harper & Row, 1988), 273–74.

6

༺ ༻

Infertility and Endometriosis

By Cathy Corman

"*I need advice and help desperately! All I ever dreamed about was one day to get married and have children, and now I feel like a hysterectomy, which also doesn't guarantee an end to this, is going to be the next step. . . . I have been dating the same man for the past three years, but he doesn't feel ready for marriage or a family at this time and tells me how guilty he feels over this, knowing my chance for children is fast running out.*"

Bobi, Virginia

"*I tried Clomid for six months and took a break since my husband says it makes me crabby. We put our house up for sale and got involved with building a new one, and wouldn't you know I got pregnant. (God has a sense of humor.)*"

Susan, Wisconsin

"*I had laser surgery and was able to conceive soon after. Unfortunately, I miscarried that pregnancy and two subsequent pregnancies.*"

Janet, West Virginia

"*I am a 36-year-old African-American female, and I know you have made an effort to reach endo sufferers in my community. I really appreciate your acknowledgment that women like me exist. So many times I feel that people don't believe or expect black women to have fertility problems. How wrong they are, and how alone we feel. When I attended an [infertility] support group meeting, I was the only nonwhite woman. I felt like I didn't belong and never returned.*

"*The people I know personally who have endometriosis include two other black women, one Cuban-American, one Mexican-American, and two Caucasian women, including my sister-in-law. People don't realize that endometriosis sufferers come in all shades. Black people haven't been excluded from experiencing all other major illness. Why would we be excluded from this one? We should be so lucky!"*

Tawnya, Los Angeles

"I am 20 years old. . . . I was finally diagnosed with endometriosis six months ago. . . . I got married a year ago and have not been able to have sexual intercourse since the first month of my marriage. So, needless to say, I'm getting very frustrated! I have such severe pain starting at the opening of my vagina, and I just can't stand it. It feels raw. Everything feels so swollen on the inside that there is no room. I use K-Y Jelly and lubricated condoms to try to help the rawness, but I still can't do it.

"My doctor doesn't seem to be concerned about my not being able to have intercourse. He says, 'We'll take care of that when it comes time to get you pregnant.'"

Melissa, Alabama

"I am fortunate enough to have had one child, but I was unable to have a second despite years of effort and medical treatment."

Brenda, Virginia

"I don't want to pass this nightmare life on to a daughter. I would rather adopt. . . ."

Sheryl, Ontario

"At age 23 my husband and I decided to have a baby. A few months went by, and nothing happened. A few more months. Nothing. The anxiety increased. I began keeping temperature charts and saw a fertility specialist. We went through several tests. . . . We tried fertility drugs and husband insemination. Nothing. Our lives were disrupted by regimented sex and the monthly devastation of not being pregnant. Our dreams of a family were shattered. When we could no longer stand the disappointment, after three and a half years of waiting for a family and much thought and prayer, we applied for a foreign adoption. In a few short months we became the parents of a nine-month-old who has delighted us in every way since."

Sandra, Illinois

"When my son was born in 1992, I sat and looked at this wonderful little person. And I realized that his birth was really due to all the information and support I had received from the association group in Vancouver and what a difference that support group had made to my life. So I decided to organize a support group here. I thought, Maybe the information and support will change these women's lives as much as it's changed mine."

Nanci, Yukon

"Although I have no children, which I always hoped for, I now find ways to be close to children through local activities and help economically disadvantaged children."

Caroline, Colorado

And she was bitterness of soul, and prayed unto the Lord, and wept sore.
I Samuel, The Holy Bible, King James Version

Because we menstruate, we women are—at least in theory—able to bear children. But for those of us with endometriosis, our menstrual cycles may actually prevent us from getting pregnant. An awful irony, to be sure. Who among us has not felt, like biblical Hannah, a bitterness of the soul so overwhelming as to bring us to our knees in grief? Although this chapter focuses on medical and surgical approaches to endometriosis-related infertility, let no one who reads it be fooled into thinking that the inability to conceive has solely physical consequences. It is important from the outset to acknowledge the emotional ramifications of this disease. We must take care of our bodies. We must take care of our souls as well.

Since endometriosis affects primarily the reproductive organs, it isn't surprising that more than one in three of us with the disease is infertile. Whether or not you are ready to start a family when you are diagnosed with endometriosis, you will want to make sure that treatments at least preserve, if not enhance, whatever chances you have to get pregnant and give birth if having children is a life goal for you. Unfortunately, there are no clear steps to take to guarantee this.

If your goal is to have babies, you may well wonder why you would want to accept the standard medical treatments for endometriosis, which are themselves contraceptive. And since recent research indicates that thorough surgical removal of endometriosis, the most effective surgical treatment for pain, may actually inhibit fertility (see clarification later in this article), you may wonder whether to worry about immediate physical well-being or what seems an abstract desire to get pregnant in the future. In addition, since the powerful drugs used to increase your odds of conception will reliably exacerbate your endometriosis and may even be linked to cancer, you will probably wonder if these drugs are appropriate no matter how much you want to experience pregnancy and childbirth.

Given all of these apparent conflicts, how do you begin to make informed choices? Reviewing recent medical literature, it is possible to extrapolate a few guiding principles, many of which may help you make decisions.

First, it is important to clarify who, specifically, is considered infertile and when, exactly, you might want to seek treatment. As with most advice concerning endometriosis, no hard-and-fast rules exist. Doctors usually deem a couple infertile if, after a year of unprotected sexual intercourse, no pregnancy occurs or no pregnancy is carried to term. Resolve, a U.S. national support group devoted to helping infertile couples, counsels women to seek help from specialists sooner than a year if they fall into any of the following categories: if they know they have endometriosis, if they have irregular menstrual cycles, if their mother took DES, or if they are over the age of 35.

If you see a specialist, typically you will go through a routine infertility work-up that relies on a variety of tests, possibly including blood tests to determine if hormone levels are normal, a complete semen analysis, a postcoital examination, a hysterosalpingogram, endometrial biopsy, and laparoscopy. Even when you know you have endometriosis, these tests can be extremely important in determining your best course of treatment.

Assuming you have been diagnosed with endometriosis, you will probably want to make decisions about fertility based on the severity of your disease. Research indicates that if you have mild to moderate endometriosis your best course of action may be "expectant management" or careful watching without any further drug or surgical treatment. Since the medications used to control the disease will interrupt ovulation and even menstruation, infertility specialists sometimes suggest that it may be wisest to leave well enough alone when damage to reproductive organs is minimal. All treatment options should include a careful consideration of quality-of-life issues: living in pain, even when you want to preserve potential fertility, is never an easy choice, even when you believe you are doing it "for a good reason."

As for surgery, *any* kind of abdominal procedure carries the risk of creating new adhesions. If you can tolerate oral contraceptives, these may offer a relatively noninvasive way to suppress further endometrial growth and may allow you to put off decisions regarding pregnancy. If, however, you have already been trying to conceive without success, you may want to think about assisted reproductive technologies, which will be addressed later.

How do you know how easy or hard it will be to get pregnant? Statistics aren't very helpful. For instance, if you have been diagnosed with stage IV endometriosis and also have a "male factor" (your partner has a low sperm count or low sperm motility), you have a 7 percent chance of conceiving. If, however, you have stage I endometriosis and no male factor, your odds of conceiving may be as good as 82 percent. The current system used to classify disease stages is somewhat unreliable, making it difficult to assess exactly where in this huge spread to place yourself. Perhaps it is most helpful to rely on the generalization that the more severe your disease (correlated to the extent of endometrial growth, not pain), the more difficult it will likely be to get pregnant. Consequently, aggressive treatments are more appropriate for severe endometriosis than for mild to moderate disease.

Regardless of the stage of your disease, you will always want to recognize that timing is an important factor in outcome. Whether or not endometriosis is a progressive disease is a source of debate among infertility specialists and research scientists. Will you have *more* endometriosis over time from menstrual blood flowing out of your fallopian tubes into your pelvis? Will the disease that you already have just get worse over time, causing more scarring and swelling? Or will whatever amount of disease you have stay put but look different as you age? In any case, if left alone without surgical intervention or medical suppression, the disease may make you *feel* worse over time. If—and only if—it is a good time in your life to have children, conventional wisdom dictates that you not postpone pregnancy. The longer you wait, the more time the disease may have to worsen. The worse the disease gets, the less chance you may have to get pregnant.

Timing is also important in deciding how soon after treatment to try to get pregnant. Many physicians speak of a "window of opportunity" after surgery that lasts about six to nine months. At the beginning of this window the disease is probably fairly quiet, giving you your best shot at getting pregnant. Doctors hypothesize that after six months of unregulated menstruation, especially if endometriosis is still present in the pelvis, it will have caused enough scarring, encysting, and adhering to interfere once again with attempts to conceive.

Doctors don't completely understand why pregnancy success rates are significantly higher during this period. They speculate that putting the disease into remission most likely gives the pelvis and reproductive organs a breather from the bleeding and scarring that interfere with normal ovulation and embryo implantation.

Doctors and researchers continue to argue whether there may be a relationship between endometriosis and miscarriage. One study with a control group found no increased risk of miscarriage in women with endometriosis. Some practitioners are inclined to believe that surgery and medication may improve chances of carrying a pregnancy to term, but no hard data exists to support such belief. More studies are needed to explore the role of endometriosis in miscarriage.

One promising study exploring this link demonstrated significant aberrations in the endometrium in some women with endometriosis that may account for an inability to implant an embryo or carry a fetus to term. A recent study at the University of North Carolina found that infertile women with mild to moderate endometriosis were often missing a biochemical cell adhesion marker responsible for effective embryo implantation in the uterus. If tissue obtained by endometrial biopsy lacks the beta-3 subunit of the vitronectin receptor integrin, or beta-3, a woman is extremely likely to have mild to moderate endometriosis and also to have trouble getting pregnant. Egg production, egg release, and fallopian tubes may be normal but if the body does not produce beta-3 six or seven days after ovulation a woman probably cannot get pregnant. Fortunately, women lacking beta-3 can be given supplemental beta-3, greatly increasing their chances of pregnancy. Just as important, the test may tell women ahead of time not to resort to advanced reproductive technologies without first seeking treatment for beta-3 deficiency. At the time of publication, this test is only being performed experimentally. With FDA approval, which may take two to three years, it may become widely available.

Which treatment holds the best promise for women with moderate to severe endometriosis who want to bear children? None of the medications currently available to treat endometriosis actually enhances fertility. Danazol, Lupron, Synarel, Zoladex, and Provera are only effective in shrinking active disease. They don't promote ovulation, nor do they correct disease-related anatomical abnormalities. By depriving the body of estrogen, these medications essentially dry up endometriosis, which is estrogen-dependent. When treatment stops and the body again produces estrogen, endometriosis is reactivated.

With what we know about the window of opportunity, however, it is important to remember that *whatever* your odds with any treatment, they will be best immediately after termination of treatment. The only effective medical (as opposed to surgical) treatment for endometriosis you'll probably want to avoid if fertility is an immediate concern is long-term Depo-Provera therapy. This drug can hang around in the body so long that it may significantly delay the resumption of ovulation. This, in and of itself, could confound attempts to get pregnant.

As for surgery, some recent research indicates that conservative laparoscopic surgery (so called because its aim is to conserve or preserve potential fertility rather than to wipe out all disease) may help women get pregnant more than other kinds of treatment. (One infertility specialist, Dr. Charles Koh, Milwaukee, points out that pregnancy rates are better after surgery for women with endometriosis than they are with in vitro fertilization.) The benefits probably last for only six months to a year after an initial procedure, especially if some endometriosis is left in the pelvis. Very aggressive surgery to remove, for example, endometriosis deep in the cul-de-sac or in the bowel is thought perhaps to damage fertility potential because of the potential for adhesions. *Any* kind of scarring (whether from endometriosis, from infection such as from pelvic inflammatory disease, or from surgery) can impair fertility since it can damage fallopian tubes and ovaries.

During conservative surgery surgeons can correct mechanical and structural abnormalities, remove endometriosis from the ovaries and reposition them and the fallopian tubes if necessary, and drain peritoneal fluid (which may temporarily counteract immune system irregularities that may be related to endometriosis-associated infertility). These procedures together may help create a more hospitable environment in which to incubate an embryo. Most significant, they may also provide the chief benefits to fertility afforded by any kind of pelvic surgery without greatly increasing the odds of scar tissue formation.

Some infertility specialists suggest deep implants and bowel adhesions be left for the time being unless they present a threat to life or are causing serious problems, agreeing that if you are not pregnant within a reasonable amount of time—possibly six months— you will need to think about more surgery. Other gynecological surgeons argue just the opposite, insisting that complete removal of endometriosis is the very best way to boost fertility. Without this complete removal, you will not be relieved of your pain. Trying to weigh physical misery against the possibility of pregnancy, you may feel that you have been firmly wedged between the proverbial rock and a hard place. Remember: just because you *can* tolerate intense pain, doesn't mean that you *should*.

Surgeons also debate the relative merits of a variety of techniques they use to remove endometrial implants. Studies indicate that all commonly used techniques—laser, excision, and electrosurgery—can effectively remove endometriosis in the hands of a *skilled* surgeon. (See the surgery articles in Chapter 2 for more information.)

Given that your best odds to conceive will be in the few months after therapy, how do you make the most of this time? Again, severity of disease may be the best indicator when determining a plan of action.

If you have mild disease, are not yet 35 years old, and have no other complicating factors, you probably have more time to play with when trying to get pregnant. You therefore may choose to rely on relatively low-tech methods to maximize the possibility of conception. These include basal body temperature thermometers and ovulation prediction kits. What you will try to do is figure out when you are most likely to ovulate, timing intercourse so that it coincides with the maturation and release of an egg from an ovary.

As stated earlier in this chapter, it is difficult to know when to consider yourself infertile, especially when many variables come into play. But if you fall into any of the categories putting you at a disadvantage for getting pregnant, you may want to proceed more quickly to more invasive techniques. Intrauterine insemination, or IUI, is usually considered the least invasive of all artificial methods used to increase odds of conception. To undergo IUI, you would chart egg production and release, probably by relying on an ovulation prediction kit. At the appointed time a physician would inject specially treated, concentrated sperm from your partner or a donor into your uterus. Nature is allowed to take its own course from there, as it would after intercourse. IUI will not, in and of itself, make endometriosis worse; no step in the procedure would encourage more endometrial growth or scarring, and no drugs that might exacerbate the disease are necessary.

If you have severe endometriosis, and especially if you already have documented infertility, these noninvasive techniques will not be included on your list of preferred treatments. Current medical opinion would have you run, not walk, to more aggressive procedures. You will want to think carefully about whether you want to lace up your jogging shoes and enter the race.

Return to our by-now-oft-cited principles: time and timing are of the essence. Instead of using assisted reproductive techniques as treatments of last resort, infertility specialists argue, it makes more sense to try them as soon as you've completed endometriosis treatments, before your best chance to conceive is gone. Given financial concerns and health risks, it may make perfect sense to proceed cautiously from basal body temperature thermometers to IUI to in vitro fertilization (IVF). But with severe endometriosis, argue infertility specialists, what's the point? If you already know your tubes and ovaries have been damaged, you already know your chances to conceive have been reduced drastically.

There are a variety of options you may want to consider as you think about trying to conceive, but many of them will be appropriate only if your tubes are undamaged. These options include ovarian hyperstimulation combined with IUI, as well as a range of in vitro fertilization techniques, such as gamete intrafallopian transfer, or GIFT, and zygote intrafallopian transfer, or ZIFT. All would involve treatments with one or more of the medications Clomid, Pergonal, Humegon, and Metrodin, and some would also include GnRH drugs and human chorionic gonadotropin (HCG).

Clomid, an ovarian stimulant, and Pergonal, Metrodin, and Humegon, follicle-stimulating hormones, work by convincing your ovaries to produce and ripen more than one egg during a single menstrual cycle. Often doctors use GnRH drugs in the early part of the cycle, before beginning ovarian hyperstimulation, to help control and predict most accurately the maturation of eggs. Doctors will frequently rely on HCG to time the precise release of the eggs from ovaries before procedures are to take place.

If your fallopian tubes are in reasonably good shape, most commonly where little or no endometriosis is present, you may try IUI just as your ovaries release mature eggs. Or you may undergo laparoscopy so that a surgeon can remove the ripe eggs from your ovaries and immediately place them in your fallopian tubes along with sperm (this is GIFT). Surgeons can also retrieve eggs transvaginally, using an ultrasound probe to guide a hollow needle through the vaginal wall up to the ovaries, where they can aspirate, or suck out, ripe eggs. These eggs, combined with sperm in a dish or "test tube," will grow into zygotes, or preembryos, which can be placed into your fallopian tubes during laparoscopy (this is ZIFT). Because embryos develop inside your tubes and can travel on their own into the uterus, as they would have without technological intervention, they may be more likely to settle in for the duration, causing pregnancy.

For most women with severe endometriosis, however, each of these three options is risky since each one relies on open, working fallopian tubes. Badly scarred tubes may not be able to deposit embryos smoothly into your uterus. In fact you may so significantly run the risk of ectopic pregnancy, where developing embryos become trapped in your fallopian tubes and can cause hemorrhaging and even death, that you may be advised not to consider any of these techniques. For you standard IVF may be the best option. Here eggs and sperm are combined outside the body to produce embryos, which, placed in a tiny catheter, are inserted through your cervix into your uterus.

Should you venture into the world of advanced assisted reproductive medicine, you will be surrounded by a swirl of mind-boggling statistics and odds. A few words to the wise: because, at the time of this printing, fertility specialists are unlicensed and IVF clinics are unregulated, it is vitally important that you choose practitioners with utmost care. A single round of IVF at the time of this printing can cost anywhere from $6,000 to $10,000, enticing unsavory, unqualified characters into the business for purely pecuniary reasons. Remember that success rates for pregnancy with any of these techniques are low, somewhere in the 15 to 20 percent range, and remember that pregnancy is not the same thing as live birth. You will want to ask how many patients wind up with live babies, not just how many wind up pregnant. Centers touting higher-than-average success rates may be manipulating more than their numbers. Look for well-respected clinics, often attached to teaching and research hospitals, where volume is high enough that you won't be one of only a few women with endometriosis seeking treatment. If at any time you don't feel comfortable, don't proceed.

Even in the best clinics you will open yourself up to possible risks, many of which can be minimized if you limit the number of times you try any of these procedures. The high doses of Clomid, Pergonal, Metrodin, and Humegon used in any kind of assisted reproductive medicine can lead to ovarian hyperstimulation syndrome, in which your ovaries swell to dangerously large sizes, and you can, in extreme cases, wind up in shock. Careful monitoring is vitally important to prevent dangerous complications from occurring.

These high doses of hormones can boost estrogen levels to a point where you will run the risk of exacerbating your endometriosis. If you get pregnant, the endometriosis will, for the duration of the pregnancy, probably go into remission. Otherwise you may develop endometriomas (cysts) and other by-products of unchecked endometrial growth. In addition, since you will doubtless produce and ripen more than one egg during one cycle while taking these medications, you will also run the risk of implanting more than one embryo. Carrying more than one fetus during pregnancy increases the risk of miscarriage and premature birth.

The most alarming data concerning these drugs have linked Clomid, in particular, to ovarian cancer. It is possible that any of the drugs used to hyperstimulate the ovaries could be involved with cancer, but data do not presently exist to verify this presumption since long-term studies have not yet been completed. In one study researchers found that women who used Clomid for more than 12 cycles and who had never been pregnant and did not subsequently become pregnant were 27 times more likely to develop ovarian tumors than fertile women who had not used the drug. In addition, the study found that ovarian tumors were twice as likely to develop in infertile women with ovulatory abnormalities as in infertile women with other types of abnormalities. Infertile women who used Clomid and conceived were not found to be at any increased risk for developing ovarian cancer. Obviously more study is needed.

If we factor endometriosis into the equation, especially if we assume that with the endometriosis comes some degree of lessened fertility, should we conclude that Clomid and drugs like it are especially dangerous for us? Infertility specialists don't think so. Since 85 percent of all pregnancies associated with Clomid occur in the first three ovulatory cycles taking the drug, physicians suggest limiting the use of Clomid and similar drugs to six cycles or fewer. You probably won't greatly increase your chance of getting pregnant using these drugs past six cycles, but you apparently will increase your risk of developing cancer. Again, be on the lookout for new evidence and new studies following the use of these drugs.

Another way to protect yourself is to consider natural-cycle procedures. In these procedures no drugs are used—instead, a single egg is harvested from the woman's ovary and used in assisted reproductive procedures.

Association advisor Deborah Metzger, M.D., Ph.D., states that it's important to remember through all this soul-wrenching decision making that you *do* have some control in what feels like an uncontrollable situation. The way to maintain some control is to decide, as a couple, how much time, money, and emotional resources you will invest in infertility procedures. What is best for any one couple will depend on many factors, including age, feelings about technological interventions, emotional comfort, insurance, and financial issues.

Finally, some women have meditated on what it means to carry endometriosis and what it might mean to pass it on to future generations. Do we women with endometriosis harbor some harmful genetic material that will damage our children? Is it possible that pesticides and environmental contaminants have so polluted our bodies that we are passing on some of these toxins or mutations that will ultimately harm our children? We do not know the answers to any of these questions at this point. Each of us must come to terms with these potential dangers and continue to educate ourselves and our families about their implications.

In your struggle to become pregnant, remember that it is your body having trouble becoming a parent, not your soul. Only you can decide how far to pursue pregnancy. Only you can make decisions that you find acceptable, that are within your value system, that keep in mind what's best for your body, your family, and the child you might someday parent (whether through birth, adoption, foster parenting, or stepparenting).

Opting not to undergo assisted reproductive procedures is not an indication of a lack of desire to parent. And trying a round or two of IVF isn't a folly-filled delusion stalling inevitable defeat. One way or another, if it is something you care about, you will find a way to become a parent. Maybe the only silver lining to endometriosis's curse of infertility is that once you become a parent you will not be able to take for granted what it means to have children.

Selected Bibliography

Hintz, S., and Ballweg, M. L. "Fertility and Pregnancy Considerations." *Overcoming Endometriosis: New Help from the Endometriosis Association*. New York: Congdon & Weed, 1987, 74–80.

Laurence, L., and Weinhouse, B. *Outrageous Practices: The Alarming Truth About How Medicine Mistreats Women*. New York: Fawcett Columbine, 1994.

Lessey, B. A., Castelbaum, A. J., Sawin, S. W., Buck, C. A., Schinnar, R., Bilker, W., et al. "Aberrant Integrin Expression in the Endometrium of Women with Endometriosis." *Journal of Clinical Endocrinology and Metabolism* 79 (1994), 643–49.

Martin, D., M.D. "Infertility or Endo Pain—Which Do You Treat?" *The Endometriosis Association 10th Anniversary Conference Audiotapes*. Milwaukee: Endometriosis Association, 1990.

Martin, D. "Telephone Interview Concerning Clomid and Ovarian Cancer, Dan Martin and Cathy Corman." March 1995. Notes in the possession of the author.

Olive, D. L., M.D., and Haney, A. F., M.D. "Endometriosis-Associated Infertility: A Critical Review of Therapeutic Approaches." *Obstetrical and Gynecological Survey* 41, no. 9 (1986), 538–55.

Redwine, D., M.D. "Telephone Interview Concerning Endometriosis as a Progressive Disease, David Redwine and Cathy Corman." April 1995. Notes in the possession of the author.

Rönnberg, L. "Endometriosis and Infertility." *Annals of Medicine* 22 (1990), 91–96.

Rosen, G. F., M.D. "Treatment of Endometriosis-Associated Infertility." *Infertility and Reproductive Medicine Clinics of North America: Endometriosis* 3, no. 3 (July 1992), 721–30.

Rossing, M. A., D.V.M., Ph.D., et al. "Ovarian Tumors in a Cohort of Infertile Women." *The New England Journal of Medicine* 331, no. 12 (September 22, 1994), 771–76.

Serta, R. T., M.D., et al. "Minimal Endometriosis and Intrauterine Insemination: Does Controlled Ovarian Hyperstimulation Improve Pregnancy Rates?" *Obstetrics and Gynecology* 80, no. 1 (July 1992), 37–40.

Thomas, E. J. "Endometriosis and Infertility." *Modern Approaches to Endometriosis*. E. J. Thomas and J. Rock, eds. The Netherlands: Kluwer Academic Publishers, 1991, 113–27.

Tulandi, T., M.D. "Do Fertility Drugs Cause Ovarian Cancer?" *Infertility Awareness Association of Canada, Special Edition no.* 1 (October 1994), 49–50.

■ *Cathy Corman is the full-time mother of two-and-a-half-year-old triplets, a part-time grad-uate student in American studies at Yale University, and a member of the Endometriosis Association. She has worked as a full-time and freelance reporter.*

Pregnancy, Labor, and Postpartum Experiences of Women with Endometriosis

By Mary Lou Ballweg

Women with endometriosis have frequently been assured that if they can become pregnant their pregnancies will be normal. Although early studies suggested that women with endometriosis had a higher risk for miscarriage and for ectopic pregnancy, later studies have been unable to verify those findings—some have found a higher rate of these complications, some have found that other factors make clear conclusions impossible at this time. Thus, the true rates of both complications in women with endometriosis are still unknown. Because miscarriage and ectopic pregnancy have a major physical and psychological impact on women, we think doctors should avoid glib reassurances about pregnancy for women with endometriosis.

It's a shock to realize that these reassurances that one's pregnancy will be normal—with the "exceptions" of possible higher rates of miscarriage and ectopic pregnancy—have been made without scientific study of the actual pregnancy experiences of women with endometriosis. So, when association member Carolyn Ansell, a master's degree student at the Yale School of Nursing Midwifery, wrote us asking if there were any topics for research of burning interest to the association, I responded eagerly that we indeed had some needs that could be answered well by someone with Ansell's credentials:

- Do women with endometriosis experience more (frequency, severity, and duration) morning sickness with pregnancy?
- Do women with endometriosis experience other difficulties with pregnancy?
- Do labors of these women differ from those of other women on the average?
- Do women with endometriosis experience more postpartum depression?

These questions arose out of my concern that pregnancy and labor seem very difficult for many women with endometriosis. Although this was only an informal observation, I was amazed by how frequently I hear reports of severe morning sickness, for example. A study that addressed these issues would be very valuable.

Ansell had been through her own "battle" with endometriosis and decided to go into women's health care because of it. She wrote that she believed research on endometriosis could "best be accomplished by the women who have a personal stake in finding the pieces of the puzzle." Ansell and colleague Catherine Gorchoff carried out an extensive review of the research literature and writings on endometriosis. "Most of the existing literature addresses the issue of treating endometriosis so pregnancy can be attained," they write in their final report on the study. "Once the pregnancy is achieved, the research ends. However, it is important for clinicians to be able to answer questions about the course of pregnancy in the woman who has endometriosis. What can she expect? Will the pregnancy be 'normal' or different? Are the common discomforts exaggerated?"

Ansell and Gorchoff developed a questionnaire to address this lack of research. The questionnaire was then published in the association newsletter, and 187 women with proven endometriosis who had been pregnant, regardless of outcome of the pregnancy, responded with completed questionnaires.

Their study of the pregnancy experiences of women with endometriosis, the first of its kind, found multiple discomforts during pregnancy, a high incidence of dysfunctional labor, high rates of postpartum depression, and a faster return of symptoms in those who did not breast-feed. These are new findings. Reconfirmed findings were a statistically significant rate of miscarriages and ectopic pregnancies.

Ansell and Gorchoff explored many aspects of pregnancy and endometriosis in this study. They asked if the diagnosis of endometriosis had influenced respondents' decisions to attempt to become pregnant—55 percent of the respondents said it had.* Forty-four percent said it had not. A high rate of medical interventions (surgery, danazol, Clomid, oral contraceptives, Pergonal, and other treatments for endometriosis and infertility) was required to attain pregnancy. Over half of those responding to the questionnaire stated that they had required these types of medical assistance to achieve pregnancy. Many had multiple treatments. The average length of time within which pregnancy occurred after beginning treatment was 11.9 months.

A total of 334 pregnancies were reported by these women. Not all study participants filed complete data on all pregnancies; in some cases participants were pregnant at the time of completing the questionnaire and so could not file data on the end of their pregnancies or postpartum. Information on 187 pregnancies is reported here.

A higher rate of miscarriage, 34 percent, occurred than the 15 to 20 percent thought to prevail in the general population. A higher rate of ectopic pregnancies was also evident: 3 ectopics or 1 per 62, compared to an estimated risk of 1 per 125 women to 1 per 300 women in the overall population.

On the good-news side, there was a low incidence of premature birth (.01 percent). Unfortunately, our foray onto the good-news side of things can only be brief. Nausea and vomiting ("morning sickness") was reported by 73 percent of the study group. Most of the women reported this in the first trimester, but for some it occurred in the second and third trimesters also. The authors note that there is no body of literature on general incidence of nausea and vomiting with pregnancy for comparison purposes. (Author Tracy Hotchner in *Pregnancy & Childbirth: The Complete Guide for a New Life* writes that one-third of women are affected by vomiting or digestive disturbance in the first three months of pregnancy.)

---

*Percentages may not always add to 100 due to rounding.

Ansell and Gorchoff cite a study by S. F. Gould published in *Fertility and Sterility* 39, no. 4 (April 1983), on the nausea and vomiting in women with endometriosis during pregnancy and depression after pregnancy: Gould and his colleagues proposed that there is an abnormality in estrogen control in women with endometriosis. Gould notes that if the estrogen receptors do not 'shut down' during pregnancy, but allow high levels of estrogen to accumulate, they may lead to a higher incidence of the side effects associated with estrogen excess: nausea and vomiting, headaches, and depression.

Other problems experienced by the women during pregnancy included early contractions of the uterus (26 percent); bleeding (16 percent); and cramping (12 percent). Again there are no numbers from the general population for comparison, note Ansell and Gorchoff.

When asked about endometriosis symptoms during pregnancy, the majority of questionnaire respondents reported none. Those who did experience symptoms cited pelvic pain as most common, experienced by one-fourth of the women. Nine percent reported bowel symptoms (pain immediately prior to or during defecation, rectal bleeding, severe diarrhea, or constipation). "It appears that the women in this study identify the presence of endometriosis through menstrual period symptoms; they often noted on their questionnaires that familiar symptoms occurred with the resumption of menses," note the researchers.

Besides the "problems" the women reported, a variety of "complications" was reported, including dysfunctional labor (26.7 percent), fetal malposition (12.1 percent), fetal distress (10.7 percent), preterm labor (9.3 percent), premature rupture of membranes (5.9 percent), preeclampsia (5.3 percent), false labor (5.3 percent), placental problems (3.3 percent), cephalopelvic disproportion (CPD) (2.7 percent), and other complications (13.9 percent). Seventy-eight percent had at least one complication; 20.8 percent were free of complications. One hundred forty-five of the babies born were apparently healthy (43.4 percent); 2 were stillborn (.6 percent), and 11 had some type of morbidity (disease or sickness) (3.3 percent). The remaining pregnancies were terminated or resulted in miscarriages or ectopic pregnancies.

The average length of labor for women in this study was 14 hours. The average length of labor in the general population is 12 hours for a woman having her first baby; 7 hours and 15 minutes for subsequent babies. Using weighted averages, allowing for those with first and second pregnancies should have resulted in an average labor of 11 hours in this group (108 of the pregnancies carried to term were first pregnancies, and 27 were second pregnancies). Ansell and Gorchoff point out that there is potential difficulty with the figures in the study since women mark the time labor starts differently.

The most frequent complication of labor was dysfunctional labor, a term applied to labors that exceed certain time parameters established by the researcher E. A. Friedman or that come to a halt before the infant is born. The causes of dysfunctional labor noted by the authors of this study are "malposition of the fetus (such as the fetal head presenting posteriorly or in the transverse diameter of the maternal pelvis), prolonged or premature or early rupture of the membranes surrounding the fetus, an unripe cervix (resistant to dilation), disordered uterine function, and cephalopelvic disproportion (Friedman, 1978).

"It is reasonable to speculate that endometriosis would not be a cause of either malpositions or CPD (cephalopelvic disproportion) since both of these conditions usually result from mechanical abnormalities such as contracted pelvis, lax maternal abdominal musculature, uterine anomalies such as fibroids, or fetal abnormalities. It would be more likely that the dysfunctional labor is a result of hormonal imbalance leading to uterine dysfunction. Decreased levels of progesterone which have a quieting effect on the uterus combined with increased levels of estrogen, lead to prostaglandin synthesis and increased myometrial activity (Speroff, 1978). There is a large body of evidence which supports the theory that prostaglandins play an essential role in labor. If prostaglandin levels are elevated in women with endometriosis as proposed by Williams (1976); Meldrum, Shamonki & Clark (1977); and Weed (1980), one would anticipate a lower incidence of dysfunctional labor (in women with endo). Our findings of a 26 percent rate of dysfunctional labor are theoretically consistent with the speculations of Gould, Shannon & Cunha (1983) who suggested that endometriosis patients may have an abnormality in progesterone receptors. It would be intriguing to conduct a study focused exclusively on the duration and course of labor in women with endometriosis to observe whether this high incidence of dysfunctional labor persists."

A woman with dysfunctional labor is often given hormones to stimulate contractions, most commonly a drug called *pitocin*. Consistent with the findings of a high rate of dysfunctional labor was the finding of a high rate of use of pitocin in these women (26.7 percent). This is a startling and somewhat disturbing finding, given the controversy surrounding use of drugs such as pitocin, due to oxygen deprivation that can occur in the fetus when the mother is given the drug. Oxygen deprivation can result in brain damage and cerebral palsy. Besides dysfunctional labor and use of pitocin, other complications of labor were not significantly higher or lower than found in other groups, report the authors.

Possibly the most startling finding of the study is that 54.6 percent of the women in the study reported postpartum depression. "True postpartum depressive illness, differentiated from short-term spontaneously remitting three-day 'blues,'" note the authors, has been characterized by research as "having an onset between two and eight weeks postpartum, being at least partially disabling, and persisting for a period of at least two weeks." By these criteria postpartum depression is found in 11 percent of the general population of women after giving birth. The average length of depression of women in this study was an amazing 8¾ weeks.

The cause of postpartum depression is not known absolutely but is thought to be related to the drastic drop in levels of estrogen and progesterone after delivery, hormonal imbalance, or hormonal sensitivity. The finding of high rates of postpartum depression is consistent with the evidence of some hormonal imbalance or problem in women with endometriosis.

It is also thought that unresolved problems related to pregnancy/childbearing issues contribute to postpartum depression. As Ansell and Gorchoff point out, the feeling of not being in control of one's life, especially concerning pregnancy/childbearing decisions, was expressed by many of the women in the study, a very natural outcome of a disease like endometriosis. They note that the high rate of postpartum depression could also be influenced by numerous stresses experienced by this group. These stresses included lack of control over pregnancy/childbearing decisions, inability to control timing of conception, feeling pressured to attempt conception before childbearing and child rearing decisions were fully made, the medical interventions required to become pregnant, the numerous discomforts of the pregnancy itself experienced by these women, the dysfunctional labors, and the additional medical interventions faced because of it.

Endometriosis symptoms returned within a year after the birth of their babies for the majority of the women in the study. The average length of time before symptoms reappeared was 10 months. "These data refute the concept that pregnancy serves to cure endometriosis," write the authors. This information is not new to most members of the association, of course, but bears repeating because of the common misperception in the public and medical community. It's obviously of the utmost importance that women with endometriosis not make pregnancy, childbearing, and child rearing decisions based on the expectation that pregnancy will cure their disease. (The decision to bring another human being into the world is too important to be made for that reason!)

"There was a significant difference in the time that symptoms reappeared between the women who breastfed and the women who bottlefed," write Ansell and Gorchoff. A very high percentage of women in the study breast-fed, probably because of their awareness of the possibility of suppressing ovulation with breast-feeding (which would mean no periods and no return of the worst symptoms of endometriosis during that time) and also possibly because of the desire to get the most out of the pregnancy/infancy experience after the difficulties faced in attaining it. Nearly 83 percent of the women in the study breast-fed. (Hotchner, in the book cited earlier, notes that in the overall population only 30 percent of babies have been breast-fed since 1950.) The average length of time spent breast-feeding was nine months.

The researchers studied the relationship between breast-feeding and the return of endometriosis symptoms and found that women who breast-fed had significantly later onset of symptoms. The researchers also noted that many women reported no symptoms until they stopped nursing—indeed the relationship between the average length of time spent breast-feeding (nine months) and the average return of symptoms (10 months) is striking.

In addition to the numerical data from the study, the researchers extrapolated data on the *quality* of pregnancy-related experiences for women with endometriosis. They used open-ended questions such as "How do you feel the experience of having had endometriosis affected your pregnancy?"

Ten common themes of emotional response were found in these answers. Six of the themes (anger, loss of control, body dysfunction/failure, guilt, relationship to authority, and "miracle" baby) find support in the literature on the emotional aspects of infertility, the authors note. The other four themes identified by the authors were fear, concerns about use of hormonal therapy, pregnancy as a cleansing/curative experience, and pain tolerance.

"Fear was a central theme," note Ansell and Gorchoff, "and included fear of both the known and the unknown aspects of having endometriosis." Fear of miscarriage was expressed by 47 percent of the respondents. "Many of the respondents had experienced one or more previous miscarriages, others experienced bleeding or cramping, while still others had no signs or symptoms of a problem with pregnancy, but were responding instead to a generalized fear of 'something' going wrong." Ansell and Gorchoff quote a couple of the women on the fear theme:

"I was so cautious and held my breath the first 3–4 months. I had just begun to relax and think "Maybe it's all finally coming true" when I miscarried. At 20 weeks, I really thought I was safe.'

"I was extremely nervous that my pregnancy would not go full term. I had tried for so many years to get pregnant that when I finally was, I was paranoid that something would happen. . . .'"

Ansell and Gorchoff also note that "Fear of an ectopic pregnancy secondary to the scarring from endometriosis and/or surgery was also a commonly expressed concern." Some of the women had experienced a prior tubal pregnancy and were frightened by the fact that they had only "one chance" left.

"I am now afraid to try again, because I do not want to go through another tubular pregnancy. After having the laparotomy to remove the tubular pregnancy, the doctor said my left tube looked good. The only way I think I would try again is if they can tell me which side I am ovulating on.'"

Anger was another emotional response of the women. "Anger at self, at the medical establishment and at the general situation of being diagnosed with and/or dealing with endometriosis were most frequently expressed." Ansell and Gorchoff note that in this category were some of the strongest statements received:

"'First came diagnosis. Accompanying this was guilt, anger, depression, pity, rage, violence . . . I hated myself and my body.'

"'Again, life is full of disappointment, frustrations, and anger at my body.'

"'When I couldn't conceive after surgery and with the aid of Clomid and a temperature chart I felt cheated and robbed of my womanhood. I was very angry and frustrated.'"

"We were particularly impressed," the researchers write, "with the total 'gestalt' of the comments: these were spontaneous expressions, some appearing in context following the answer to a question, while others were literally scrawled in large, sloppy handwriting, across the bottom of the page:

"'Too bad I nearly lost my mind and health because I was a "neurotic hypochondriac" who "enjoyed my misery" and "didn't want to become pregnant!?"'

"'I wonder if any other women like me had to bear the labels, "selfish," "immoral," "irresponsible" and be accused of a "deep-seated ambivalence toward motherhood and/or being a woman?"'

"'(re: hysterectomy after delivery): I mentioned this to my doctor, who said "You're young— don't make this kind of decision without thinking." My God! With endo, I didn't HAVE a life!'

"'In the last 10 years, doctors all over three or four states I have lived in have called my endo "nonexistent," or "all in my head—see a psychiatrist" or "get a hysterectomy now; you'll need one later anyway." I haven't yet. Or "let's use you as a guinea pig for danazol.'"

Ansell and Gorchoff write that the statements of anger were sometimes linked to past events that might have been different with more knowledge about endometriosis. Wrote one respondent:

"'If my doctor had adequately informed me about endo and infertility problems, I think I wouldn't have had that abortion—honestly.'"

There was also anger or frustration expressed at the fact that endometriosis imposed a timetable on the important decisions surrounding pregnancy and the loss of control in planning conception.

"'The most difficult aspect for me has been planning the pregnancies. I simply did not feel ready for a child at age 22 and for a long while afterwards, but of course I didn't want to risk not having a child. The pressure was hard to cope with and strained my relationship with my husband for a time.'

"'I was rushed into a pregnancy during a time I had a dysfunctional relationship.'

"'I felt an incredible urgency to conceive—something I had imagined I could put off indefinitely . . . marriage then became an issue, given my family's attitudes. . . .'

"'Having endo forced me to have a child earlier than I probably would have. Since I had trouble conceiving I feel I can't wait another 3 or 4 years to have another, which is how I would like to space my kids. . . .'"

But there were also women who felt endometriosis helped them in making life decisions:

"'I was glad to be "forced" into deciding whether to have kids or not. . . .'

"'. . . definitely propelled me into deciding to finally get pregnant. . . .'"

The category of emotional response surrounding the feeling that the woman's body has failed her, note the researchers, "included comments which revealed a dysfunctional body image secondary to the respondent's experience as an endometriosis sufferer. The respondents' poor self-perceptions included all aspects of their reproductive abilities":

"'Endometriosis has resulted in my feeling very much like a "loser" in that part of my body, confirmed by the difficulty to get pregnant, the loss of my first pregnancy, and the need for second surgery before I could get pregnant again. . . .'

"'There were other pregnant women at my place of employment who had "easy" pregnancies, working up to the last week of their pregnancies, while I was struggling to make it another day. I felt that my body was somehow not up to par; it was inadequate.'

"'I remember wondering if I could even be a good nursing mother, since that was part of my poor reproductive system. . . .'

"'[Endometriosis] made me fearful and distrustful of my body; that it would betray me again, that something would go wrong. . . .'"

The authors cite the work of other researchers who have found that impaired self-image is often part of any chronic illness. In addition, certain body parts have specialized meanings to people. "The reproductive organs," Ansell and Gorchoff write, "are charged with the significance of generation of offspring, creation, and continuation of life. It is therefore not surprising that damage or perceived damage to these organs would result in altered self-image and the view of oneself as 'defective,' 'inadequate' or, in the words of one respondent, 'a loser.' The significance of this altered self-image is inestimable in its potential impact on all aspects of the endometriosis sufferer's life."

A particularly fearful part of the anxiety over a woman's body failing her was the fear expressed by some of the respondents that their bodies might not be able to produce a normal baby or that hormones used prior to conception would harm the baby. The authors note that concern about the health of her baby is common to most women but that for these women there was the added concern that any abnormality would in some way be related to endometriosis. Recognizing that the long-term effects of drugs used for endometriosis and infertility are not known added to the concern:

"'I am hoping and praying I will deliver a normal child. I feel more nervous than my friends who are pregnant that never had endo. I'm afraid you get used to your body failing you.'

"'I'm scared . . . of the long-term effects of drugs like Danocrine or Depo-Provera on the baby and myself.'

"'I would really like information on any research done regarding the effect of danazol on the future birth/child conceived soon after treatment. I guess one can't help but be in fear of another DES.'"

The most surprising theme found by the researchers, in my opinion, is the guilt expressed by some of the women who were able to conceive when others could not:

"'I felt so guilty because I'd managed to conceive where others couldn't.'

"'I felt guilty about my good luck when around other infertile friends.'

"'Later on I felt "guilty" that I was able to conceive when others could not.'"

Another theme expressed by respondents in the study was that their pregnancies had a cleansing or curative effect related to their endometriosis. Only 5 percent of the women expressed statements of this type, but the authors found them important because they illustrate that the idea of the "therapeutic baby" (having a baby to supposedly cure a disease) still exists in the minds of some caregivers and women with endometriosis. Given the recurrence rate of endometriosis after pregnancy, the authors caution against this unfounded belief.

"'I was relieved to be pregnant, knowing that it would retard the growth of my endometriosis. . . .'

"'I would not have had a second pregnancy . . . if I was not led to believe the pregnancy would "cure" the endometriosis. . . .'

"'. . . endo was the main reason for the pregnancy. . . .'

"'I wonder if I wanted a baby or if I just wanted the pain to stop.'"

"Some women," write the authors, "expressed the same notion that their pregnancy had provided either a temporary cure or respite from the disease, but expressed it in more positive tones":

"'I had a feeling of my body being cleansed while pregnant.'

"'I had such total relief of symptoms while pregnant I was actually sad I was early. . . . I felt so good pregnant, my body and I were actually getting along.'

"'I'll be breastfeeding this baby too, so I'll be going almost 3 years without a period and am hoping this will keep the endometriosis in remission for a few years.'"

Ansell and Gorchoff report that some of the women stated they had "never felt better" than while pregnant, while another commented, "Everyone said being pregnant is when they felt their best. I think that is a joke!"

Another theme expressed by 5 percent of the respondents in the study was that endometriosis had prepared them for the pains and discomforts of pregnancy and labor.

"'The horrible pain I had with endometriosis made labor probably easy for me, as I had experienced severe pain—not unlike that experienced during delivery.'

"'Contractions were no worse than pain from endo. I felt more ready than my friends to handle a difficult birth, if I had one—not scared of surgery!'

"'I was actually looking forward to labor and delivery to see if it was worse than endometriosis (it's not).'"

About 10 percent of the respondents made comments about the physician-patient relationship. "Some of the comments were complimentary of the care received, some reflected a dissatisfaction, but what struck us was the sense of power that these women ascribed to their physicians," allowing them an enormous amount of control in attempts to conceive and in their pregnancies. Examples Ansell and Gorchoff give are statements by doctors about the woman's chances of conceiving ("'I was told I had only a 35 percent chance of conceiving.' 'He said my chances were one in ten thousand.'"), which reflect, given our current state of knowledge on endometriosis and fertility, guesswork. But the women seemed to cling to these statements, giving them much more credence than they warranted. (Part of this is due, I would add, to the assumption by some people that everything a doctor says is based on science and that science knows a lot more about endometriosis and infertility than it does. Part of it also represents, I believe, a grasping at straws in the hope of pinning down something concrete in a maze of unknowns—percentages in particular sound so solid and scientific!)

Because of these feelings, the authors were not surprised to find that some of the women regarded their babies as "miracle babies." As people become aware that more women with endometriosis are fertile than infertile (current statistics are that 30 to 40 percent of women with endometriosis are infertile or, conversely, that 60 to 70 percent are fertile), the miracle baby idea may change.

Ansell and Gorchoff conclude from the "miracle baby" comments and others on emotional response that "these women who suffer from endometriosis share in the feeling that they are in some way 'different' from other women, with special needs and concerns not shared by women who have not had this disease."

Ansell and Gorchoff also came to other conclusions: "Throughout our analysis of this data, we were impressed by some of the comments which suggest that, indeed, there are 'holes' in the information available to caregivers with regard to just what differences, if any, *do* exist between the endometriosis patient and the 'normal' gravida. . . . *The importance of continued quantitative and qualitative data-gathering in this area cannot be overemphasized.*

"The comments were fascinating, sometimes surprising, often desperate in tone. The 'gestalt' reflected a tremendous need on the part of the respondents to vent their feelings of frustration, anger and confusion. With all that is known about the disease, why are so many questions unanswered? Why is it so difficult for these women to receive the help and support they need? A recent advertisement created by the Endometriosis Association (headquartered in Milwaukee, Wisconsin) described the symptoms of endometriosis and urged women who suspected the condition to contact the association for information. The average number of responses in the first month of publication was over 2,000 per day. Even given the inevitable number of women who may have responded and do not, in fact, suffer from endometriosis, this represents a large population of women whose needs are presumably not being met by the providers of the women's health care."

Ansell and Gorchoff note that their study provides the groundwork for any number of valuable research projects on the pregnancy-related experiences of women with endometriosis. "There is a need to pursue these questions pertaining to fertility and pregnancy, chances of conceiving, of carrying a normal pregnancy to term, and complications that can be expected, in order that we may begin to dispel some of the myths and misinformation which some physicians and caregivers continue to provide."

Notes (from the Ansell/Gorchoff Report)

Carolyn Jean Ansell and Catherine Cardwell Gorchoff, "A Descriptive Investigation of the Perinatal Clinical Courses of Women with Endometriosis" (Yale University School of Nursing, 1987).

E. A. Friedman, *Labor: Clinical Evaluation and Management*, 2nd ed. (New York: Appleton-Century-Crofts, 1978).

S. F. Gould, J. M. Shannon, and G. R. Cunha, "Nuclear Estrogen Binding Sites Seen in Foci of Endometriosis," *Fertility and Sterility* 39, no. 4 (April 1983).

D. R. Meldrum, I. M. J. Shamonki, and K. E. Clark, *Prostaglandin Content of Ascitic Fluid in Endometriosis: A Preliminary Report*, 25th Annual Meeting of the Pacific Coast Fertility Society, Palm Springs, California (1977).

L. Speroff, R. H. Glass, and N. G. Kase, *Clinical Gynecologic Endocrinology & Infertility*, 3rd ed. (Baltimore/London: Williams & Wilkins, 1983).

T. J. Williams and J. H. Pratt, "Endometriosis in 1000 Consecutive Celiotomies: Incidence and Management," *American Journal of Obstetrics and Gynecology* 129 (1977): 245.

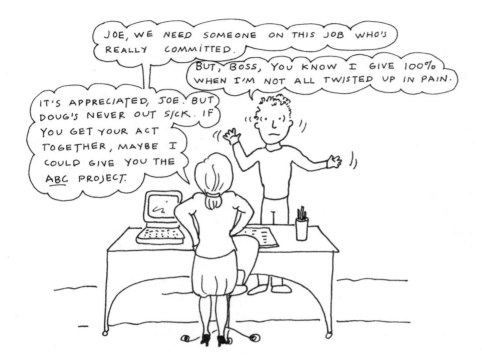

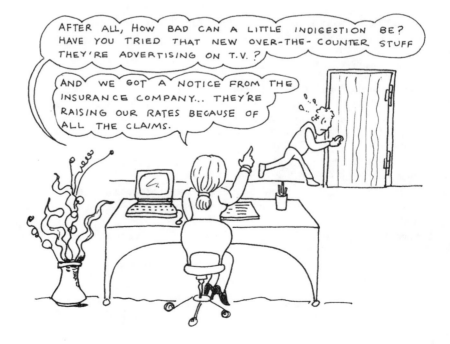

7

◉◉

Traditional Chinese Medicine and the Treatment of Endometriosis

By Arthur D. Shattuck, Dipl. Ac. NCCA

"*Not many years ago I was desperately in pain with no more medical options. My only thoughts at that time were to give up and take illegal narcotics. Just by chance I happened to hear of Dr. Ni. When I first met him, I felt I could completely trust him—he was very communicative, supportive, and caring. I thought since there was nothing to lose and there were no side effects to this unusual treatment I would commit for a six-month period, and if it did not work, I would simply give up on life entirely.*

"*Once a week I visited Dr. Ni's clinic for acupuncture, and three times a day I drank a strong and horrible-tasting but nourishing tea. My acupuncture was not at all painful; the fine wirelike needles did not hurt. After the treatments I felt an immediate wonderful sense of well-being, a nice, natural high. It was not until a few months had passed that I felt any relief of my chronic pain and not until several months later did I find complete relief from my severe and incapacitating menstrual pain. There were times I felt worse with what may have been detoxification and times my hormones shifted and gave me strange cravings. After about a year I started to ovulate, and at that time I felt better than I can ever remember in my entire life.*

"*My lifestyle has certainly changed. Traditional Chinese medicine was not a panacea, not a cure-all for what had ailed me. Yet I was assisted and guided. I learned that I was the only one responsible for the management and prevention of my condition. With the support from both Dr. Ni and the Endometriosis Association, I now feel privileged and blessed that in my illness I have had the opportunity to have learned to live well while still in my youth. Now 40 years old, I will live a long and healthier life. I have also realized that it all could have been worse; it could have been fatal and final.*"

Kathleen JoHanson, California

"*I am a new member who has benefited from the knowledge and support inherent in the newsletters I receive. As they say, knowledge is power—something I've learned since being diagnosed with endo during a laparoscopy last year. Another source of power is taking control of your life and treatment. It is an exhausting, hard thing to do, but only this way can we obtain the results we are looking for. . . .*

"*I decided to try acupuncture. The treatment was suggested to me by my sister, who had success with allergies and head colds. No one else I knew had tried it before—but I knew its effects would be less hazardous than hormones. . . .*

"*The treatments are not painful—but can make you feel like years of tension have been released from your body. I had six treatments over the summer and had the second laparoscopy in late August. My doctor found my condition to be much more favorable than either of us thought it would be. . . .*"

"*I also experienced a drastic decrease in pain (which had been getting progressively worse after surgery number one) during acupuncture treatments. . . .*"

Laura, Massachusetts

"*Before choosing surgery I got treatment from a Chinese herbalist/acupuncturist. Through diet, herbs, meditation, writing, and prayer, we shrank my ovarian cyst. My Western doctor called it miraculous. Had it not been for the fear of cancer I might have avoided surgery. . . .*"

Betty, California

"*Late last winter or early last spring, I read* Overcoming Endometriosis. *On pages 98–100, Mollie Ridout describes her experiences with acupuncture and dietary changes. I read that account over and over and paid close attention to the line 'Treatment is aimed at reestablishing normal hormone production levels by reducing stress, controlling diet, and using acupuncture.' After reading this account I started my search for a physiotherapist with knowledge of acupuncture. . . .*

"*Eventually I found a traditional Chinese medicine acupuncturist in Halifax. . . . I went to meet with him and asked about the possibility of acupuncture being able to stabilize estrogen/progesterone levels. He agreed that it was possible and began to treat me weekly for the myriad side effects that I was experiencing with Lupron. I should add that my gynecologist encouraged me in my search for an acupuncturist and continues to be very positive about the treatments, referring other women with endo to my acupuncturist. . . .*

"*I have to digress a bit to outline changes in diet that helped me to cope as well. The Lupron created many problems that other members of EA have outlined. Like others, I was plagued by painful, recurrent atrophic vaginitis. In addition to using nystatin cream, I went on a very strict antiyeast diet. I cut out sugar, including fruits, stopped eating flour, dairy products except for yogurt, and ate lots of veggies, some eggs, nuts, and seeds. After a month or so I added brown rice. I am a vegetarian and infrequently ate salmon, halibut, and eggs. Even now, 10 months after the first Lupron injection, I continue to stay away from yeast,* white sugar (I use blackstrap molasses in bran muffins), white flour, and other Candida-encouraging foods. I do slip up, but for the most part diet changes have helped so much I am drawn back to eating sensibly.

"During August and September of 1991 I went for weekly acupuncture treatments. During each session my acupuncturist also used myofascial massage to help scar tissue 'pullings,' especially inguinal pain and sacral pain. He used moxibustion during most sessions as well. . . . [Moxa is an herb that is burned over the point of the energy meridians, stimulating the flow of chi or energy.] Between my sessions I used moxa. . . . The intent of the moxa treatment was to move stagnated blood and chi and to reduce abdominal pain.

"The treatments helped me survive the rigors of Lupron and got me through a painful summer. I have continued to go for regular but less frequent treatments. . . .

"I continue to take vitamin and mineral supplements as outlined for the treatment of endo in a book called Prescription for Nutritional Healing by James F. Balch, M.D., and Phyllis A. Balch, C.N.C. Like your book, this valuable work has led me to a lot of useful self-help strategies. The sections about yeast infections, immune disorders, and endo are very useful (helpful for allergy-induced asthma also). . . .

"In closing, I'd like to add that TCM, nutritional healing, and the compassionate understanding of my acupuncturist and gynecologist have all offered me hope and help. Above all, it is important to know that we all have alternative options for treatment—some of which we can apply and monitor ourselves. Overcoming endo means overcoming the often pervasive feelings of helplessness and pessimism. TCM and nutritional healing are not 'fly-by-night' approaches to endo. They are practical, positive approaches from which all can gain some relief from (and control over) endo."

Debra, Nova Scotia

EDITOR'S NOTE: For more information on other alternative treatments, including nutritional approaches, see *Overcoming Endometriosis*.

In Chinese medical schools and clinics, *Fu Ke,* or gynecology, is a subdivision of *Nei Ke,* or internal medicine, which is also synonymous with herbal medicine. The diagnoses of the various gynecological disorders are discussed according to the differential diagnosis of *Bian Zheng,* or patterns of disharmony. Chinese medicine as a whole has existed for thousands of years, with gynecological pathologies being recorded in numerous texts such as *Fu Ren Da Quan Liang Fang (Complete Effective Prescriptions for the Diseases of Women)* by Cheng Zi-Ming in 1270.

The closest mention of a complete syndrome that may be comparable to endometriosis that I have found to date in Chinese medicine would be *Zheng Jia Ji Ju,* which means the formation of masses in the abdomen. These masses may be either fixed or movable and are often accompanied by fullness, distension, and pain. Literally, *Zheng Jia Ji Ju* means not only a hard lump with a fixed location and localized pain but also a movable, formless, and invisible accumulation within the belly.

Zhang Jing-Yue (circa 1563–1640) was the author of several books on gynecology. He felt that abdominal lumps resulted from a variety of causes, one being accumulated residual blood not discharged during menstruation or childbirth. If we complete a differential diagnosis on abdominal masses, we find no fewer than 11 different treatment strategies using acupuncture and Chinese herbs in conjunction with dietary advice.

All of the Oriental therapies are based on a system of regulating and balancing energy in the body. This energy, called *chi* (chee) in Chinese,

Professional Designations Used in Traditional Chinese Medicine:

Dipl. Ac.: Diplomate of Acupuncture; nationally certified.
Dipl. C. H.: Diploma of Chinese Herbology
L.Ac.: Licensed Acupuncturist; most of the states use this designation for those who have passed the state exam.
D.O.M. or **O.M.D.**: Doctor of Oriental Medicine or Oriental Medicine Doctor; usually involves some advanced training.
C.A.: Certified Acupuncturist; requires passing a more vigorous exam than the National Commission for the Certification of Acupuncturists (NCCA) exam; some herbal knowledge.

is the basic energy of the body. It flows in particular pathways called *meridians*. The meridians interconnect the entire body and all its systems both internally and externally. *Chi* follows various daily, monthly, and yearly cycles and can be assessed and affected via the points along the acupuncture meridians. When *chi* follows its prescribed paths and cycles, there is health and peak bodily performance. Where it becomes impeded or weak, ill health, pain, and discomfort occur. By restoring and maintaining the proper balance and flow to this energy system, one can often enhance health and well-being.

Methods of Diagnosis

In evaluating a person's *chi*, the diagnostic procedures of Chinese medicine are unique. Observation, listening, questioning, and pulse taking are known as the four diagnostic methods in traditional Chinese medicine. The case history and clinical symptoms and signs gained through the four diagnostic methods are the basis for further differentiation of the syndrome.

The two pillars of Chinese medicine, however, are the observation of the tongue and pulse taking. Indications of the nature of a disease can be learned by observing the color, form, and condition of dryness or moisture of both the tongue proper and its coating and the motility of the tongue.

Taking the pulse is such an important feature of China's medicine that Chinese patients often speak of going to the doctor as "going to have my pulse read." Chinese pulse theory gives meaning to the pulse as it is felt in each of its positions on each wrist. Disharmonies in the body leave a clear imprint on the pulse. Classical Chinese texts reflect a centuries-old effort to classify the basic pulses with their associated disharmonies. Twenty-eight general pulses are recognized by most practitioners. They are called *general* because an individual's pulse is most often a combination of types.

Diagnosis of Endometriosis

The Western diagnosis of endometriosis is too broad a diagnosis for the practitioner of Chinese medicine. Chinese medicine is more symptom-specific in its diagnosis and treatment. While one woman may complain of painful cramps before her periods, another may complain of pain during her periods, while yet another may complain of pain before and during her periods plus fatigue, low-back pain, and constipation. Each might be diagnosed with endometriosis in Western medicine, while in Chinese medicine these three patients would receive quite different diagnoses and very different treatment strategies. This is called *differential diagnosis* and is the key to understanding Chinese medicine. The Western diagnosis of endometriosis doesn't give the practitioner of Chinese medicine very much information about the patient.

Since there are so many different manifestations of this one disease, it is only after a differential diagnosis has been formulated that treatment can proceed. For this reason there is no singular acupuncture or herbal treatment for all endometriosis patients. Many different treatments and combinations of treatments must be considered once the differential diagnosis is obtained.

Following, I have given an example of the beginning of a differential diagnosis for *one* possible symptom of one patient with endometriosis. While Western medicine recognizes painful menstruation as dysmenorrhea, Chinese medicine would classify it into different symptom pictures, each to be treated differently. Remember that most patients present with more than one symptom. Each symptom must be taken into account and separated according to its individual manifestations.

Dysmenorrhea: Excessive pain associated with menstruation.

1. pain before menstruation
2. pain occurring before and during menstruation
3. pain felt at the end of menstruation
4. pain relieved somewhat by warmth
5. pain aggravated by warmth
6. pain rather than distension, which subsides to some extent once menstruation has started
7. distension rather than pain

From a complete symptom history, in conjunction with the four diagnostic methods, a pattern would develop that would allow us to complete our differential diagnosis and proceed with a treatment strategy. A treatment strategy is formulated with the intention of restoring and then maintaining the proper flow and balance of one's *chi*. The strategy would include one or more of the treatment modalities.

1. Acupuncture

Acupuncture is a relatively painless form of therapy, contrary to many people's fears. The treatment involves insertion of very thin steel needles into energy points along the meridians. The needles, which are perhaps as thick as three human hairs, generally do not go deeper than ⅛ to ¼ inch, although when a fleshy, muscular area of the body is involved, the needle may be inserted more deeply. The sensation elicited by the needle insertion, unlike the kind of pain associated with hypodermic injection, most often amounts to a slight sting or at times an ache or a slight heaviness.

Every energy point has a specific therapeutic effect on a related organ, specific effects on the body area covered by a meridian, and a general effect on the body's vital energy through the entire meridian complex. Although as few as 1 or 2 needles may be used in the course of treatment, more commonly 8 to 12 are inserted and left in place for 20 to 45 minutes. People almost always feel very calm and relaxed after the completion of an acupuncture treatment, a feeling that quite often can last for the rest of the day.

Acupuncture often can be used to cure diseases of the internal organs as well as relieve painful symptoms in bones, muscles, joints, and skin. In some cases acupuncture can bring about dramatic changes in health very quickly, even after one or two treatments. However, because the body works its way step by step from illness to health and because healing is a process that is constantly ongoing, most disorders commonly require a series of 10 treatments to effect a true change in the illness. In cases of chronic illness even more than 10 treatments may be required. Treatments are generally scheduled once a week, but if schedules permit, twice a week would be optimal.

2. Chinese Herbal Remedies

Your practitioner may decide to recommend certain Chinese herbs that will further enhance the treatment. Traditionally Chinese herbs come in their raw form, sliced root or bark, etc., and have to be boiled for a period of time and then drunk as a tea. In our fast-paced life, it is often difficult to find the time, and the tea itself is an acquired taste.

Fortunately, most herbal formulas are available in pill, capsule, or powdered form as "patent formulas" from mainland China or from a variety of reputable firms now in the

United States. The patents are valuable as adjunctive therapy to acupuncture and therapeutic massage.

Daily ingestion of an appropriate patent will allow healing to take place at an accelerated pace. The majority of pills are of a fairly standard size, to be taken 6 to 10 at a time. While Westerners are often surprised at the number to be taken, it must be understood that aside from the fair amount of honey or other binders making up the pills, the natural herb material contains large amounts of cellulose, starch, sugars, and other inactive ingredients so that larger amounts need to be taken than with modern drugs.

3. Dietary Advice

Chinese medicine is a holistic practice. Acupuncture and the use of Chinese herbs are two of the treatment modalities. The daily activities of eating are also included not only in the treatment but also in the prevention of illness. An entire realm of treatments are dietary in nature.

The pioneer Chinese diet classic was published in A.D. 652 by Sun Shu Mao (581–682), a Chinese physician. We can look to his work and that of many others for changes in our eating habits that will have a positive impact on our health status. These changes may be as easy as changing the way we prepare certain foods. More often they will entail adding foods to and/or deleting them from our diet.

4. Massage Techniques

Chinese massage techniques are simple and effective. Massage clears the meridians of blockages, stimulates circulation of blood and energy, loosens stiff joints and muscles, and raises vitality and resistance to disease. There are many massage techniques, but the most common and effective focus on the nerve centers and meridians that run down to the heels, especially along either side of the spinal column. Massage therapy is often followed up with herbal poultices and pills. These techniques are often taught to clients and their family members so that they may be utilized at home when the need arises.

Study Results

Preliminary results from studies I have been conducting found that traditional Chinese medicine appeared to offer 65 percent of women with endometriosis some element of pain management. Some women experienced a slight reduction of pain; others were able to go off all pain medications. In addition, when aggressive therapy was started immediately following laparoscopic surgery, nearly 70 percent had no further surgery for up to 4.2 years.

We are still following the group to see how long the surgery-free time can be extended. Pain maps and pain descriptions developed by Dr. Arnold Kresch (see Chapter 2) and daily symptom diaries were used to track symptoms.

One of the Chinese herbal formulas used in this study is called Neiyi Wan #1. In a study from the *Chinese Journal of Integrated Traditional Western Medicine* 1, no. 9 (1991): 524–26, which involved 76 women with endometriosis, immune measures were conducted before and after treatment with Neiyi Wan #1. After treatment 41 of the women monitored had normalized T8 cell levels. (T cells are immune cells, blood cells—lymphocytes—that destroy abnormal cells in foreign material. T8 cells are a type involved in turning off antibody production or in attacking abnormal or foreign cells.)

In addition, of 73 patients checked for immunoglobulin (antibody) levels, 53 showed abnormal levels that normalized after treatment. Prostaglandins involved in endometriosis also declined markedly. "The indicators are consistent with an autoimmune type of process that is alleviated by the herbs," according to Subhuti Dharmananda, Ph.D., director of the Institute for Traditional Medicine and Preventive Health Care, Portland, Oregon. Dharmananda said there has been a lot of interest in autoimmune diseases in China.

The treatment was particularly effective in relieving menstrual pain (89 percent of those reporting this symptom experienced relief). Other symptoms reported on in the study were improvement or resolution of pelvic pain (67 percent) and relief of pain with intercourse (72 percent).

An expansion of this study had to be discontinued due to lack of funding. It is my hypothesis that the treatments will be even more effective in preventing recurrence of the disease for some years when aggressively pursued following laparoscopic removal of existing lesions. This is where my research will focus in the years to come.

■ *Arthur D. Shattuck, Racine, Wisconsin, is a practitioner of traditional Chinese medicine and a nationally board-certified acupuncturist and has been in private practice for more than eight years.*

Traditional Chinese Medicine and Endometriosis: An Interview with Daoshing Ni, L.Ac., Ph.D., D.O.M., Dipl. C.H.

By Kathleen JoHanson

EDITOR'S NOTE: As the foreword to the book *The Web That Has No Weaver: Understanding Chinese Medicine* states, if one tries to interpret Chinese theory through Western terms, the central Chinese concept of medical patterns and disharmonies is disturbed—you're forcing the concept into terms that don't fit it. The author of the book suggests that upon encountering concepts that are difficult the reader just keep reading: "Greater familiarity with the material and hence the thought process behind it will bring the reward of greater clarity." For definitions of terms in this interview, see the Glossary.

In a talk with the Los Angeles chapter of the Endometriosis Association, Dr. Ni noted that endometriosis is seen as a *new* disease in traditional Chinese medicine and there is research and interest in China on what is causing it.

KJ: What is traditional Chinese medicine (TCM)?
Dr. Ni: Traditional Chinese medicine is a natural medical system developed by the ancient Chinese Taoist sages. Acupuncture and herbal therapies, which are known to many Westerners, are parts of this ancient medical system, which developed through the observation of nature.

The ancient sages believed that the human body is like a miniature universe or microcosm that functions in a similar harmonious pattern on universal principles. Our bodies subscribe to the laws of nature, and when there is disease or illness it is because our universe has a certain imbalance. To treat an imbalance, an introduction of traditional Chinese medicine therapy to the body can help bring the body back to balanced homeostasis.

The ancient sages also believed that the human body does not function on its own; it is a reflection and a coordination of our spirit, mind, emotions, and physical body. No one aspect can function alone; we cannot be separate from ourselves. Separation of the spirit from the physical body can create or can be seen as a condition of death. TCM was developed not only to treat the physical body but also to understand and balance the mental conditions.

TCM has been tested, proved, and accepted by the Chinese people for more than 5,000 years. Only in the last decade has this system become more known throughout the Western world. It has gained an increasing acceptance, especially by those who have not been able to find relief from conventional medicine.

Because the principle of TCM is to assist the body in bringing back its own balance and homeostasis, the body does not become dependent on it. Nor does TCM destroy or remove any parts of the body. We call this *regenerative* or *constructive medicine*.

Many people have found that TCM is a very good tool in obtaining optimal health and preventing illness. When one part of the body is imbalanced or ill, it can eventually affect the other parts of the body with a domino effect. When treating an illness, TCM does not treat just one part of the body. It treats the system where the weaknesses arose.

We also treat other systems that have been affected by a particular imbalance. For example, if someone who has an acute knee injury does not or did not treat the knee properly or allow it to heal, when it becomes chronic it can start to injure other parts of the body. It will cause stress and injury to the tendons, the ligaments, the liver, and the kidney system, where it may create back pain. It can affect and create weaknesses of the legs and lower extremities, weakness of the hips, urination weakness, irritability, restlessness, excessive anger, eye problems, and blurry vision. This is how we see one imbalance affecting and weakening the other parts of the body within the system.

TCM sees the human body as a network of energy channels, where the energy of the body flows and circulates throughout these channels. Within this network, an imbalance in a certain area of the body can create blockage or stagnation in that channel or meridian. This blockage of energy (or *chi*) is seen as an illness and/or pain. When acupuncture is utilized, fine needles are inserted to stimulate certain points on a meridian to unblock the circulating energy of the body and allow the bodily energy to flow freely. This rids the body of the imbalance and illness.

Modern scientists have found that some of these points have physical and biochemical properties. They have found that when stimulating these points there is a physiological and nervous reaction throughout the body and an unblocking of stagnation. It also has been found that acupuncture stimulates the brain's production of endorphins, which causes a decrease in inflammation, promotes healing, and creates a sense of well-being.

KJ: What is herbal medicine?

Dr. Ni: About 6,000 years ago a leader among the Chinese tribes made the first attempts to discover and utilize natural substances such as plants and minerals to heal people. He is considered the Father of Herbology and Agriculture, and his name was Shen Nung.

He was a virtuous man who devoted his life to developing the agriculture skills that were to be followed for many centuries. At the same time, he personally tried and tasted different plants and developed a system of three grades of herbs. Superior grade are edible herbs that promote health, longevity, and spiritual well-being. Premium grade are medicinal herbs used to alleviate sickness. The majority of herbs fall within this category and should be prescribed by a doctor of traditional Chinese medicine or an herbalist. Last are toxic herbs, which are administered only by a doctor and used in extreme circumstances.

Shen Nung's commitment to the search for herbs to treat illnesses was great, and because of his persistent spirit he was able to develop an herbal system composed of 360 herbs. These herbs were initially utilized by the ancient sages to maintain health and achieve longevity and were called "the immortal foods."

In this modern day approximately 5,000 herbs have been utilized and listed in a pharmaceutical dictionary of the Chinese government. Many of these herbs are grown in different locations throughout China and in many other parts of the world.

KJ: What is traditional Chinese medicine's view of endometriosis?
Dr. Ni: Endometriosis is a multisymptom disease generally characterized by dysmenorrhea, although pain and many other symptoms may be experienced throughout the menstrual cycle. In TCM endometriosis is seen as an imbalance of yin and yang, the female and male life forces that run throughout the whole body.

The cause of this imbalance might be due to several different factors: an imbalanced or irregular lifestyle; excessive stress or emotional disturbance; infection (especially of the reproductive or genital areas of the body, which become more vulnerable with sexual activity during menstruation); poor dietary intake; injury; or the introduction of chemicals into the body.

Endometriosis is also a condition of stagnancy of both *chi* (energy) and blood—especially in the lower abdominal area—and can lead to symptoms of dysmenorrhea, hesitant or profuse flow, clotting, infertility, hormonal imbalance, or PMS. (Some common symptoms of PMS include water retention, chills, fatigue, night sweats, irritability, restless sleep, poor appetite, constipation, sluggish and difficult urination, poor concentration, and others.)

KJ: How does TCM view the relationship of the immune system and endometriosis?
Dr. Ni: Endometriosis is viewed as an imbalance of yin and yang and a condition of stagnancy that can be caused by the factors just listed. These factors come from outside the body as well as inside. When there is an imbalance or an inadequately nourished body, there is a depletion of *chi* (energy) and a weakened immune system, which can create a vulnerability and probability of endometriosis and stagnancy.

KJ: How can TCM diagnose endometriosis?
Dr. Ni: TCM has its own unique procedure that diagnoses imbalances according to a system referring to syndromes, not simple disease names. Disease or syndrome of the liver

system would include those areas of the body the liver is associated with, such as the blood and circulatory systems, the immune system, and the nervous system. An imbalance in the liver would manifest itself in conditions of the eyes and nails and headaches.

KJ: How does TCM specifically treat an endometriosis condition?
Dr. Ni: The treatment for endometriosis is basically to bring the yin and yang of the body back into balance and to disperse and dissolve any kind of stagnancy. This will enable and facilitate the flow of the menstrual period, disperse pain, and implement regulation of the female and pituitary hormones. The two major treatments TCM applies are acupuncture and herbal therapy.

Acupuncture is a treatment that utilizes fine needles inserted into the different meridian points of the body to facilitate the *chi* (energy) flow. This helps disperse and dissolve any kind of blockages there may be in those meridians.

Herbal therapy's major focus is to improve the regulation of hormones. It does not take the place of the body's natural hormones but rather mimics the hormones and their function at the same time it stimulates the body to bring back its own hormonal balance. Because the source of endometriosis is deep in the endocrine system, the treatments a patient undertakes must be strong, thorough, and deep enough to correct the imbalances.

KJ: Can TCM work along with modern Western medicine?
Dr. Ni: Yes. In fact, in most hospitals in China there are modern medical doctors working side by side with TCM practitioners in the best interest of the patient.

There are conditions where modern medicine works well while TCM does not and vice versa. Especially in chronic conditions TCM offers more relief than modern medicine. Still other conditions are much better managed and treated with a combination of TCM and modern medicine. An example is cancer. Where chemotherapy destroys the good cellular structure of the human body, TCM can work to replenish that damaged cellular structure.

With endometriosis TCM works very well along with modern medicine, especially in severe cases where surgery is indicated. TCM can follow surgery and facilitate the recovery process. The TCM treatments do not interfere with most modern pharmaceuticals.

KJ: How can one find a good TCM practitioner?
Dr. Ni: In this country many states have different laws regarding the TCM practices with state board exams and certification requirements before one can practice. To find a good practitioner you first need to contact the local state acupuncture association, which can supply you with a directory in your area. Then you can interview each practitioner to find out his or her background.

Good TCM practitioners usually will have a comprehensive education of no less than two to three years of training in acupuncture and no less than five years in herbal training. At the same time these doctors will have many years of clinical experience working in a busy setting such as a clinic or hospital.

KJ: In TCM's view, what can a patient do to help herself?

Dr. Ni: There are many different ways that her lifestyle can help the endometriosis sufferer manage and prevent further symptoms from occurring.

With proper gentle exercise, the *chi* (energy) and blood flow is activated, the stagnation disperses, and the blood flow becomes better and smoother. This can bring about a change in menstrual pains.

Diet is another important aspect. Heavy meats, foods with a high fat and protein content, spicy foods, raw foods, dairy products, and cold foods are difficult to digest, and the body will spend more energy to digest them. This can create a burden on the reproductive system and in turn increase its imbalances and symptoms. Cooked vegetables, grains and beans, and cooked fish, for example, do not burden the digestive system.

A positive outlook and enjoyment of life is of absolute importance for the endometriosis sufferer. This can make a big difference in how a patient lives a more fulfilling life with the pain she is under. A certain amount of counseling or self-help reading and self-nurturing is necessary to develop a good mental outlook and attitude for the patient to cope with her sufferings. In a severe condition, Chi Gong therapy is advised. This is a breathing and imaging therapy in which the patient learns a meditative exercise that can help move and circulate the body's own energy deep within.

Remember the Chinese proverb "One disease, long life; no disease, short life." Those who *know* what is wrong with them can take care of themselves accordingly and will tend to live a longer and healthier life than those who neglect their weaknesses and their limitations. That's an example of a positive outlook on endometriosis.

■ *Daoshing Ni*, *L.Ac., Ph.D., D.O.M., Dipl. C.H., Santa Monica, California, is the 38th generation in a line of traditional Chinese healers. He was trained by his father, the eminent master Hua-Ching Ni, and earned his doctorate in Oriental Medicine at Samra University in Los Angeles. He also has received advanced training in mainland China. In addition to teaching and practicing Chinese medicine for the last 13 years, he is president of Yo San University of Traditional Chinese Medicine in Santa Monica, California.*

Kathleen JoHanson, *Napa, California, has been an Endometriosis Association member for over 10 years. She helped in the chartering of the Los Angeles chapter and has served as its vice president and president in those years. Her experience with traditional Chinese medicine for endometriosis is described in her letter at the beginning of the preceding article.*

Tips to Protect Yourself

Subhuti Dharmananda, Ph.D., director of the Institute for Traditional Medicine and Preventive Health Care, suggested these tips for women with endometriosis seeking help through traditional Chinese medicine:

1. Go to a licensed practitioner. In states without licensing, seek a nationally board-certified practitioner. Seeking a practitioner who is a member of local and national Chinese medicine/acupuncture associations is also something of a protection. Such membership shows some commitment to the profession, and associations generally have a code of professional ethics that members promise to uphold.

2. Obtain your herbs from a licensed practitioner. Don't just go to a store or mail-order company. It's important to obtain herbs from a reputable source since a few of the herbs from China are mislabeled or, in a few cases, Western-type prescription drugs are incorporated into the herbs. (In China, companies may produce both drugs and herbal preparations.)

3. Dharmananda said traditional Chinese medicine should produce substantial improvement within three to six months. Very complicated cases could take longer, but in general, he stated, one should not have to wait years and years for results.

4. Be sure you feel comfortable with the practitioner. Also ask for references from previous patients treated for similar problems.

Overcoming Endometriosis Through TCM

By Gail Toussaint

I am writing to share with you my success in overcoming endometriosis. I hope that what I have learned might help you in your struggle with this disease.

My gynecologist discovered my endometriosis in 1983, when I was 27, during a tubal ligation through laparoscopy. Since I was asymptomatic, I did not pursue treatment. Three years later, in 1986, my periods became very painful with sharp stabbing pains. I then went to my gynecologist for information on the treatment options. At the same time I discovered the Endometriosis Association.

I was dismayed at the information I found. There were no reliable treatments for the disease, nor were the drugs used in treatment necessarily FDA-approved at that time for treatment of endometriosis. The side effects of some of the drugs were deplorable. I could not justify the potential gains from taking any of them against their known side effects. I also did not want to endure conservative or radical surgery at age 30 and most likely have the disease return. The Endometriosis Association was an invaluable source of information, help, and support for me at this time.

My doctor prescribed codeine to help manage the pain while I researched the treatment options to determine a safe one to pursue. Three years later, in 1989, the pain had become excruciating, and I was at a point where I could not tolerate it much longer. But I still had not found a desirable treatment. I knew there had to be an answer, so I began looking toward holistic approaches for treatment.

I knew about holistic healing because I had been in a serious car accident in 1982 and incorporated a holistic approach to healing during that recovery. It was a long recovery but successful because the treatments I pursued were aimed not only at physical healing but also at many other facets, including mental, emotional, and spiritual. The human body is regenerative, meaning it will heal itself and return to a healthy balanced state if given the proper conditions. Holistic, alternative treatments encompass all facets of healing and use the body's natural regenerative ability to overcome disease and maintain health.

To research alternative treatments for endometriosis, I learned everything I could about diet, nutrition, herbalism, massage, homeopathy, etc., and their application to women's diseases. I began eating a healthy vegetarian diet with proper fatty acids, omitted caffeine, and began using different herbs to control the pain. I investigated different cultures' (Native American and Chinese) approaches to health care. I found that much in our contemporary diet, lifestyle, and socialization contributes to an imbalanced state in our lives, and this can promote disease.

I became very interested in traditional Chinese medicine (TCM) and acupuncture. TCM recognizes there is seldom only one factor involved in the etiology of endometriosis.

I went to see a woman in Minneapolis where I live, a board-certified acupuncturist, who suffered from endometriosis and was helped by acupuncture treatments.

When looking for an acupuncturist, it is important to find someone certified by the National Commission for the Certification of Acupuncturists (NCCA), even if he or she is an M.D. Someone who is not board-certified in acupuncture through NCCA might have only enough knowledge to use it to do simple pain relief. Much knowledge is needed to get at the underlying cause of the disease. Not treating the underlying cause can mean soon after treatments cease the pain and endometrial implants return. Acupuncturists refer to this type of treatment as *cookbook acupuncture*. TCM is complex, requiring a wide knowledge base to use the techniques to heal and not just treat symptoms.

I started weekly acupuncture treatments, began taking Chinese herbs, and had regular shiatsu massage (the Japanese equivalent of acupressure) treatments to correct the energy stagnation. I continued to eat a vegetarian diet. I also made some definite changes in my lifestyle to alleviate stress and removed myself from some unhealthy emotional dynamics. The results have been incredible because, after seven months of weekly treatments, my periods have returned to normal and the symptoms of the endometriosis are gone. I no longer take codeine for pain, nor do I need regular acupuncture treatments. I am healthier from eating a better diet. I no longer suffer from PMS because of the acupuncture, and I am more energetic. My overall health is better.

I do not feel the need to know the theory behind TCM and understand how it works because I have gotten results from it without harmful drugs or mutilating surgery. Western medicine does not hold all our answers to endometriosis. We need to look beyond the sanctioned, orthodox treatments for endometriosis to overcome it. Most important, we must not be looking for a single cause and a single cure. In our struggle to overcome this disease, we must not be afraid to guide our own healing, since each of us is different. We must be willing to examine ourselves and our lives. We must help ourselves by opening up to different options and by making the changes in our lives as needed.

■ *Gail Toussaint, St. Paul, Minnesota, is a member of the Endometriosis Association.*

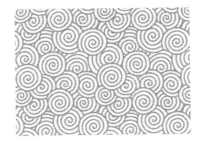

PART III

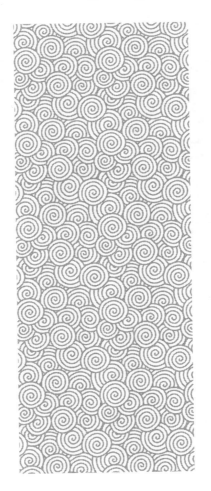

Coping

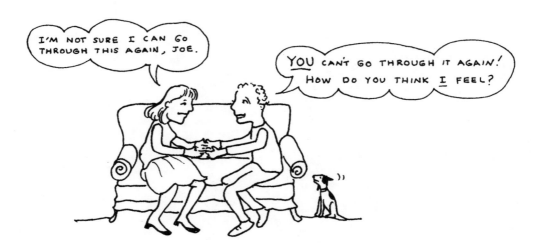

8

Learning to Cope with Endometriosis

By Lynn S. Schwebach
(Research additions by Mary Lou Ballweg)

"*I have just found out that I am not the only person in the world dealing with the pain and frustration of endometriosis! What a wonderful feeling to know that there is a group of people who can help me understand what's happening to my body. . . .*

"*Dealing with physical pain has been (and continues to be) difficult for me. But even more traumatic has been suffering without understanding the cause. Endometriosis seems so intangible. So many of the doctors I saw were unable to pinpoint a reason for my pain. As a result, feelings of frustration have led to serious personal questioning. . . .*"

Beth, Alberta

"*You learn a lot when you are chronically ill. You learn to smile when you hurt, to laugh when you feel despair, to act with strangers, to take one day or sometimes one minute at a time, but most of all you learn how to survive. People who have suffered know the dark side of life, which makes them appreciate the good all the more.*"

Linda, New York

"*Could you do more on emotional support or dealing with the results of illness? Taking the Provera, I have a problem with being tired. I have discovered that if I sleep large chunks of Saturday and Sunday I can work without getting every infection that comes along and missing too much work and getting so tired that it all suffers. My dad is very ill now, and the added stress has me sleeping a lot. It interferes with my life a lot.*

"*I have lost three relationships now from endo/fatigue issues. I've read things from you on marriage problems, but it's definitely a problem to be single. One man wanted to spend more time with me. One man I asked not to call until late on Saturday and Sunday, so he*"

277

just didn't call me anymore at all. One man wasn't willing to be gentle with the lack of lubrication/easy infection side effect of Provera."

Joy, Florida

"*I am deeply touched by EA's recent newsletter dealing with the most real and important issue people with a chronic illness face: 'Who is responsible for the emotional and mental support?!'*

"*After living with endo my entire adult life, I thought I had dealt with all possible facets of this disease. After reading this recent issue I realize . . . the most difficult pain with which to cope is the emotional pain and the lack of support and disbelief of those who have no knowledge of what it's like to live with a chronic disease.*

"*I learned through my trials with endo how important support, true support, is to one who has a chronic disease like endo. Not always was I successful in obtaining support. Not always was my doctor able to provide support. During the early days of my disease I felt, at times, my doctor was holding information back from me, not telling me everything about this disease. There was so much I had to find out for myself. My doctor's support didn't come until a few years later, when I finally knew a little bit more about the disease and could speak up for myself, assert myself comfortably.*

"*The part of the equation that deals with the physical traits of the disease can be solved with public awareness, better-educated doctors, and research. The remaining equation, the equation for the emotional traits of the disease, can be solved only by us, the patients. . . ."*

Jodie, Minnesota

"*It's impacted my relationships, finances, vacations, lifestyle, and my dreams. I even recently lost a job when the manager . . . refused to tolerate my absences."*

Mary Ann, Texas

"*People really don't understand that hormones can change your personality and make you feel lousy in the bargain. It's strange, because I'm sure if you asked someone directly if they thought hormones could affect moods, etc., they'd agree that they could. When it's someone close to them, though, all this goes out the window (or it does in my case anyway). Maybe it's because they're too close and are so alarmed to see you having a bad time that they forget logic. I don't know.*

"*I came very close to hitting someone one night (I'm not usually like that, but she really pushed me too far). I went to a party with people I work with. Well, one of the women had a bit too much to drink. . . . She told me that I had to learn to deal with my illness myself. She said this as if it was some kind of divine revelation that only she'd been privy to. I told her I knew that. She then started telling me how I'd wasted a year of my life by letting this disease take over my life. That's when I got angry. I told her that I didn't waste a year of my life—SOMETHING STOLE IT FROM ME!! I also told her I'd had to endure idiotic doctors, surgery, trips to distant cities just to see a gynecologist who was a moron, hormones, night sweats, and that I really wasn't too keen on any of it. I've had to join associations I didn't want to join, have surgery I didn't want to have, read books I didn't want to read, and cope with a whole load of feelings that I just didn't want to have. . . . Of course, none of this made sense to her (it's not like you can die from it, so what's the big deal? ARRRRGH!). . . .*

"The trauma of all that has happened to me still keeps me up at night sometimes. I've been having a bad time lately, which is why I've been doing so much writing about it. I was afraid to write about it before because I was trying to forget everything. . . .

"I got to the point where I couldn't stop crying (definitely not me), so I phoned one of the crisis call helpers from the Endometriosis Association. I told this very patient woman everything I'd been feeling, and she said it was definitely the danazol. . . .

"Since stopping the drug, I have felt much better mentally and physically, although my periods are still bad. The rest of the month is relatively pain-free, although there are bad days. I seem to be in the middle of a 'remission.' . . ."

Anne, Québec

EDITOR'S NOTE: We urge readers experiencing depression to get help. Anne called an association crisis call listener, a volunteer who has received training to help or at least listen in times of crisis. Members can also call local support group leaders or headquarters. It is important to find someone who hears what you are going through when feeling overwhelmed, depressed, and alone in your pain. Depression is a potential side effect of danazol, and GnRH drugs as well as of persistent pain.

"On the psychological end of things, my relationship with my disease has been a continuous challenge. At first I felt guilty and blaming about it. I thought I had brought it on myself somehow. . . . I thought I was being punished. I was very angry with myself about the whole thing. And my mind would create worst possible scenarios.

"A turning point came when I started to meet and talk with other women who have endometriosis. Shock: the first woman I talked with had a child. She still had endo and had much, much worse symptoms than I. The second woman I talked with had five children. She also had had a hysterectomy. And she still had symptoms . . . terrible pain! Woman number one was beautiful. The main thing I got from talking with her was 'Look, this is just the way it is. Some people have club feet, other people wear eyeglasses, some people get in car wrecks. . . . We have endometriosis.'

"It started to become a very matter-of-fact thing. And then I really began to learn what a common thing it is for women and, again, the isolation, feelings of guilt, and impending doom lessened. Shock number two: when I finally told my mother about this, she said, 'Oh, yes, I used to get terrible pains . . . ,' the same kind. That hastened the healing process for me, learning that. Suddenly I realized the possibility that it was simply hereditary. My mother had it; I have it. What to do? It certainly didn't kill her. And she doesn't have it any-

more. Hmm, I thought, that means it's likely I won't get worse as I age, but better. Whether it's true or not, it's a much healthier, happier, nourishing thought than the opposite. And nice to have a living example of improvement. . . .

"While this disease has brought with it a good deal of physical pain over the years, it has also been a 'poke in the ribs,' always reminding me to look carefully at my life. At the most fundamental level it reminds me of my mortality, it encourages me to meditate, it tells me to look carefully at the question of kids, relationships, and my own form as a woman. It tells me when I'm under too much pressure, and it thanks me when I find places and spaces where my whole being can relax."

Linda, Colorado

"The disease has turned everything upside down in my life, and the only comfort my husband and I found was in each other and your organization."

Karen, Ontario

Somehow in today's trendy world the concept of *coping* has become distorted. Quick-fix marketers, overzealous fitness promoters, and self-help authors all aid in the distortion. They propose easy answers, checklists, and menus for coping with many of life's hardships. But those who have suffered with a chronic illness like endometriosis know there isn't one simple solution.

Coping with endometriosis is very complicated, says Rona Silverton, Ph.D., a psychotherapist in private practice in New York City who has endo herself. "There isn't a prescription for coping," she says. "People use a number of strategies to cope, and different strategies work at different times."

When asked to define coping, many longtime sufferers of the illness hesitate. "Cope?" asks Carol Kendall of Sandstone, Minnesota. "I don't know, maybe I coped; I think maybe I just existed." After pausing for a brief second, she reconsiders her definition and talks of the strength and support she receives from her children, husband, church, and a support group. She says that acupuncture has eased some of the pain and talks about becoming more aggressive with the medical establishment. All of these things, she supposes, have helped her "cope."

A 16-year sufferer who wishes to be identified only as Loretto from Toronto says of coping: "You do and you don't." She finds her strength in a close friend, the Endometriosis Association, and some personal lifestyle changes.

To many women the word *coping* signifies something different from how they actually live their lives. They don't imagine themselves as having it all together, living life as if the disease didn't exist. Instead they search constantly for more effective ways of living with the disease.

Dr. Silverton offers a better definition for coping: "It's the thoughts and the methods used to manage stressful events," she says. "While most of us may conceive of coping as the ability to overcome major problems in life, it may be more helpful to view coping as a process made up of a variety of strategies called into play when facing stressful events."

Given time and reflective thought, most women can tell others how they managed through years of pain, discomfort, and even depression. Many women share fundamental coping strategies, and most feel that something can be gained from hearing how other women live with endometriosis.

Each woman interviewed for this article, for instance, emphasized the need to become an active participant in health care relationships and medical treatments. Most agree that friendships and a support network, including support groups, are essential. And many find comfort in spiritual practices. In conjunction with traditional medical care, many recommend alternatives such as acupuncture, keeping a journal, healthy eating, and visualization.

But many caution against enthusiastically diving into only one approach or alternative treatment. It takes finding the correct balance of several techniques for most women to cope successfully. The idea, according to these women and psychologists specializing in this area, is to pick and choose and find what works for each individual.

Taking Control of Your Medical Treatment

Over the last 20 years many women with endo have, unfortunately, experienced the worst of the health care system. They have endured the trials of misdiagnosis, been told that the pain is "all in their head," and undergone emotional and financial stress from endless tests, medications, and surgeries.

In addition many women have hesitated to question their doctors about surgeries, medications, and alternatives to prescribed treatments. The physical and emotional aspects of dealing with the disease weigh heavily, they have discovered, when they have not adequately investigated treatments or searched for answers. Only the individual woman knows how endo has affected the most personal aspects of her life, and only she can bring order back into a life that appears to have been turned inside out.

Peggy O'Brien from South Dennis, Massachusetts, says that she was told from age 14 that menstrual pain was "just something women had to buck up and learn to live with. I was told that this was a woman's lot in life and once you got married and had a baby you wouldn't have to worry about these nasty little menstrual cramps."

O'Brien, now 41 and unmarried, was first diagnosed with endometriosis at age 29. Finally, 12 years after her first diagnosis and after 27 years of vomiting and painful periods, she has found a good doctor. The first doctor to diagnose her disease was not a communicator; he did the diagnostic laparoscopy and found the disease "to kind of shut me up," she says.

But back then she did not take an active role in her health care; she simply followed the doctor's lead. Things have changed. "Now I'm an active partner. I'm hungry for any information at all about the disease. This enables me to make the best decision possible for myself. The doctor advises, and I listen, but ultimately I make the decision."

Carol Kendall, quoted earlier, was finally diagnosed with endometriosis at age 46, after being misdiagnosed and treated for interstitial cystitis (IC) for 18 years. IC is a chronic inflammation of the bladder and shares many of the symptoms of endo. (See Chapter 5, "Endometriosis and the Urinary Tract.") "I was in so much pain that I couldn't eat and I couldn't sleep. I couldn't even function; I couldn't live with the pain it was so bad," Kendall says with a strain in her voice.

One doctor told Kendall that she had "phantom" pain; another told her that she wanted stroking from her husband. She went from doctor to doctor until, at age 46, she was told that she didn't have IC. The shock of this discovery after 18 long painful years was overwhelming.

In two years she had five surgeries relating to endometriosis, one of which was a hysterectomy. Once a passive person, Kendall says that she doesn't take "garbage" from doctors anymore. "They are either kind to me, or I don't go back, or I tell them what I think," she says.

Deborah Every, Psy.D., a clinical psychologist in Oceanside, California, who has endo, encourages women to take control of their doctor-patient relationship. Women with endo lose so much control over other aspects of their lives that it's imperative they try to take hold of what they can.

Researchers agree. Caryn E. Lerman, Ph.D., a health psychologist and researcher at Fox Chase Cancer Center in Philadelphia, has studied the relationship among better health, feelings of control, and psychological adjustment. She conducted a study measuring breast cancer patients' perceptions of their communication with doctors and their psychological adjustment. Patients who had a more positive outlook and perceived themselves as more assertive adjusted better to medical treatment. Those who perceived themselves as less assertive were more pessimistic and felt less in control; they adjusted less well to treatment.

"People who score high on an assertiveness measure are people who, in a variety of situations, are able to ask for what they want as opposed to being more passive. If somebody does something that upsets them, they'll be more likely to say something about it or try to change the situation," Lerman says.

Another study of women with breast cancer found that those who confronted the disease with a fighting spirit survived longer than those who responded with stoic acceptance. And a study of melanoma patients found that assertiveness and the ability to express emotions seemed to improve their chances for survival.

Peggy Chumbley of San Francisco has had endo for 16 years and says that once she got past the daunting task of doing her own medical research she felt ready to fight. For many the arduous task of sorting through a world of scientific terms and articles is overwhelming. But, Chumbley says, after finding her way through the library, she was "ready for war."

Over the years Peggy wrote to each doctor and health care provider for copies of her medical records. Once she found a statement in a surgical report that said she was highly addicted to drugs. She went to the surgeon and told him that he was "absolutely wrong," and she successfully demanded that he take it out of the report.

Peggy says that she visits doctors armed with information. "I take comfort in doing research on endo and becoming educated. I tell the doctor, 'Look what I've found; I want you to tell me about this.'"

Any woman who characterizes herself as a passive person should take a friend or relative with her to her doctor's appointments. Sometimes an impartial ear can help sort through the facts and emotions. If she can't say what she feels to a doctor's face, writing a letter can help. Some women advise taking a tape recorder to the doctor's office so that they can go back later and review the conversation.

Finding Support and Support Groups

Those who choose to take a friend or relative with them to the doctor must find someone who truly understands the serious nature of endo. Dr. Every says that perhaps more than other illnesses endo elicits inappropriate responses. Some people classify endo as one of those "female problems," which undoubtedly leads to bizarre statements like "Just relax; you worry too much" or "Don't give in to your pain."

Acknowledging that there is pain is a positive first step in dealing with it. You can't deal with something if you don't acknowledge it exists. Some people fear that accepting the existence of pain will lead to a life of isolation or loneliness. In reality, however, it helps lead to a new life with an awareness of what you can and cannot endure. You can plan for and around the pain if you're aware of it, and you can work to obtain relief if you acknowledge it. Comments such as "Don't give in to the pain" are stressful and will only make you feel worse. Therefore it's important to seek help only from someone who can view endo realistically.

Providing friends and family members with articles about endo may help, advises Dr. Every. "However, you might have to exclude those who don't understand, remain uneducated, or continue to make unsettling remarks," she says.

Women with endo must find people who understand and listen to them. The disease causes such emotional distress that no woman can cope totally on her own. This is where support groups such as those sponsored by the Endometriosis Association can help.

Peggy O'Brien started a support group in Massachusetts in 1991. Fortunately she receives a lot of support from family, friends, and co-workers, but women from the group have given her a lot of strength and courage as well. She finds great strength when she can help another woman by listening and empathizing. "They give me the drive to keep going, to get the awareness out there, to keep the education going, to keep trying to reach out," O'Brien says.

Association member Jodie Peschl of St. Cloud, Minnesota, wrote: "Little did I know I was going to get as much out of the support groups as I was giving."

When San Francisco member Peggy Chumbley found out that other women suffer with endo, it changed her life. In 1986, after suffering for 11 years, Chumbley was watching an evening medical show. The doctor talked about endometriosis and provided the address of the Endometriosis Association. "I can't tell you how happy I was that I was not alone. Up until that point I thought I was the only person in the world with this disease. Discovering that I wasn't was the most awesome feeling I've ever gone through."

Contacting the association and using it as a resource helped Chumbley through a "low point" in her life. Support groups can help women through the rough times that many endo sufferers experience. These groups provide a setting for women to feel that they're not abnormal, that others have the same feelings, emotions, and personal struggles. It's a gathering not to garner sympathy but to try to regain self-esteem. As a *Washington Post* article on the rapid growth of the self-help movement noted, "What self-help groups seem to be good at doing is imparting a sense of control, and helping participants feel 'normal.'" They do this, notes the article, in part by making the person affected by the problem the key player rather than the more passive patient or client that traditional group therapy with a professional leader does.

Seeing others in the group who cope successfully helps give group members the confidence it can be done. Discovering that there are many wonderful women with endo also helps restore self-esteem. The traditional model is simply a repeat of the self-esteem-destroying medical model that has hurt so many women with endo.

Sally Berg, co–executive director of SHARE, a U.S. national support and educational program for women with breast and ovarian cancer, says support groups are important for everyone, even those who receive a lot of support from family. "Just talking to someone who has survived the disease and who is familiar with the medical treatments is terribly reassuring. . . . It's a place to come where people truly understand what you are going through. No matter how supportive your family is, it's not the same thing as sitting next to another woman who has lost her hair [due to cancer treatment]."

Support Groups Appear to Improve Physical Health

Some researchers believe that there may be an important link between support groups and overall physical health. David Spiegel, M.D., professor of psychiatry and behavioral sciences at Stanford University, studied 86 women with breast cancer, half of whom received standard medical care plus attended support groups for a year, and half who just received standard medical care. The women in the support group were encouraged to share their feelings and also learned self-hypnosis for pain control. Dr. Spiegel found that the women who were randomly assigned to a support group lived almost twice as long as those who did not attend a support group. The women who attended the support group were also less depressed, felt less pain, and had a more positive outlook than the women who received only conventional treatment.

In another study, reported in the *Washington Post* article on self-help groups mentioned earlier, high-risk patients with chronic emphysema, bronchitis, or asthma who attended a self-help group were hospitalized less frequently and for fewer days than a comparable group of people who did not attend the self-help group. In a study sure to bolster the spirits of those struggling with infertility, the University of Massachusetts Medical School studied 102 infertile couples over three years and found that participation in a support group significantly increased the likelihood of pregnancy, regardless of the reason for infertility or the treatment course pursued.

Helping others also may help strengthen the immune system, certainly good news for women with endo. One study found that even a film clip of Mother Teresa helping the sick and dying in India temporarily boosted the immune systems of students who watched it. A number of psychologists in a *Psychology Today* article say there is mounting evidence that helping others strengthens the immune system. More scientific studies are needed on this intriguing connection.

A more subtle benefit of support groups occurs when women begin to feel that they are, in some way, helping other women cope with the disease. Kenneth Maton, Ph.D., associate professor of psychology at the University of Maryland, has studied support group dynamics for many years. His research indicates that individuals who are highly involved in the groups as both givers and receivers of support benefit most from them. Such participants reported "greater well-being than those who are only on the providing or the receiving end of support," says Maton.

Many researchers have found that those who have meaningful roles in groups regain self-esteem and a feeling of purpose in life. "It just helps people feel good to help others," Maton says.

Another benefit is that sharing ideas, advice, and experiences helps people solidify their own coping mechanisms. Sharing coping strategies increases their own commitment to those adaptive strategies.

"And just giving to others helps them feel connected to the group; it helps them feel a sense of community and a sense of belonging," Maton says. All these benefits probably help explain why an estimated half million self-help support groups exist in the U.S. alone according to the previously mentioned *Washington Post* article.

Stress and the Mind-Body Connection

Support groups help women deal with the stress associated with endo, but for many years stress was unfortunately called the culprit of this disease. Many doctors believed that stress diabolically left its imprint with endometriosis, which had the devastating effect of making women feel responsible for instigating the illness.

"Women shouldn't hold themselves responsible for this disease," advises Dr. Silverton, "yet they do. More than any other disease, endo elicits feelings of self-doubt, self-blame, and guilt. Even when women know that the disease was physiologically induced and that it wasn't stress-related, they feel, psychologically, that they somehow brought it on themselves."

Women blame themselves for past abortions, inadequate feelings about sex, their high-powered careers, their decision to put off marriage and family. But there is no scientific evidence of a link between stress or any one life event and the onset of endometriosis.

On the other hand, endo *causes* extreme stress. It plays havoc with relationships, careers, marriages, pastimes, and fertility. And the stress that affects almost every aspect of a woman's life exacerbates pain. A woman may, for example, tense her muscles while in pain or in a stressful situation, causing more pain.

Because of the physical reactions associated with stress, scientists have engaged in a relatively new field of research to find the link between emotions and health. In a study examining the link between the immune system and negative emotions, researchers found that those who confronted traumatic experiences by writing about them had better-working immune systems than those who did not write about such experiences.

The study, conducted by Janice Kiecolt-Glaser, a psychologist at Ohio State University College of Medicine; Ronald Glaser, an immunologist and associate director for research at the same school; and James Pennebaker, a psychologist at Southern Methodist University, was groundbreaking. Fifty undergraduate students were divided into two groups and asked to write about either personal traumatic experiences or superficial topics. For four consecutive days the students wrote in journals. Blood was drawn the day before they started writing, after the last writing session, and again six weeks later. Students writing about traumatic experiences were directed to (1) just vent their emotions, (2) just write down the facts, or (3) write about facts and emotions at the same time. They wrote for 15 minutes a day over four days. The immediate impact was often painful for the students, some of whom cried as they wrote, but after a few hours or days they felt better.

"The findings were unequivocal," wrote Pennebaker in an article for *American Health* magazine. "People who wrote thoughtfully and emotionally about traumatic experiences showed heightened immune function compared with those who wrote about superficial topics." Pennebaker said that "writing seems to produce as much therapeutic benefit as sessions with a psychotherapist."

In the months following the writing sessions the researchers found that the trauma-writing students visited the health center for illness less often than the others. Only the students who had written about *both* facts and emotions experienced this healing benefit, while the students who wrote only about their emotions surrounding a trauma or only about the facts did not. Researchers concluded that by confronting upsetting events participants no longer felt as if they were holding these experiences in, thereby reducing long-term stress. It also allowed these participants to put the event in perspective, reframing it, making it more manageable, and finding some meaning for it. The researchers found significantly higher levels of T cells (immune cells) among people who wrote about traumatic experiences.

"By translating the experience into language," Pennebaker says, "people begin to organize and structure the surge of overwhelming thoughts. Once organized, they are easier to resolve." Many women write the association long letters sharing both the facts and emotions of their endo experiences. Perhaps this study helps explain why sharing their stories helps.

What boosting T cells might mean in a disease such as endo, where the T cells themselves are involved in some way, is obviously an important question that we cannot answer yet.

Drs. Kiecolt-Glaser and Glaser have continued intensive research into the link between the mind and the immune system. Recently they studied 90 couples who were asked to resolve a disagreement. In a laboratory setting blood was monitored continuously for 24 hours. Those couples who showed a lot of hostility and negativity during the discussions showed a drop on eight immune measures for the next 24 hours. In another case they studied medical students during the stress of final examinations and found that students who had close relationships with others had stronger immune responses to vaccinations.

Another researcher, Dr. Sheldon Cohen, psychologist at Carnegie-Mellon University in Pittsburgh, found in a study of macaque monkeys that "affiliation protects animals from the potentially pathogenic [disease-causing] influence of chronic stress." Monkeys that engaged in affiliation behaviors—touching other monkeys, grooming them, or simply sitting close to them—were found to have stronger immune responses after a period of stress, while the most hostile and aggressive monkeys had the poorest.

All these studies showing that there is a connection between the mind and the immune system do *not* show that humans can prevent or cure diseases, researchers in the budding new field of psychoneuroimmunology (the study of the links between psychological states and the immune response) point out. "To claim that negative thoughts somehow cause disease or that happy thoughts can heal by helping the immune system is premature," says Robert Ader, the scientist who coined the term *psychoneuroimmunology*. "There's simply not the slightest scientific evidence that it's true." But the studies do seem to show that certain responses help us cope with disease better. It may be, an article on the subject in the September 1992 *Hippocrates* magazine states, that patients with a fighting spirit push themselves harder to do the things that help them survive.

Stress and Pain Management

So how do women with endo relax, handle stress, and relieve pain? Besides traditional drugs and therapy, many have turned to alternative health care practices. Carol Kendall of Minnesota visits an acupuncturist about once every three weeks. She says that this ancient Chinese treatment gives her energy while helping her relax.

Helen Beer of Matthews, North Carolina, says that she has stopped taking over-the-counter and prescription pain relievers. She has started eating more healthily, taking gamma-linolenic acid, an essential fatty acid that promotes healthy skin and teeth and the integrity of cell membranes, and taking vitamins and other supplements. (A section on evening primrose oil as a source of certain essential fatty acids appears in the association's first book, *Overcoming Endometriosis*.)

To help her cope with pain, she keeps a daily medical diary. "It's a pragmatic description of what's happening with my body so I can go back and say, 'OK, that lasted only a couple of hours, and it passed.'" There's a real cycle to her pain, Beer says, and once she started recognizing the pattern it was a lot easier to handle. Pain doesn't come as a surprise to her any longer. If it's day 18, she realizes that some pain may start occurring. She also uses the diary as ammunition when visiting the doctor.

Angie Perrault of Orion, near Detroit, claims that a form of creative visualization helps her deal not only with endo but with many other aspects of her life as well. She made an "image board," a collage of images of the way she wanted to be: pictures showing healthy people and inspirational sayings. It hangs on a wall where she can look at it every day.

Perrault believes strongly in the image concept. Because she had been taking Depo-Provera, a drug that can possibly prevent the return of menstruation, she was worried that she would never get her period again. Only 27 and unmarried, she still hopes to have children someday. After eight months without menstruation, her period returned the day after she hung her board.

She also incorporates the concept of positive self-talk. "The more you concentrate on anything, that's what you get more of. So instead of concentrating on 'I don't want endo,' concentrate on 'I want to be healthy. I will have normal cycles.'" Using negatives only causes women to tense their muscles and experience more pain, she says.

And finally, Peggy Chumbley visits a pain clinic once or twice a week for acupuncture treatments and electro stimuli therapy, a heat therapy to help with the pain caused by adhesions from her prior surgeries. She also has started taking vitamin B_{12} shots, which she believes increase her energy level.

Each of these women states that simply using these techniques does not make the pain disappear but does help take her mind off the pain or the anticipation of it. Angie Perrault emphatically believes that a woman must give her full faith and effort for the practice to have a fair chance to work—in other words call on the power of positive thinking.

Reaffirmation of Healthy Functioning

Trying to address all the aspects of life affected by endo often leaves women and their families overwhelmed. Yet many women come to appreciate the strength they gain from having to conquer and cope with these changes in lifestyle, career, and family plans.

Dr. Rona Silverton conducted one of the most comprehensive psychological studies to date on coping with endo. She studied a group of 30 association members who were suffering with endo: 10 were chronically ill despite treatment, 10 were experiencing a recurrence after remission or treatment, and 10 had recently been diagnosed. She uncovered 13 coping strategies in this sample group (enumerated in the next article in this chapter). Of these 13 strategies one coined by Silverton as "reaffirmation of healthy functioning" was used by 35 percent of the women.

These women employed a "take charge" approach to dealing with endo; they were active despite pain, possessed a positive attitude, and appeared better adjusted than those showing no signs of this response. Silverton says the attitude is characterized by eating healthily, exercising, or relying on other stress reduction techniques, and focusing on well-being with appropriate self-care actions.

"Some of the women with the most severe symptoms used the reaffirmation strategy, and they seemed to do better," Silverton says. Overall these women were less depressed and anxious. Within reason these women focused their thoughts on being functional, on doing as much as possible. They focused less on the fear of becoming dysfunctional. They took action by getting involved in their medical care and by trying to live healthy lifestyles. Although Silverton is quick to point out that her study didn't clearly state that the reaffirmation of healthy functioning caused a better outcome, it suggests that the women using this strategy had a better adjustment.

Perhaps a better adjustment is what each woman with endo hopes to achieve. Many have reaffirmed their commitment to living lives as rich and functional as possible. They have determined that life, after all, is worth living—with or without endo.

■ *Lynn S. Schwebach, Laramie, Wyoming, is a freelance writer and desktop publishing specialist. After several years of misdiagnosis, pain, and infertility, she was correctly diagnosed with endometriosis in 1991.*

Silent Enemy

By Michelle Walden

Endo what?
Endometriosis.
No, you're not in my mind
You're in my body
Your long tentacles reaching into every nook and cranny of my body
First you seem to invade small parts of my body and life
Then progress insidiously to take and take
Organ by organ
You ruin my love life
I have to cut you from my flesh
I have to swallow drugs to fight you
And all the while you're only naked through machines
Invisible to the human eye.

I have some relief from you now
Now that you have my uterus, fallopian tubes, ovaries, appendix
And not yet my bowel
Although you tried to get it.
May no one have to know you, *my silent enemy*
Oh! I forgot you took my most important need
My opportunity to have a child
Is there anything you won't do?
You give me pain, surgery, drugs
You, my silent enemy.

May you be exposed to the human race for the monster of the deep that you are.
No, you will not take my sanity,
My faith in the Lord or
My kindness to humanity.
You will not make me bitter and twisted.
I will fight to protect people from you and with research my ambition is
To immobilize you
You, my silent enemy.

■ **Michelle Walden** *is a member of the Australian Endometriosis Association.*

Coping Strategies Used by Women with Endometriosis

By Lynn S. Schwebach

Dr. Rona Silverton, a psychoanalyst with a doctorate in clinical social work and member of the association, studied women with endo to learn more about how they cope. She uncovered the 13 strategies listed here from a range of women coping with endo. These 13 strategies clustered into two groups: a type of passive-dependent coping associated with poorer adjustment and a type of active-independent coping associated with healthier adjustment.

Dr. Silverton cautions women, however, not to simply categorize these strategies into positive or negative ways of coping. One strategy may be helpful in one context and hurtful in another. For example, avoidance or social withdrawal can help a woman feel better when experiencing acute pain or sickness; however, such strategies could be detrimental if they lead to giving up and not seeking the necessary medical treatment or social support.

The four most frequently used strategies were problem solving, seeking out social support, tension release, and avoidance. As stated in the preceding article, about 35 percent of the women studied used the "reaffirmation of healthy functioning" strategy, a more active approach to coping that also was associated with better adjustment. Helplessness/passive resignation, social withdrawal, and negativism (passive-dependent strategies) were associated significantly with worse adjustment. Overall, Dr. Silverton's study suggested that women who employed active coping strategies "rose to the challenge," felt more in control, and had a more enhanced ability to live with the disease.

The 13 coping strategies identified by Dr. Silverton in the study "Psychological Adjustment and Coping Strategies of Women with Endometriosis" are:

1. **Denial**. Some women used this strategy to cope with particular aspects of the disease, such as threat of recurrence, concerns of chronicity, or infertility. Women using this method delayed getting medical treatment or more information about the disease and tended to deny the chronic nature of the disease.

2. **Optimism**. Women displayed a "hopeful, positive attitude" or "looked on the bright side."

3. **Negativism**. Women dwelled on bad consequences and anticipated the worst outcome.

4. **Acceptance**. Women were hopeful while at the same time realistic about the disease; they displayed a balanced outlook.

5. **Selective Ignoring**. Women focused on the positive consequences of having the illness, a strategy characterized by attitudes such as "I have endo, and it's a big problem, but this crisis brought me closer to my family or friends."

6. **Reaffirmation of Healthy Functioning**. A global mental attitude that changes women's perceptions about the threat of this disease. Women placed emphasis on staying healthy and functional rather than focusing on the fear of becoming dysfunctional. Women displaying this strategy acted in ways they felt were health promoting, such as eating healthily, exercising, and relying on stress reduction techniques. This strategy helped women build an internal image of being in control.

7. **Avoidance**. Women who used this coping strategy tried to relieve pain or anxiety-provoking aspects of endo by distracting themselves or pushing endo-related stress out of their minds. Activities to escape, such as reading, sleeping, and watching television, were used.

8. **Tension Release**. Some women had to "let go" or "vent their emotions." Having a good cry is an example of this strategy. Tension release was used to let out anger, sadness, and despair over stresses such as delays in obtaining a diagnosis, physical pain, and interference with goal achievement.

9. **Withdrawal**. Taking to bed, avoiding friends, family, or other women with the illness, was typical of this strategy.

10. **Seeking Out Social Support**. Women who displayed this strategy would attend support groups and/or seek support from friends, family, doctors, and co-workers.

11. **Passive Resignation**. Women employing this strategy demonstrated helplessness and passivity. They wanted to be taken care of by family, friends, and their physicians. In extreme cases they relied on others to make decisions for them.

12. **Problem Solving**. Several women who used this strategy adopted an active "take charge" attitude toward their own medical care and treatment. They typically became walking encyclopedias on the illness. They also were willing to try nontraditional treatments, such as acupuncture, diet, and creative hobbies. These women tried a variety of behaviors that they believed would master stress and worry.

13. **Reordering of Priorities and Goals**. The illness is used to change something about what is important to the woman in her goals such as the time frame for major decisions about childbearing, marriage, relationships, or career planning. In some cases the woman described making a concerted effort to achieve childbearing goals earlier or balancing them with career goals.

How to Get Sick

- Don't pay attention to your body. Eat plenty of junk food, drink too much, cut short your sleep—and, above all, feel guilty about it. If you are overstressed and tired, ignore it and keep pushing yourself.
- Think of your life as meaningless and of little value.
- Do things you don't like and avoid doing what you really want. Follow everyone else's opinion and advice. See yourself as miserable and "stuck."
- Be resentful and hypercritical, especially toward yourself.
- Fill your mind with dreadful pictures and then obsess over them. Worry most, if not all, of the time.
- Avoid deep, lasting, intimate relationships.
- Blame other people for all your problems.
- Do not express your feelings and views openly and honestly. Others won't appreciate it. If at all possible, don't even know what your feelings are.
- Shun anything that resembles a sense of humor. Life is no laughing matter!
- Avoid making any changes that would bring you greater satisfaction and joy.

How to Stay Well (or Get Better)

- Do things that bring you a sense of fulfillment, joy, and purpose. See your life as your own creation and strive to make it a positive one.
- Pay close and loving attention to yourself, tuning in to all your needs. Take care of yourself, nourishing, supporting, and encouraging yourself.
- Release all negative emotions—resentment, envy, fear, sadness, anger. Express your feelings; don't hold on to them. Forgive yourself.
- Hold positive images and goals in your mind, pictures of what you truly want in life.
- When fearful images arise, focus on images that evoke feelings of peace or joy.
- Love yourself and love everyone else. Make loving the purpose and primary expression in your life.
- Create fun, loving, honest relationships, allowing for the expression and fulfillment of needs for intimacy and security. Try to heal wounds in past relationships.
- Make a positive contribution to your community through work and service that you value and enjoy.
- Make a commitment to health and well-being and develop a belief in the possibility of total health. Develop your own healing program, drawing on the support and advice of experts without becoming enslaved to them.
- Accept yourself and everything in your life as an opportunity for growth and learning. Be grateful. When you screw up, forgive yourself, learn what you can from the experience, and then move on.
- Keep a sense of humor.

■ *"How to Get Sick" and "How to Stay Well (or Get Better)" are reprinted by permission from* Surviving and Thriving with AIDS: Hints for the Newly Diagnosed, *by Steven James (New York: The People with AIDS Coalition, Inc. 1987). New People with AIDS Coalition of New York, 50 West 17th Street, 8th floor, New York, NY 10011.*

9

⊚⊚

"It's All in Your Head"

By Mary Lou Ballweg

"*I am 27 years old. My endometriosis was discovered when I was 13. So for the past 14 years (over half my life) I have been living with it. Fourteen years ago very little was known about the illness. Also because I was so young, the doctors couldn't believe I had it. From the age of 13–17 they called my problem cystic ovaries, Stein-Leventhal syndrome [polycystic ovarian disease], and multiple other names.*

"*They didn't tell me I had endometriosis because they thought this occurred only in 'career women' and not in young girls. They did, however, suggest to my mother that I have a complete hysterectomy. When she refused, they gave me birth control pills—all this at the age of 13. One doctor asked how often I had intercourse. I didn't know what that meant; I still played with dolls. When I was 13, we were still kids, not like the 13-year-old girls today.*

"*I had multiple pelvic exams when I was 13. It hurt and scared me. It made me feel dirty. Sometimes they let my mom be with me during the exams and hold my hand, but most of the time they wouldn't.*

"*Also between the ages of 13 and 17 they [the doctors] decided I had a mental problem—a conduct disorder. The doctors said I was using this pain as a way to get attention. They told me this was all in my head—even after several laparoscopies that showed I had the disease. I was hospitalized in a mental hospital twice. I was given antipsychotic medication and heavy doses of tranquilizers. The doctors told my parents that I had a fear of menstruation, and they [doctors] told them I became hysterical when I had my monthly period. Yet all along the medical doctors knew I had this physical problem.*

"*When I was 17, I was referred (again) to another doctor. This doctor did a laparotomy that lasted three hours. He said I had the worst case of endo he had ever seen. . . . He told me my pain was real and not in my head.*"

Susan, Texas

"*In my case it took eight internists, two gastroenterologists, and five gynecologists before my endo was diagnosed even though I had 'visible' symptoms (a high fever for five months, constant vomiting, diarrhea, and internal bleeding). Although I had not seen a doctor in 15 years, I was given the gamut of diagnoses from hypochondria to cancer to anxiety attacks to my age and marital status being a factor and was even told at one point that I had these problems because I did not have a date for that Saturday night! . . .*"

Karen, Pennsylvania

"*One physician told me that in his 20 years of clinical practice he had found that 90 percent of his patients' menstrual complaints were due to psychological problems. He informed me that if I got married and had a child, my symptoms would go away (I am in my early thirties). Finally, I found a female internist/endocrinologist specializing in infertility who listened carefully to my history (a first). . . .*"

Robin, New York

What do the following symptoms describe?
- pain during menstruation
- irregular menstrual periods
- excessive menstrual bleeding
- pain during sexual intercourse
- pain in the abdomen (other than when menstruating)
- nausea
- bloating
- diarrhea
- intolerance of several different foods
- back pain
- pain during urination
- urinary retention

They describe endometriosis, right? Wrong. According to the American Psychiatric Association, these symptoms, taken together or in combination with others not listed here, describe a mental disorder called *somatization disorder*.[1] Somatization disorder occurs, according to the psychiatrists, when the patient has underlying psychological factors or conflicts causing the symptoms rather than true physical disease. It affects primarily females, according to the standard diagnostic manual used by mental health practitioners, and "occurs only rarely in males in the United States."[2] The manual is called the *Diagnostic and Statistical Manual of Mental Disorders (DSM)*,[3] and is considered the bible of the profession. A patient can be diagnosed with somatization disorder, according to this manual, if a doctor finds no physical reason for the patient's symptoms.

The *DSM* does acknowledge that the symptoms on its list[4] could be caused by lupus, multiple sclerosis, hyperparathyroidism, and porphyria and that those diseases are in the differential diagnosis. (*Differential diagnoses* means a physician should, in theory, rule the other diagnoses out before the mental diagnosis is made.) But in real life little attention seems to be given to ensuring accurate evaluation. No specific measures are noted to be sure the physician has even considered those diagnoses; some of the medical articles on the disorder fail even to mention these physical diseases (none, of course, mention endometriosis at all); and no awareness of the great difficulty in diagnosing multiple sclerosis and lupus, for example, is indicated. One article written by psychiatrists for the *Journal of Family Practice* even states: "Only a one-hour outpatient evaluation is required to make the diagnosis [of somatization]."[5] Nor is there any indication of awareness of the studies showing that women are not given the same legitimacy in the medical system as men.

Who Does Somatization Affect?

Somatization disorders are said to affect up to 2 percent of women. The *DSM* states, "Symptoms usually begin in the teen years or, rarely, in the 20s. *Menstrual difficulties may be one of the earliest symptoms in females*"[6] (emphasis added). There is also said to be a family pattern to the disorder—the *DSM* says the disorder is observed in 10 to 20 percent of female first-degree biologic relatives (daughters, mothers, and sisters) of females with somatization disorder.[7] In an amazingly illogical statement, the revised third edition of the *DSM* also states, "Although most people without mental disorders at various times have aches and pains and other physical complaints, they rarely bring them to medical attention."[8] Does this mean that only people with mental disorders seek medical attention? Or that symptoms of endometriosis, lupus, and multiple sclerosis are trivial "aches and pains"?

Given the symptoms listed in the *DSM*, the long delays most women face in obtaining a diagnosis of endometriosis, and the frequent lack of knowledge about endometriosis, it would be easy to label most women with endometriosis, especially before diagnosis, with "somatization disorder." Any unfortunate girl or woman with these or other complaints listed in the *DSM*, who has sought medical help for her symptoms but not been diagnosed (even if she has not had a laparoscopy), could be labeled with this mental disorder. The consequences of this label, as seen in the introductory quotations, can be devastating.

In fact, even a woman or girl who has been diagnosed with endometriosis could be given the label if her complaints or social or occupational impairment is judged "in excess of what would be expected from the history, physical examination, or laboratory findings."[9] We are all aware of the lack of a consistent direct relationship between the amount of misplaced endometrial tissue and symptoms of endometriosis (that is, some women with lots of lesions have few symptoms and some with tiny or few lesions have many or severe symptoms).

Even if a woman or girl with endometriosis doesn't have enough of the symptoms listed for somatization disorder, she could be labeled with "undifferentiated somatoform disorder." To meet these criteria, symptoms must persist for six months or longer. According to the *DSM*, "this is a residual category for those persistent somatoform presentations that do not meet the full criteria for Somatization Disorder or another Somatoform Disorder."[10]

And, should she not yet have the symptoms for at least six months, she can still be "diagnosed" with "somatoform disorder not otherwise specified"—which will cover just about anything that doesn't fit the criteria for the other diagnoses![11] (Where there's a will, there's a way: slap on a label and bill away.)

When I first stumbled across articles in medical journals on somatization disorder many years ago, I was horrified. No wonder, when a physician sent a woman with symptoms of endometriosis to a psychiatrist or psychologist (who is likely to know even less about endo than the referring physician), the woman often is told that her problems are in her head. (Of course the referring physician has already come to that conclusion or presumably would not have sent the woman to a mental health practitioner.) And no wonder that so many gynecologists and family practitioners dismiss women with endometriosis without thorough evaluation—in addition to limited teaching about endometriosis and exposure to it during training, the climate of dismissal of these symptoms and judgmental labeling is strongly reinforced by mental health specialists.

Some 70 percent of women coming to the association have been told at least once, in one form or another, that their symptoms are in their heads. Nancy Petersen, R.N., manager of the Endometriosis Treatment Program in Bend, Oregon, has also noted that about 75 percent of the program's patients have been told that their symptoms are in their heads. And a study carried out at the Institute for the Study and Treatment of Endometriosis in Chicago found that the majority of women were told they were overreacting to the pain and their symptoms were psychological in origin.[12]

According to the psychologists, "patients with somatization disorder experience emotional discomfort and psychosocial distress, which are expressed as primarily physical symptoms."[13] Why would these patients express emotional discomfort through physical symptoms, according to the psychiatrists? First, to obtain "gratifications that the patient finds otherwise unobtainable. . . . Somatizations are viewed as defense mechanisms to resolve conflicting emotions (e.g., dependency versus autonomy) or as manifestations of a latent need for nurturance and support, which the patient obtains from the medical community."[14] Obviously the people who came up with this idea have spent little time in the typical busy doctor's office—what precious little support might rarely be available in a few doctors' offices is certainly not worth the price. Few people would take time from work and other parts of their lives, wait for long periods of time to see the physician, pay the high costs involved, sometimes even put up with ignorance and rudeness, share intimate and taboo symptoms, and subject themselves to a pelvic exam unless they had the motivation of painful, life-disrupting symptoms driving them to seek answers.

A second explanation given for why patients somatize is they exaggerate or misinterpret their perceptions of normal bodily sensations. This explanation ties in with the general medical community's belief that women are not accurate reporters of their own symptoms and are more likely to have psychogenic disorders. The most famous study of this problem, reported in the *Journal of the American Medical Association*,[15] found that when women and men reported the very same symptoms, physicians gave the men significantly more extensive work-ups than the women. Many other studies have shown that physicians prescribe tranquilizers and other psychotropic (mind-altering) drugs for similar problems as much as two to three times as often for women as for men[16] and that the rate is significantly higher for male physicians than for female physicians. (In fact, following the association's first analysis from our data registry in the early eighties, we were horrified to discover that some women with endo were being prescribed tranquilizers and told the drugs would help with their symptoms.)

Third, "somatizing patients view complaints of bodily suffering as a means of establishing and maintaining relationships."[17] The "somatization pattern becomes a form of communication, a means of expressing emotion and a way of controlling the environment," according to the article "Somatization Disorder in Family Practice," which appeared in *American Family Physician*.[18]

Avoiding Blame, Blaming the Patient

The article also suggests that somatization allows patients to avoid blaming themselves for their problems "as in the patient who is convinced that her pain is due to some disease and that the physician is at fault for not diagnosing the disease." (Seems to me that the blame avoidance is among those who can't properly diagnose even the most obvious cases of endometriosis. Rather than being blamed for not knowing or keeping up with the needs of patients, physicians who label patients with a psychiatric "diagnosis" thus exonerate themselves!) The somatization literature itself notes that 25 percent of the patients given a "diagnosis" of somatization disorder are later found to have an organic basis for their symptoms.[19]

The authors of *Womancare*, an encyclopedic work on women's health, note that the all-in-your-head diagnosis is used all too readily by doctors for women's problems:

> If, however, the doctor's tests fail to explain your condition, you, along with those women seeking treatment for premenstrual syndrome, menstrual cramps and menopausal problems,* are apt to find yourself up against the old it's-all-in-your-head-dearie diagnosis or the I-can't-figure-out-what's-wrong-with-you-so-you-must-be-crazy syndrome.

Consider, for example, what an edition of one of the most widely used gynecological textbooks in this country has to say about the diagnosis of puzzling cases

---

* With the growing interest in menopause in recent years and the frequent prescription of hormones for menopausal problems, it's hard to even remember that not very long ago physicians passed off menopausal problems as psychological. Now some even call it "estrogen deficiency disease" and believe all menopausal women should be given estrogen replacement.

of amenorrhea [absence of periods]. After pointing out that even the most exhaustive tests administered by the most conscientious doctors will sometimes fail to pinpoint a cause for amenorrhea, the authors conclude, "It is undoubtedly incorrect to classify all such cases as of psychogenic origin, but such a practice is not uncommon and, until additional evidence is available, no more satisfactory solution can be suggested."

"Psychogenic" means "of emotional or mental origin"—in other words, it's-all-in-your-head. The authors of this widely-read textbook, who apparently feel that it's perfectly all right to diagnose a woman as neurotic just because they have failed to find out what's wrong with her, are obviously suffering from the I-can't-figure-out-what's-wrong-with-you-so-you-must-be-crazy syndrome. These women aren't even given the benefit of the traditional judicial principle, innocent until proven guilty; instead they are to be judged crazy (or to put it in more polite, medical terminology, as having problems of psychogenic origin) until "additional evidence" proves otherwise. The doctors who authored this text can't suggest a "more satisfactory solution" to their inability to diagnose the cause of a woman's amenorrhea, but we can. How about a simple, honest, "I don't know"?

If this sort of thing happened only after doctors had performed exhaustive tests and given women the benefit of what medical science had to offer, it wouldn't be such a problem. Women could perhaps learn to recognize this as one of the peculiar foibles to which doctors are prone and take such a diagnosis with an appropriate grain of salt. But all too often these attitudes prevent doctors from giving their women patients proper medical care.

Menstrual cramps, which have traditionally received the psychogenic "diagnosis," are an excellent example of how this works. One woman we know had cramps and vomited each time she had her period. Her gynecologist (who had no psychiatric training) decided she was neurotic and referred her to a psychiatrist. After extensive and expensive therapy, in which her male therapist helped her explore "her rejection of her femininity" as symbolized by her menstrual problems, she finally consulted another gynecologist. This doctor did not assume her problems were psychogenic and performed a thorough diagnostic work-up, including a laparoscopic exam. It was then discovered that this woman had a condition known as endometriosis that was affecting her bowels. We don't know whether she ever got around to accepting whatever it was she'd been rejecting, but once the endometriosis was treated she did stop vomiting and having pain each month. This is just one example of the ways in which doctors' prejudices and assumptions can negatively affect the health care a woman receives. . . .

If, after a thorough diagnostic work-up, your doctor is unable to identify the source of your problem, don't allow yourself to be made to feel that you have psychological problems. In all likelihood, the problem is that medical science just hasn't advanced far enough yet to understand your condition.[20]

The classic of the women's health movement, *Our Bodies, Ourselves*, describes the same problem in this way:

> In a strange way, a doctor often feels personally attacked or threatened when he cannot find any physical cause for the symptoms you report, and this can cause him to become hostile and use a label of "neurotic" or "psychosomatic" as a weapon when in fact he has no evidence of psychological symptoms and isn't qualified to diagnose them anyway. In other words, it is false reasoning to diagnose a problem as psychological merely by ruling out other, physical causes. It becomes a weapon of convenience, used whenever the doctor cannot deal with the situation in his accustomed way, and frees him from having to take the complaints seriously any longer.[21]

What happens once someone is labeled with somatization disorder? Given that the label is a psychiatric one, it's surprising to find that the medical literature, especially for family practice physicians, advises them to "manage" the patient. Essentially, the literature directs, the physician should work to establish trust with the patient by scheduling regular office visits and then gradually use that trust to get the patient to accept a psychiatric referral. "Billing patients for their medical symptoms—headache, chest pain—may help with third-party reimbursement," one article helpfully confides.[22] So even though the physician does not believe the patient has a medical basis for the symptoms and is not a psychiatrist or psychologist, strangely, some of the articles imply that the doctor may be able to carry out counseling.[23] ("Longer, counseling-length visits may be required when you are ready to do psychological work in the area of core conflicts."[24])

How is it possible that simple logic doesn't dictate to a professional group such as psychiatrists that if a diagnosis is found to affect primarily women some real discrimination might be occurring? Or that the well-publicized gaps in research on women's health problems would be expected to result in lack of understanding of some of women's ailments? How is it possible that professionals in the medical field would not understand that modern medicine does not yet have explanations for all physical symptoms and that simply because we don't yet have the medical understanding does not mean the patient's problem is all in her head? Even laypeople with the most rudimentary understanding of science generally know this. An article on the weaknesses in current diagnostic techniques noted a study showing "psychiatrists who referred patients to a psychiatric outpatient program failed to recognize major physical illness in 48 percent of their referrals, while medical doctors missed major physical conditions in 32 percent of their referrals."[25]

Psychologizing Medical Problems

Indeed, however, the psychiatric profession has shown an interest in taking over areas not yet explained scientifically. By doing so, the profession can justify the billing of patients, insurance companies, governments, and others who pay for psychological "care." (Those working on health care reform and ways to cut astronomical costs should look closely at this area.) There are many recent examples of this tendency to "psychologize" medical problems:

- *Ulcers* were for many years chalked up to "stress" and supposedly occurred in high-strung, anxious people who secreted too much stomach acid, which ate through the lining of their stomachs or intestines. Then scientists found that a particular bacterium caused inflammation of the stomach and intestinal lining leading to ulcers. Treatment to kill the bacteria was found to heal the ulcers and significantly reduce recurrence.[26]

- *Fibromyalgia,* a painful condition of the fibrous connective tissue that sometimes affects women with endo, was considered a psychosomatic disorder until recent studies. "Even now," one researcher noted in an article on the subject, "it retains that outdated association for many physicians who are unaware that current studies have failed to show neuroticism, hypochondriasis, somatization, depression, or similar psychological abnormalities in the majority of individuals with fibromyalgia."[27]

- *CFIDS or chronic fatigue immune dysfunction syndrome* (some people think CFIDS and fibromyalgia are facets of the same underlying abnormality) has frequently been diagnosed as somatization disorder and depression, according to Dr. Jay Goldstein, a leader in CFIDS research. Dr. Goldstein wrote in the *CFIDS Chronicle*: "Each time many of us in the clinical research community believe that we have convincingly dismembered, exploded, or immolated the notion that CFIDS is due to depression, unwary or foolhardy physicians somehow manage to resurrect this destructive superstition. These unenlightened physicians resemble those foolish teenagers returning for another 'fun' summer at Camp Crystal Lake, only to find—to their 'surprise'—a depressed Jason ready to wreak havoc on rational thought and scientific data."[28] Studies have shown distinct physical abnormalities in CFIDS so that those who formerly labeled CFIDS a psychosomatic disorder have had to admit they were wrong. Dr. Goldstein notes that many CFIDS patients are depressed (who wouldn't be with a debilitating illness that can make it impossible to work or even leave home, that people don't understand, and that may last for years?) but that the depression occurs *because* of the disease rather than *causing* the illness. (Women with endo appear to be at special risk for CFIDS. An article in a past association newsletter addresses CFIDS and endo.)

- *Postpolio syndrome,* a recurrence of polio symptoms many years after the initial bout, was also ascribed to psychological problems until research showed the disease definitely recurred in some survivors. One expert who has treated more than 500 such survivors reported that more than 90 percent of them come to his clinic frustrated and angry because "their doctors said the problem was all in their heads."[29]

- *Severe PMS (premenstrual syndrome),* the constellation of symptoms such as anxiety, moodiness, abdominal cramping, bloating, breast tenderness, headache, and cravings for sweets and high-carbohydrate foods, which some unfortunate women experience in the 7–10 days before menstruation, was added recently to the *DSM*. The move was controversial. While the cause of PMS is not yet known, most studies of the disorder have presumed a physical basis. (Some professionals working with candidiasis have noted the many symptoms the two conditions have in common and wondered if *Candida albicans* could be a factor in PMS. In fact one article in the somatization disorder literature points out that chronic candidiasis has a marked similarity to somatization disorder and that some patients currently labeled with somatization disorder could well be erroneously diagnosed and may respond to treatment for chronic candidiasis. See *Overcoming Endometriosis*[30] for more information on candidiasis.)

The Boston Women's Health Book Collective has pointed out that there is no parallel category for men, "no suggestion that the well-documented mood and behavior changes that result from variations in 'male hormone' changes should be given the label of a mental illness (no 'testosterone-based aggressive disorder')." And the head of the committee that decides what goes into the *DSM* acknowledged that psychiatrists have no effective treatment for PMS. So why create a mental label that could seriously hurt women in work situations, custody proceedings, and other parts of their lives? (The label probably also hurts all women with its reinforcement of the idea that women's "raging hormones" cause mental problems.) The answer seems to be that labeling the disorder a mental one allows psychiatrists, psychologists, and others in the self-described "helping" professions (they must mean helping themselves?) to bill for "treatment," thus increasing their incomes.

Toronto psychologist Paula Caplan, Ph.D., says that PMS is the only hormonally based diagnosis in the DSM that affects only one sex. If the American Psychiatric Association was not being discriminatory against women, it would also be proposing classifications for hormonal disorders that affect men. (The APA claimed in its news release that "premenstrual dysphoric disorder" is not the same as PMS. The APA description of "premenstrual dysphoric disorder" emphasizes the typical mood changes, irritability, and emotional aspects of PMS rather than the physical symptoms. But it's unlikely there will be keen awareness of such subtleties for most people.)

The American Psychiatric Association had also listed homosexuality as an official disease until 1974, "when gay and lesbian groups finally got the point across that if there's any genuinely hazardous ailment that begins with the letters h-o-m-o, it's homophobia," according to *Ms.* magazine, January/February 1989.[31]

- *Poison ivy, "chronic abdomen," and food poisoning,* as well as many other disorders, have been labeled psychological. In fact, as noted earlier, anything not readily explainable with the knowledge available at the time has been labeled "in the head." It seems by now that the lesson should have been learned!

An example of the ease with which people are labeled "mental cases" is the 1985 botulism outbreak (a type of severe, life-threatening food poisoning) that occurred among individuals who ate at a popular restaurant in Vancouver. At least 37 people from three provinces and two foreign countries were poisoned, according to a report that appeared in the January 1992 issue of *Hippocrates*.[32] "Many were tourists, who had gone on to take their baffling symptoms to hometown doctors who misdiagnosed their ailment. *At least three people spent time on psychiatric wards, assured that their muscle weakness, agitation, or paralysis had psychosomatic roots*" (emphasis added).

In hindsight, these diagnostic disasters are sometimes funny, such as the report in a British medical journal[33] in the last century on "hysterical rash," a new disease contracted only by women. As it turned out, the rash was caused by poison ivy brought back to England by visitors to North America who planted it in their gardens because of its beautiful fall colors.

In other cases the hostility shown by physicians toward patients in their psychiatric labeling makes it hard to laugh, even years later. The article on so-called chronic abdomen, "The Abdominal Woman," later in this chapter, is an example.

How These Attitudes Hurt Women with Endometriosis

Besides fighting the inappropriate use of endometriosis symptoms as diagnostic criteria for a mental disorder, women with endometriosis need to be ever vigilant for how these attitudes affect their care, treatment, and research on the disease. Examples abound.

Some time ago, for instance, one of our medical advisors sent me an article that had appeared in a magazine that goes out to every ob-gyn in the U.S. and suggested that a physician interviewed in the magazine needed to be reeducated on endometriosis. The physician claimed that "most patients with mild or moderate endometriosis have no pain at all, because the disorder does not usually cause pain."[34] He also used the fact that women with endometriosis are sometimes not better after surgery or hormonal treatment as an argument for his belief that the chronic pelvic pain these women experienced (which he nicknamed "pelvalgia") was not caused by their endometriosis or other problems such as adhesions or cysts but rather by psychological factors, primarily "a history of major childhood and adult physical and sexual abuse." Strangely, the studies used to justify these ideas about endometriosis had no women with endometriosis in them! As in the past, endometriosis seems to continue in its role as a lightning rod for those intent on "psychologizing" symptoms.

The physician then described the program of behavior modification he used to "treat" these patients. (We're not disputing that women with endometriosis need and deserve coping help or that a wellness program focused on nutrition and exercise would be beneficial. But to offer no medical care—only counseling—to control symptoms is at best inadequate and may well be grounds for malpractice.) Furthermore, efforts to convince the patient her symptoms are not physical, when indeed they are, could seriously undermine her self-esteem and her confidence in the medical profession.

He also claimed that patients with "pelvalgia" or chronic pelvic pain were more likely to have somatization disorder, with four times as many "unrelated" items from his somatization scale (different from the *DSM* scale) as controls. The "unrelated somatic symptoms" included headache, low-back pain, pain with urination, premenstrual syndrome, nausea, bloating, vomiting, diarrhea, constipation, fatigue, palpitations, vaginal discharge, and other symptoms. These symptoms were apparently considered "unrelated" to the women's pelvic pain because they were not, according to the article, specifically gynecologic.[35]

For another example, consider the impact on attitudes toward women with endometriosis of a recent professional pronouncement. At the Fourth World Congress on Endometriosis, held in Salvador, Brazil (May 1994), we were shocked to hear a Brazilian psychologist assert that endometriosis is the result of modern woman's conflict over her role in society. Using slides of Salvador Dali's surreal art and lyrics from a Beatles' song to illustrate his point (no, I'm not kidding—I wish I were!), he asserted that women with endometriosis experience severe conflict over menstruation and sexuality and express this conflict in the form of endometriosis.

His unsubstantiated statements reminded me of other psychological pronouncements we've had to fight over the years. In 1984 a Kalamazoo, Michigan, newspaper[36] reported that a psychologist, in her 1979 Ph.D. study, had found that women with endometriosis "viewed themselves negatively because they were female and wished they could change their sex, *an attitude that began with the onset of menstrual life at about age 12*" (emphasis added).

"The duration of this unfavorable sexual identity persists into adulthood and manifests itself in painful sexual intercourse and continued menstrual difficulties as dysmenorrhea (painful menstruation) and hypermenorrhea (excessive menstrual bleeding)," she said. "She has feelings of being limited and pressed by social and vocational aspects of her life space, is oversensitive and experiences pervasive and generalized resentment and hostility. She expresses this hostility in an indirect fashion toward men."

The newspaper article on her work continues: "Complaints of painful intercourse were often used as a way of avoiding intercourse," she said, noting that "endometriosis is a nice protection for some women who do not want children." (What a hurtful statement for women with endometriosis who have desperately wanted children. This person needs to read the book *Blaming the Victim* (William Ryan, New York: Random House, 1971), a classic work showing how society blames those unfortunate enough to be victims of inequalities in society rather than address the inequalities.)

"Although women with endometriosis may 'display an image of extreme femininity, this posture appears to be overcompensation for the resentment directed toward her sexuality and/or a reflection of her incapacity,'" the article continues. The psychologist then goes on to state that the psychological pressures at work in the mind of women "who fit the endometriotic personality" lead to the organic disease. And, the article asserts, psychological therapy can help some women regain their fertility! Appallingly, these extremely prejudicial judgments were publicized although the study was based on tests of only 20 women with endo from one small group in one clinic in one city, with most of the women being one religion (Catholic).

At least this article received no further notice, but we will not be so lucky with the Brazil talk. The proceedings of the Fourth World Congress will be published, and then, unscientific as these ideas are, the mere fact of publication may lend them some credence as well as spread them around the globe. Our only hope is to continue working together worldwide to fight these insidious ideas wherever they arise and to insist that research continue to determine, in a scientific way, what is causing the disease. Given the dual challenge of having a disease not yet understood (by society or science) and the deep-seated taboos involved in the disease (menstruation, female sexuality, and, to a lesser extent, infertility), it is going to remain very tempting for psychologists and physicians to continue the hundreds-of-years-old tradition of chalking these problems up to psychological disorders.

Even our own specialists fail us at times in this regard (the pressures of treating patients who do not get better are huge), but at least we've seen improvement in the last 10 years. A study presented at the American Fertility Society annual meeting in 1985, for instance, found that infertile women with endometriosis experienced much more stress than infertile women without endometriosis. Because the person doing the study assumed endo was just another reason for infertility rather than understanding it as a chronic, painful disease, the conclusion that women with endometriosis have psychological problems was inevitable. It's almost inconceivable that such a study would be presented at a meeting of the same society (now known as the American Society for Reproductive Medicine) today because of much better understanding of the disease in these circles.

The "Science" of Somatization Studies

Reading the studies purporting to show how women with chronic pelvic pain are somatizing or the relationship of childhood physical or sexual abuse to adult chronic pelvic pain is a *nauseating* experience. (Whoops . . . did I say "nauseating"? Better watch out—I'll be accused of somatizing.) Many of the studies are done poorly, with small numbers, and with all types of pelvic pain lumped together as if it were all one entity. The sweeping generalizations made from the small amounts of hard data are hard to *stomach*. (Oh dear.) And the knowledge of endometriosis displayed (when the authors even bother to break out the numbers with endo in their samples) is *dizzyingly* simplistic. (I give up.)

Moreover, the study designs and tools used are often very unscientific. Scales often have not been validated.[37] An interesting article on a controversy in the American Psychiatric Association in the mid-1980s over a proposed new diagnostic category that members of the Committee on Women of the APA believed would be discriminatory to women and other subordinated groups noted that the new diagnosis ("Masochistic Personality Disorder") could not be rejected for lack of scientific evidence because "if rigorous scientific standards were imposed, not only this category but many other diagnoses in the manual would have to be scrapped."[38] In fact a book by Toronto psychologist Paula Caplan, *They Say You're Crazy* (Reading, Massachusetts: Addison-Wesley, 1995), describes the unscientific process by which "diagnoses" are added to the *DSM*.

In addition to lack of validation, the measures used for "diagnosing" psychological disorders often include physical symptoms that are part and parcel of medical illnesses. As shown by the authors of a very interesting study on how standard psychological tests make infertile people look as if they have psychological problems, removal of a single item on the Minnesota Multiphasic Personality Inventory (MMPI)—"The idea that something serious is wrong with your body"—changed the score for females from being interpreted as a moderate *elevation* in the psychoticism scale to *average*. In other words, if you have a disease or are infertile and truthfully agree with the statement, you automatically are rated higher on the psychoticism scale. In fact, 44 percent of the infertile men in the study and 52 percent of the infertile women met criteria for being classified as psychiatric cases, primarily because the tests failed to account for typical side effects of drugs such as Clomid and for the stresses infertile people experience.[39]

The use of inappropriate psychological measures, including symptoms of endometriosis and related health problems, also may have slanted the results of another study of the supposed psychological status of women with endo. The study was based on interviews (a method that in itself is considered more subjective since it depends on the judgment of the interviewer) of only 16 women with endo and used the *DSM-III* criteria, which still allowed inclusion of physical symptoms in making a diagnosis of depression. The study concluded that a significant number of the women had mood disorders—both manic episodes and major depressions.[40] (A manic episode, or mania, is defined as a "disordered mental state of extreme excitement"—*Dorland's Medical Dictionary*.) While mood disorders are certainly possible in women with endo (and might be linked to possible hormonal imbalances), a much more sophisticated study than this will be needed to separate out the physically based symptoms from psychological ones. (As a humorous aside, the article notes that one patient suffered a manic episode while at the clinic: "she blew bubble gum in the face of a senior physician and addressed the head of the clinic by pet nicknames of her own choosing."[41] The patient might indeed be manic, but some readers might think her reaction appropriate to the treatment so many women with endo receive!)

Either those administering these tests to people with physical problems believe there are no genuine physically caused problems in this world (and there are some such people), or they are very thoughtless in using tests designed for physically healthy people to assess those with medical problems. Psychotherapist and association member Deborah Schwallie has pointed out that there are tests designed for people with chronic illness that do not include physical symptoms, but they don't often get used due to lack of awareness or insensitivity on the part of the investigators. (Aside from chronic illness, how is it possible that all people react the same physically so that a person's tiring more easily can be assumed to be a measure of psychological functioning rather than simple biological diversity?)

On numerous occasions the association has had to remind researchers seeking access to our members for psychological or coping studies that their results would be invalid if they used standard psychological scales incorporating symptoms of endometriosis. It's clear that if the association had not been involved these "studies" (which serve only to point out the lack of scientific standards in the field) would have gone ahead and found, based on their biased data, that women with endo were more psychologically unbalanced than women without the disease.

Some progress is being made, however. As noted in a recent article from the journal *Psychosomatics*, "*DSM-III-R* refines the *DSM-III* criteria for major depression by stating that a symptom cannot be 'due to a physical condition' in order to be counted."[42]

In addition, often little or no effort is made to separate cause from effect, to recognize that having a chronic, painful (physically or, as in the case of infertility, psychologically painful), misunderstood disease or problem might *cause* psychological stress. The infertility study just mentioned points out: "Some symptoms ordinarily indicative of psychopathology [mental disease] can represent normal side effects or reactions to infertility treatment, thus causing spurious [false] estimates of pathology. Alternatively, item analyses revealed a profile of infertility strain reflecting tension, depressive symptoms, worry, and interpersonal alienation frequently occurring among both male and female infertility patients. The concept of infertility strain is suggested as a vehicle for understanding the functioning of infertile patients and to circumvent the stigmatizing effects of psychiatric labels while providing appropriate intervention."[43]

Three studies (one for chronic pelvic pain and two specifically for endo) show that psychological profiles return to normal or near normal after patients are successfully cured of their pain or, in endo studies, after the endo is removed. These studies lend strong support to both the physical basis of the pain complaints and the physical basis of the supposedly "psychological" profiles (because of the inappropriate inclusion of symptoms on the psychological tests).[44-46]

Other studies, especially those purporting to find a relationship between childhood sexual abuse and later development of chronic pelvic pain, seem very shortsighted in their conclusions. All the chronic pelvic pain patients tend to be lumped together, which, given the inclusion of women with endo and adhesions as well as endo symptoms from the *DSM* somatization disorder criteria, calls all the findings into question. And the bias that chronic pelvic pain must be due to *gyn* reasons further leads to the impression that *female* functions are being singled out or that the authors are weak in their understanding of what's in the pelvis besides the female organs.[47]

The majority of those with endometriosis or adhesions or chronic pelvic pain are *not* found to have had prior sexual or physical abuse in the studies, but the authors inevitably fail to question what might have caused endometriosis in the majority. Instead they postulate all kinds of psychological reasons for development of the disease in the minority with prior abuse histories. It reminds one of the saying "When all you have is a hammer, the whole world becomes a nail."

The fact that a group of gynecologists subspecializing in what is called *psychosomatic gynecology* even exists, while there is no comparable subspecialty in, say, *psychosomatic urology*, smacks of pure discrimination against women.

What Should We Do?

What's to be done about this situation, which is obviously hurting women with endometriosis? Readers, we turn to you to let us know what steps you think the association should take. What are you willing to do? Should we work to have endometriosis added to the list of diseases physicians and psychiatrists are supposed to rule out before diagnosing someone with somatization disorder? Or should we work to have the entire category looked at for its discriminatory impact on women and girls, perhaps in coalition with other organizations serving those with diseases and symptoms like those in the *DSM* for somatization? Or should we petition women in psychology and psychiatry to take up this cause? Please write us with your ideas, stories about your own experiences along these lines, and, if you are interested, any contributions to help in our ongoing battle to change all-in-the-head attitudes about endometriosis!

Notes

1. *Diagnostic and Statistical Manual of Mental Disorders (DSM-IV)*, 4th ed. (Washington, D.C.: American Psychiatric Press, 1994): 446–50.
2. Ibid., 447.
3. The APA has issued four major revisions of the *DSM* since 1950. The most recent revision, *DSM-IV* (1994), actually makes it easier to label a woman with somatization disorder if she presents with the symptoms listed at the beginning of this article. The same symptoms may also earn her a new label, Pain Disorder Associated with Psychological Factors or Pain Disorder Associated with Both Psychological Factors and a General Medical Condition (Codes 307.80 and 307.89), if "psychological factors are judged to play a role in the onset, severity, exacerbation, or maintenance of the pain." This extremely open-ended wording allows psychiatrists to bill for treating a mental disorder without any objective substantiation.

4. As well as the symptoms listed at the beginning of this article, eligible symptoms for somatization disorder are "a history of pain related to . . . head, abdomen, back, joints, extremities, chest, rectum . . . food intolerance . . . menorrhagia, vomiting throughout pregnancy . . . in men, erectile or ejaculatory dysfunction . . . impaired coordination or balance, paralysis or localized weakness, difficulty swallowing or lump in throat, aphonia, urinary retention, hallucinations, loss of touch or pain sensation, double vision, blindness, deafness, seizures; associative symptoms such as amnesia; or loss of consciousness other than fainting." *DSM-IV*: 449–50.

5. G. R. Smith, "Toward a More Effective Recognition and Management of Somatization Disorder," *Journal of Family Practice* 25, no. 6 (1987): 551–52.

6. *DSM-III-R* (third ed. rev., 1987): 262.

7. *DSM-IV*, 448.

8. *DSM-III-R,* 262.

9. *DSM-IV*, 450.

10. Ibid., 452.

11. Ibid., 450.

12. P. Pepping, L. Halstead, L. Haile, and W. P. Dmowski, "Women's Experiences with Endometriosis: Delay and Disbelief," presented at the Third World Congress, Brussels, June 1992.

13. N. Rasmussen and R. Avant, "Somatization Disorder in Family Practice," *American Family Physician* 40, no. 2 (August 1989): 206.

14. Ibid., 208.

15. K. Armitage, L. Schneiderman, and R. Bass, "Response of Physicians to Medical Complaints in Men and Women," *JAMA* 241, no. 20 (May 18, 1979): 2186–87.

16. L. Taggert, S. McCammon, L. Allred, R. Horner, and H. May, "Effect of Patient and Physician Gender on Prescriptions for Psychotropic Drugs," *Journal of Women's Health* 4, (1993): 353–57.

17. Rasmussen, 208.

18. Ibid., 208.

19. C. Ford, W. Katon, and M. Lipkin, "Managing Somatization and Hypochondriasis," *Patient Care* 27, no. 2 (January 30, 1993): 31–44.

20. L. Madaras and J. Patterson, *Womancare: A Gynecological Guide to Your Body* (New York: Avon, 1981): 571–72, 573.

21. Boston Women's Health Book Collective, *Our Bodies, Ourselves* (New York: Simon & Schuster, 1979): 349.

22. Ford, 41.

23. Ibid., 42.

24. Ibid., 41.

25. S. Spitz, "Diagnostic Dilemmas," *Science for the People* (July/August 1987): 19–22.

26. "Killing *H. Pylori* Heals Ulcers and Reduces Recurrences," *Consultant* (August 1992): 104.

27. "Sharpening the Focus on Fibromyalgia," *Emergency Medicine* (April 30, 1988): 28.

28. J. Goldstein, "CFIDS Is Not Depression!" *CFIDS Chronicle* (January/February 1989): 17.

29. "Postpolio Syndrome Spurs Action," *Medical World News* (April 10, 1989): 33.

30. M. L. Ballweg, "The Endometriosis-Candidiasis Link," *Overcoming Endometriosis: New Help from the Endometriosis Association* (New York: Congdon & Weed, 1987): 228–31.

31. B. Ehrenreich, "Sick Chic," *Ms.* (January/February 1989): 28–29.

32. D. Franklin, "The Case of the Paralyzed Travelers," *Hippocrates* (January 1992): 32–34.

33. N. Vietmeyer, "Science Has Got Its Hands on Poison Ivy, Oak and Sumac," *Smithsonian* (August 1985): 89.

34. I. Gottesfeld, "Chronic Pelvic Pain: Stalking a Clinical Enigma," *Today's Woman* (October 1991): 10.

35. Ibid., 12–14.
36. B. Krasean, "Psychologist Finds Psychological Roots in Endometriosis," *Kalamazoo Gazette* (May 3, 1984).
37. R. Kathol et al., "Diagnosing Depression in Patients with Medical Illness," *Psychosomatics* 31, no. 4 (Fall 1990): 434–40.
38. J. L. Herman, "Masochism Unmasked," *The Women's Review of Books*, no. 5 (February 1986): 10.
39. B. Berg and J. Wilson, "Psychiatric Morbidity in the Infertile Population: A Reconceptualization," *Fertility and Sterility* 53, no. 4 (April 1990): 654–61.
40. D. O. Lewis, F. Comite, et al., "Bipolar Mood Disorder and Endometriosis: Preliminary Findings," *American Journal of Psychiatry* 144, no. 12 (December 1987): 1588–91.
41. Ibid., 1590.
42. Kathol, 434.
43. Berg and Wilson, 654.
44. R. Sternbach and G. Timmermans, "Personality Changes Associated with Reduction of Pain," *Pain* 1 (1975): 177–81.
45. A. E. Reading, L. C. Chang, D. Randle, D. Meldrum, and H. L. Judd, "Psychosocial Correlates of Response to Treatment of Pain Associated with Endometriosis," Poster presentation, International Association for the Study of Pain, 1987, Hamburg.
46. W. Y. Low, R. J. Edelmann, and C. Sutton, "Short Term Psychological Outcome of Surgical Intervention for Endometriosis," *British Journal of Obstetrics and Gynaecology* 100 (February 1993): 191–92.
47. J. Harrop-Griffiths, W. Katon, E. Walker, L. Holm, J. Russo, and L. Hickok, "The Association Between Chronic Pelvic Pain, Psychiatric Diagnoses, and Childhood Sexual Abuse," *Obstetrics and Gynecology* 71, no. 4 (April 1988): 591.

It's All in Your Head—
A Heartbreaking Story

Virginia's story, which follows, is heartbreaking. Unfortunately, her case is not an isolated one. The association has heard from others with endometriosis over the years who have been put in mental wards—teenagers seem to be the most vulnerable. See the excerpt from Susan's letter at the beginning of this chapter as one example. Another example is the young woman whose parents put her into a mental hospital because they believed the doctors who said their daughter had mental problems, not physical ones. Years later they felt very guilty and sad about this, as they explained to association staff. In another case a member in severe pain from bladder problems and adhesions had been going to the emergency room. When tests on her bladder failed to show a bacterial infection, she was put in the psychiatric ward. Another member, after having her bladder punctured during surgery, was given continual doses of a painkiller known to cause hallucinations despite her protests that she did not need it. When she began to hallucinate, she was transferred to the psychiatric ward, with a tube still going through her abdomen into her bladder. There she was not even allowed to make a phone call for three days. (At that point her father came to the hospital demanding to know what was going on and took her out.) Clearly this was a calculated attempt to discredit her (as a "psych" case) in the anticipated malpractice suit. In fact the malpractice defense attorney did use her transfer to the psychiatric ward to discredit her.

"I don't know when I began to suffer from endometriosis. What I do know is that from the beginning of menstruation at the age of 12, I seemed to suffer more pain than my girlfriends. They were able to remain active and to participate in sports when all that I could do was to sit and squeeze my abdomen seeking relief. When I complained to my mother, she told me that I would 'have to learn to live with it.' Then, she gave me a cup of tea. . . .

"My uterus and my bladder dropped during the first pregnancy. Successive gynecologists told me that I needed corrective surgery; however, I didn't have it.

"Following each pregnancy the cramps were harder and the pain was more intense. I became weaker, and I suffered from fatigue so often that I lost interest in swimming, golf, and other physical activities. At times I couldn't even make the bed. Sex with my husband became very painful. I felt like I had a hot rock inside my body grinding bits of sand. I was no longer fun to be with. My marriage was slipping away. I was a 'cripple,' and my husband was tired of it. Even my children and friends had grown weary of my complaints.

"My fourth child required special attention and medical treatment. With my pain and fatigue I could barely cope with all the responsibilities as a wife and mother. It was difficult to control my emotions, and the stress was taking its toll on my husband also. Observing this, my gynecologist told my husband that we both needed to see a psychiatrist.

"I did see a psychiatrist for the next two years, although my husband refused to do so. During those visits I underwent counseling and shock treatments. . . . My physical condition was deterio-

rating, not improving, and common sense told me that I needed something more than psychiatric counseling if I were to improve. My husband called the hospital and made an appointment, and I returned, believing I was going to receive a physical examination. To my surprise, I was placed on the psychiatric ward. . . .

"As soon as I could, I telephoned my husband and told him, 'I don't need this place. I need to see a medical doctor. I'm coming home.'

"My husband came to get me with the sheriff and my brother. They took me from the hospital directly to the psychiatric ward of a county hospital to await a commitment hearing.

"The next day I was declared to be 'paranoid schizophrenic.' I wasn't aware of what was happening to me because I had been heavily medicated prior to the hearing. I was unable to speak for myself—to say that I was acting irrationally because I hurt so badly, to tell about the lacerations I suffered from the childbirth or the irregular menstrual periods, the severe irritability, the constipation, and the diarrhea. I couldn't say all the things that had driven me to this point. I still couldn't get the medical attention that I desperately needed. It would be years before surgery would reveal that I suffered from endometriosis and other physical ailments.

"I was no longer in control of my life. I suffered great physical discomfort as well as mental distress, which was heightened by the fact that everybody thought my problems were all in my head. No one gave credence to my physical complaints.

"Within a week after my arrival I found myself committed to a mental hospital in a city far away from my home, my family, and my friends. . . .

"I don't know whether or not my commitment was the result of prior planning; but with nearly perfect timing, as soon as I had been confined in the mental hospital for two years, I was adjudged to be 'hopelessly and incurably insane.' Immediately afterward my husband filed his divorce action, alleging insanity as the only ground.

"After two years and five months' confinement in that mental hospital, my brother arranged for my release. I returned to my home city, where I lived with him and his wife until a house could be found for me. A court order prevented me from moving into my old house.

"My husband wasted no time in proceeding with his divorce action. On a Friday, I was forced to sign an agreement settling child custody, alimony, and property rights. The following Monday morning I was declared to be competent at a restoration hearing in the courthouse. That afternoon my husband was granted a divorce by another court in the same building.

"During the entire two years and five months of confinement I received only one physical examination. It occurred within the first six months in response to my nearly hysterical requests. The staff physician who performed the examination said that I needed surgery, but he didn't mention endometriosis. He prescribed knee-chest exercises and the use of a pessary to hold my uterus in place. After that I shut up about the pain.

"Restoration to competency didn't restore my former life. I had to carry the stigma of having been a patient in a mental hospital, which meant traveling an uncharted course. For example, I needed an operation, but I couldn't find a surgeon who would perform it. One said: 'We can't operate on you. You have a psychiatric overlay.'

"The chief of surgery at another hospital refused, saying, 'Your skirts are dirty.'

"There were other consequences. To mention a few: I couldn't live with my children; I couldn't buy real estate. I was limited in other financial transactions. And my former friends and acquaintances shunned me, except for those who were true.

"It was six more years before I had a hysterectomy. The surgeon discovered that I had a proliferated endometrium, an ovarian cyst, and hemorrhaging tumors in my uterus. At last, after 36 years, I was rid of my physical pain and my complaints were vindicated. Still later, when I began to understand endometriosis, I gained a definitive explanation of my condition.

"Yours is a wonderful cause, helping all the women who are doing battle with endometriosis. Through education and support they may avoid the many years of suffering that I had to endure. You, and the association, have my encouragement and support."

Virginia, Georgia

"The Abdominal Woman":
An Address on The Chronic Abdomen

By Robert Hutchison, M.D., F.R.C.P.,
Physician to the London Hospital

Portions of "The Abdominal Woman," which originally appeared in the April 21, 1923, issue of *The British Medical Journal*, are excerpted in this article. Not only does the article show the attitudes of some doctors of the time toward their women patients, but it also seems to espouse anti-Semitism and wife beating and puts down nurses!

Our surgical colleagues describe a condition which they speak of, in their clinical slang, as the "acute abdomen." There is, however, another condition more familiar to the physician which may be designated with equal propriety the "chronic abdomen," and if the one is, as we are told, a catastrophe, the other is certainly a conundrum.

The subject of the chronic abdomen is usually a woman, generally a spinster, or, if married, childless and belonging to what are commonly termed rather ironically nowadays the "comfortable" classes. To such a degree, moreover, do her abdominal troubles colour her life and personality that we may conveniently speak of her as an "abdominal woman." An abdominal man, on the other hand, is by comparison a rare bird, and when caught has a way of turning out to be a Jew or a doctor.

. . . The patient may speak of a "raw feeling inside," or of "an indescribable sensation in the stomach," or of a "dragging." Constipation of greater or less degree almost always figures prominently in the list of symptoms, and flatulence is also frequent. Amongst the commoner remote symptoms one finds a feeling of general weakness or "exhaustion" (especially after an action of the bowels), "mental and physical torpor," "inability to think," "a poisoned feeling," and "neuralgic pains all over." Headaches and insomnia are also very frequent, and a great many patients complain of undue susceptibility to cold and of a constant catarrh* in the throat. . . .

It is interesting to note at this point how medical history repeats itself. [**EDITOR'S NOTE:** Indeed!] *Writing in the eighties of last century on the abuse of gynecological operations in the treatment of visceral neurosis, Sir Clifford Allbutt said of the abdominal woman of that day:*

> *"She is entangled in the net of the gynecologist, who finds her uterus, like her nose, is a little on one side, or again, like that organ, is running a little, or it is as flabby as her biceps, so that the unhappy viscus is impaled upon a stem, or perched upon a prop, or is painted with carbolic acid every week in the year except during the long vacation when the gynecologist is grouse-shooting or salmon-catching, or leading the fashion in the*

---

* *Catarrh* is an old term for inflammation of the nasal mucous membrane.

Upper Engadine. Her mind, thus fastened to a more or less nasty mystery, becomes newly apprehensive and physically introspective, and the morbid chains are riveted more strongly than ever. Arraign the uterus and you fix in the woman the arrow of hypochondria, it may be for life."

On Visceral Neurosis, Goulstonian Lectures, 1884

On examination of a fully developed case of the chronic abdomen one will find that it has both a physical and a mental aspect, and that the latter is often the more important of the two. . . .

Her incessant demand for sympathy and understanding makes the abdominal woman a veritable vampire, sucking the vitality of all who come near her. Half an hour with her reduces her doctor to the consistence of "a piece of chewed string," and is more exhausting to him than all the rest of his daily visits put together, for she is always discovering fresh symptoms, will not admit any improvement in her condition, and has an objection to everything that is proposed. Crabbe must have had her in mind when he wrote of the patients—

"Who with sad prayers the weary doctor tease
To name the nameless ever new disease."

. . . What is to be desired here is something which will dislocate the patient's mind from its perpetual revolution round her umbilicus and set it open to wider horizons. The war cured some and loss of fortune and bereavement have cured others; but these are drastic remedies which it is not within our power to prescribe. Suffragettism undoubtedly was the salvation of some abdominal women, but the suffragettes are now experiencing the tragedy of fulfilled ambition, and probably many of them have relapsed. Marriage, and the advent of a child—even an adopted one—are often potent remedies, and the fancy religions—Christian Science, Theosophy, Spiritualism, and so forth—may be ways of escape. One of my patients, an ex-nurse (and ex-nurses furnish the most malignant types of the chronic abdomen), once consulted a palmist, who after looking at her hand said, "If I were your husband I would take a stick to you!" The advice was sound, and might often, perhaps, be effective. . . .

I confess, therefore, to some feeling of despair as regards the treatment of the more advanced cases of the chronic abdomen, and on the whole I am inclined to think that the less one has to do with them the better both for one's peace of mind and one's professional reputation. Yet, unfortunately, these cases are likely to increase in the future, for as civilization gets more complex, as fewer women in the upper classes marry, or, being married, have fewer and fewer children, all the factors which favor the development of chronic abdominalism will be more intense. It is a bleak prospect.

Chronic Pelvic Pain:
Stalking an Old Bias About Women

By Mary Lou Ballweg

A couple of years ago, one of the association's advisors sent me a copy of an article on endometriosis from *Today's Woman*, a magazine that is sent to all U.S. ob-gyns. Because of the misleading statements in the article, I wrote a letter of response, which was published along with a letter from Dr. David Redwine, another association advisor, also refuting the misstatements in the article. (Another advisor also responded with a private letter to the physician interviewed in the article.) The issues addressed in the article and in the response are ones that have caused confusion and difficulty for women with endo for many years.

Dear Editor:

The recent article *"Chronic Pelvic Pain: Stalking a Clinical Enigma"* contains some unfortunate statements about endometriosis. First, Dr. Reiter asserts that endometriosis causes pain only in advanced cases. This conclusion appears to be drawn from studies of infertility populations and applied to the general endometriosis population, which overwhelmingly presents with pain symptoms. These are two distinct populations, as so much work presented through the American Fertility Society and others has shown in at least the last five years.

The Endometriosis Association maintains the largest research registry on endometriosis in the world. In our data, which has been published widely in our literature and elsewhere, 96 percent of the women report a wide range of pain symptoms. The small group of patients in our registry who do not report pain symptoms are almost invariably infertility patients. A recent search of the pain literature worldwide by our Director of Canadian Projects, who served as Chair of the Pain Subcommittee of the Canadian Consensus Conference on Endometriosis, Society of Obstetricians and Gynaecologists of Canada, produced no papers suggesting that a very advanced case of endometriosis is necessary to cause significant symptoms.

Moreover, the debate on classification schemes for endometriosis over many years makes it clear that any designation of what represents advanced disease or early disease is suspect until we understand the natural history of endometriosis. A claim can be made that disease classified as "early" with current classification schemes could be more painful than later stages, based on the studies of Michael Vernon and others showing the earlier lesions produce more prostaglandins, known pain mediators.[1] (However, in what has been assumed to be later disease, adhesions and other sequelae* may also cause problems.) Even within the current classification schemes, frequent diagnostic errors cloud the issue. Investigators such as the eminent Robert Franklin of Baylor College of Medicine have repeatedly found mislabeling of deeply infiltrating disease—which has been linked conclusively to pain—as "mild" disease.[2]

Moreover, current classification schemes were developed for infertility prognosis. They make no claim to measure anything related to pain. The American Fertility Society, among others, is working to devise a good classification system, but, as discussion at the Third World Congress on Endometriosis in Brussels clearly showed, this will not be an easy task.[3–5]

In addition, our classification systems have tried to quantify disease based on a mechanical view of the disease, which can easily lead to statements questioning how a few spots of endometriosis could be causing so many symptoms. (Dr. David Redwine has made the comparison of the sensitive tissue of the peritoneum to the eyeball—no one finds it confusing that a tiny speck in one's eye can cause a lot of pain.) The mechanical view of the disease has tended to regard endometriosis as serious based on how much disease (defined as implants and adhesions) one can see without consideration of the biological activity occurring.

Endometriosis cannot be explained as simply a mechanical problem that interferes with anatomy or fertility—almost as if the body were a machine made up of moving parts rather than a living biologically active system. It is eminently clear from current research that endometriosis is not a disease simply involving some misplaced endometrial tissue. Rather, it is a disease involving disordered immunology with multiple consequences of that dysregulation, which are being elucidated piece by piece by investigators all over the world. Forty-four papers were presented on immunological aspects of endometriosis at the Brussels Congress alone.

The focus on reproduction has limited awareness of the highly typical global symptoms in endometriosis common to immunological diseases. These symptoms emerge very clearly in our large data registry, particularly in familial endometriosis. Often, we also see in these families and individuals related immune system–based disease.[6–8]

There are two additional reasons for overlooking the symptoms that show the immunological nature of familial endometriosis. First, superspecialization in modern medicine creates a tendency to disregard symptoms that don't "belong" to the organ system with which the practitioner is concerned. Second, symptoms reported by women in our society, especially "nonspecific" symptoms, are routinely discounted. This bias was clearly

---

* A disease condition following or occurring as a consequence of another condition or event.

demonstrated in the well-known study in which paired men and women reporting the exact same symptoms were treated differently according to gender—the physicians' work-ups were significantly more extensive for men than they were for women.[9]

As support for his psychological "treatment" for women with endometriosis, Dr. Reiter states that many of these women show no improvement with medical treatment, including surgery. (He cites a study in which fulguration alone was used, a surgical approach little used by leading endometriosis surgeons since studies have shown that only with excision can one be sure of having removed the entire lesion.) There are many diseases for which we do not have perfect treatments or cures. But the fact that modern science has not yet produced a highly efficacious treatment does not mean the disease or its symptoms do not exist. How wonderful it would be if we lived in a world in which diseases emerged only when we had treatments for them that worked! In any case, there are many studies, some placebo-controlled, showing reduction of pain symptoms in endometriosis with medical therapy and surgery.[10–17]

According to the article, all patients, whether they have a physical cause for their symptoms or a psychogenic one, are enrolled in a "broad-based program of cognitive behavioral pain therapy." This approach seems like a rather circuitous way to address pain in those with a physical cause.

In addition, it leads to a selection bias that could easily produce the "results" Dr. Reiter reports. As a simple example, think of the consequence if the next time Dr. Reiter has a toothache his dentist enrolls him in a program to teach him "coping strategies to help improve control over [his] symptoms and optimize the quality of [his life]. Relaxation techniques, a wellness program that focuses on nutrition and exercise, spouse and family involvement, and education and lifestyle adaptations are all part of a pain management prescription with management options and needs prioritized according to individual patient needs." I suspect Dr. Reiter would take himself to another dentist posthaste (even if his toothache was chronic). And the dentist would certainly be suspected of dreaming up a fabulous money-making venture for not only himself but also his psychiatric colleagues.

If he did remain in the study, we'd have to conclude he felt he was going to benefit and that he suspected a psychogenic cause for his chronic toothache. The result: a selected population group. It is no more indicative of the truth of endometriosis to draw general conclusions based on a behavioral modification sampling than it is on an infertility population.

Fortunately for women with endometriosis, progress is being made in understanding this disease. Recent studies in monkeys showed the spontaneous development of endometriosis when the animals were exposed to dioxin, PCBs, or radiation.[18–22] The Endometriosis Association is funding additional research on the monkeys with dioxin-induced endometriosis. Thus far, a perfect dose-dependent relationship between dioxin exposure and the occurrence and severity of cases has emerged.

Interestingly, the monkeys exhibit clear pain behaviors indicating abdominal distress, as well as depression, and they stop eating while in pain. Fortunately for women with endometriosis, the animals cannot be accused of somatizing.

In all the decades since Freud, women have been told their symptoms are in their heads. For the majority of the millions of women with endometriosis, the kind of thinking presented in "*Chronic Pelvic Pain: Stalking a Clinical Enigma*" is simply a new twist on that old bias about women.

Notes

1. M. Vernon et al., "Classification of Endometriotic Implants by Morphologic Appearance and Capacity to Synthesize Prostaglandin F," *Fertility and Sterility* 46 (1986): 801.
2. R. Franklin, "Intestinal Tract Endometriosis," Third World Congress on Endometriosis, 1992.
3. V. Buttram, "Evolution of the Revised American Fertility Society Classification of Endometriosis," *Fertility and Sterility* 43 (1985): 347.
4. A. Acosta, V. Buttram, R. Franklin, and P. Besch, "A Proposed Classification of Pelvic Endometriosis," *Obstetrics and Gynecology* 42 (1973): 19.
5. J. W. Betts and V. Buttram, "A Plan for Managing Endometriosis," *Contemporary Obstetrics and Gynecology* 15 (1980): 121.
6. K. Lamb, R. Hoffman, and T. Nichols, "Family Trait Analysis: A Case-Control Study of 43 Women with Endometriosis and Their Best Friends," *American Journal of Obstetrics and Gynecology* 154, no. 3 (March 1986): 596–601.
7. K. Lamb and T. Nichols, "Endometriosis: A Comparison of Associated Disease Histories," *American Journal of Preventive Medicine* 2, no. 6 (1986): 324–29.
8. T. Nichols, K. Lamb, and J. Arkins, "The Association of Atopic Diseases with Endometriosis," *Annals of Allergy* 59, no. 11 (November 1987): 360–63.
9. K. J. Armitage, L. J. Schneiderman, and R. A. Bass, "Response of Physicians to Medical Complaints in Men and Women," *Journal of the American Medical Association* 241 (1979): 2186–87.
10. A. Dlugi et al., "Lupron Depot (Leuprolide Acetate for Depot Suspension) in the Treatment of Endometriosis: A Randomized, Placebo-Controlled, Double-Blind Study," *Fertility and Sterility* 54 (1990): 419–27.
11. L. Fedele et al., "Comparison of Cyproterone Acetate and Danazol in the Treatment of Pelvic Pain Associated with Endometriosis," *Obstetrics and Gynecology* 73, no. 6 (1989): 1000–1004.
12. L. Fedele et al., "Gestrinone Versus Danazol in the Treatment of Endometriosis," *Fertility and Sterility* 51, no. 5 (1989): 781–85.
13. S. Telimaa et al., "Placebo-Controlled Comparison of Danazol and High-Dose Medroxyprogesterone Acetate in the Treatment of Endometriosis After Conservative Surgery," *Gynecological Endocrinology* 1, no. 4 (1987): 363–71.
14. Ibid., no. 1 (1987): 13–23.
15. J. Salat-Baroux et al., "Laparoscopic Control of Danazol Therapy on Pelvic Endometriosis," *Human Reproduction* 3, no. 2 (1988): 197–200.
16. The Nafarelin European Endometriosis Trial Group (NEET), "Nafarelin for Endometriosis: A Large-Scale, Danazol-Controlled Trial of Efficacy and Safety, with 1-Year Follow-Up," *Fertility and Sterility* 57, no. 3 (1992): 514–22.
17. D. B. Redwine, "Laparoscopic Excision of Endometriosis by Sharp Dissection, Lifetable Analysis of Reoperation and Persistence or Recurrence," *Fertility and Sterility* 56 (1991): 628–34.

18. J. Fanton and J. Golden, "Radiation Induced Endometriosis in Macaca Mulatta," *Radiation Research* 126 (1991): 141–46.

19. J. S. Campbell et al., "Is Simian Endometriosis an Effect of Immunotoxicity?" Ontario Association of Pathologists, 48th annual meeting (1985).

20. J. Fanton et al., "Endometriosis: Clinical and Pathological Findings in 70 Rhesus Monkeys," *American Journal of Veterinary Research* 47, no. 7 (1986): 1537–41.

21. J. S. Campbell, "Is Reproductive Wastage and Failure Related to Environmental Pollution?" Health and Welfare of Canada conference: Toxicologic Pathology: Quo Vadis? 1988.

22. S. E. Rier, D. C. Martin, R. E. Bowman, W. P. Dmowski, and J. L Becker, "Endometriosis in Rhesus Monkeys (*Macaca Mulatta*) Following Chronic Exposure to 2,3,7,8-Tetrachlorodibenzo-*p*-dioxin," *Fundamental and Applied Toxicology* 21 (1993): 433–41.

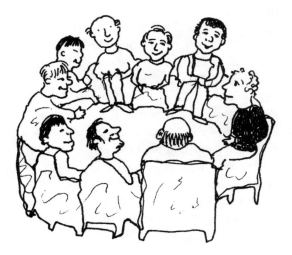

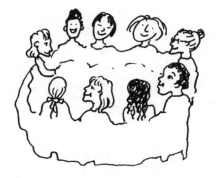

Finally, Joe finds some real hope.

Menstrual Cramps Are Not Normal

By Michael D. Birnbaum, M.D.

A young woman came to me several years ago for a routine problem. As part of my usual history I asked her whether her periods were painful and whether or not intercourse was painful. To each of these questions she responded no. I was therefore somewhat surprised to discover that on pelvic examination she was extremely tender.

I discussed the situation with her. Her husband was a sophomore medical student, and I knew it would be several years before she was in a position to begin thinking about a family. Despite her negative history, her pelvic examination was extremely suspicious for endometriosis. I therefore recommended a laparoscopy since I knew that she would be several years away from childbearing. My laparoscopy did indeed confirm the diagnosis of endometriosis.

When she came back to the office after her surgery to discuss my findings and recommendations for therapy, she surprised me with the following comment. "Dr. Birnbaum," she said, "I lied to you when I first came to the office. My periods are so painful I sometimes can't stand it, and intercourse is sometimes so painful that we have to stop in the middle." I asked her why she had not shared this information with me when I first questioned her, and her reply was astounding. She said, "I've been to two other gynecologists with the same complaints. They both told me it was all in my head. I was sick and tired of hearing that, and I was afraid that you too were going to call me a nut."

As astonishing as this story may seem, it is, unfortunately a story that I have heard repeated time and time again in my office since I have gone into practice. There is a bias that runs through the medical profession. This bias holds that women are neurotic—men are not. A recent study showed that if men and women went to a physician with identical complaints, the woman was more likely to be given a prescription for Valium, whereas the man would be taken more seriously and worked up for some illness. I have discovered in my years of practice that there is a great deal of organic disease masquerading as psychosomatic problems. While there is a common belief among some physicians that pelvic pain in women is mainly psychosomatic in origin, my experience is that very little pelvic pain is psychosomatic.

While there certainly appears to be a great deal of misunderstanding among physicians concerning pelvic pain, there seems to be an equally great misunderstanding among women. One common phrase that I hear in my office from my patients are words to the effect that "I have cramps with my period, but they are just normal cramps." *Menstrual cramps are not normal.*

■ *Dr. Birnbaum, Elkins Park, Pennsylvania, is a reproductive endocrinologist and former association advisor.*

10

ᥫᥫ

Men and Endometriosis:
What They Feel, How They Cope,
How They Can Help

By Ron Seely

"*My husband is finding it hard to understand the disease and the pain. He is optimistic that we will have a baby, and it is me that's given up hope.*"

"*For me, my husband has been honest enough to talk through the problems that have developed.*"

"*As we learned to communicate and cope with the problems, our relationship grew stronger. We would certainly like to have sex more often!*"

"*I am now separated after eight months of marriage . . . intercourse is very painful.*"

"*I have been extremely moody and depressed since on this drug [danazol]; however, my husband has been very good.*"

"*Fortunately . . . my husband is a very kind and understanding man and has been very supportive.*"

"*Trying to conceive and being unable to for four years tore us apart . . . plus the pain I suffered tore us apart.*"

"*Not married, but soon to be. My relationship did suffer some due to my pain and fears, but he's been very supportive.*"

"My emotions are always in an upheaval, and that affects my husband. When I am hurt or depressed, I tend to take it out on him. When I hurt, I cannot help do things around the house, so the tasks fall on my husband."

"I wanted more children. I've had 10 miscarriages, and I have a son. . . . Before I learned that it [endometriosis] could cause miscarriages, my husband and I blamed each other, and that caused a lot of marital stress. Support from everyone means a lot—not pity, just understanding!"

"Endometriosis has caused problems in my marriage because of infertility and pain, which led to severe depression, attempted suicide, and hospitalization in a mental hospital because I couldn't live with the pain any longer. . . . My husband is very understanding and gentle."

"Divorced from my first husband due to the illness."

"My husband divorced me because of our inability to have children."

"We have become a couple under siege. Patience and tolerance for each other decreased moderately due to the continuous tension, stress, and pain (physical and emotional) we have lived with for three years."

"My husband does not understand my frustrations and won't talk about it."

"My husband thinks I'm a sickly person . . . he will never be able to understand. He won't have sex if he knows it hurts. We are trying to have a child, so I don't want him to know."

"I feel pretty useless as a woman and think any man would feel likewise."

"Counseling might be helpful, but my husband would not go. He sympathizes with my pain, but he doesn't completely believe or understand it. He doesn't like inflicting pain on me, so he feels deprived of a normal sex life."

"I had begun a serious relationship a month after learning about endometriosis and had told him about it. Unfortunately, or rather fortunately, I learned he was nonsupportive of my plight. When I stopped taking Danocrine for three months . . . my partner balked when I asked him to use condoms until I was safe again!"

"My partner is magnificently understanding . . . endometriosis forced me to confront my lover about what our future would be—would we try to have children? . . . This experience . . . actually strengthened our relationship."

"My marriage has been critically challenged—we're working through it."

Asking a man to understand the pain and frustration of endometriosis is, I suppose, a little like asking him to understand what it's like to give birth to a child. He can never know, really, what it is like.

But a man can know and share the joy that comes with the birth of his son or daughter. And, similarly, if his wife is a victim of endometriosis, he can share in the struggle to cope with the disease. Indeed, for the sake of his wife and his marriage, he must.

I know that this is true. My wife, Doreen, has endometriosis. And I know it is true, too, because I have talked with other husbands whose wives have the disease. We have shared our stories, commiserated with one another, and agreed that sometimes when our wives most needed our support we have been real jerks. But we also shared ways in which we felt we helped our wives, making it just a little easier for them to live with such a frustrating and painful disease.

Until the fall of 1983, endometriosis might as well have been some mysterious jungle plague for all Doreen and I knew. But one afternoon I came home to find Doreen curled in a ball on the bathroom floor, wrapped in an afghan. She said the pain had started a couple hours earlier and that it felt like somebody was twisting a knife in her stomach. She could barely walk. We went to our family physician, and at first he thought she might have had a gallbladder attack. Later, however, after he discovered she was having problems getting pregnant with our second child (we'd been trying for over a year), he sent her to a gynecologist.

The gynecologist, after examining Doreen and talking to us about our hopes for a second child, put Doreen through an exhausting and often painful series of fertility tests. She had a uterine biopsy and a uterine x-ray. Eventually, he put her on Clomid, a fertility drug. She developed ovarian cysts. Suspecting endometriosis, the doctor scheduled Doreen for a laparoscopy. Through the laparoscope he saw that Doreen did indeed have the lesions typical of endometriosis. She had them on her ovaries, on the outside of her uterus, and even on her bladder. Later, in a depressing meeting in his office, the doctor told us that he suspected the endometriosis was preventing Doreen from getting pregnant.

Still, we decided to continue trying for our second child. For the next six months Doreen was on danazol. She gained weight and often couldn't sleep at night because of leg cramps—side effects of the drug, the doctor said.

After the danazol came another six months on Clomid and another futile six months of trying to get pregnant. Eventually the pain of endometriosis returned and the gynecologist took her off the Clomid and put her back on danazol.

Nothing worked. Even the danazol didn't take away the pain this time. The doctor advised surgery. He wanted to make an incision in Doreen's abdomen and cauterize the endometrial adhesions. So, early one morning in January 1985, we took our daughter, Katie, to a neighbor's and then checked Doreen into the hospital. The doctor told us the surgery would take about an hour.

Nearly three hours later I was still sitting in the waiting room, my fourth cup of coffee cooling in my hand and a *National Geographic* unread in my lap. I couldn't imagine what was happening. Had something gone wrong? Wouldn't they come out and tell me?

Finally the doctor came to the doorway in his surgical gown and signaled me into the hallway. Doreen was fine. But the endometriosis had been severe, he said. One ovary was swollen by a chocolate cyst and he had removed it. He had cauterized all the lesions he could find.

Doreen's recovery was difficult. The incision healed painfully and slowly. She hurt inside from where the ovary had been removed. And on top of it all was the knowledge that our chances of having a second child were waning. All because of this disease called endometriosis.

Sometimes during all of this I was everything a husband should be—supportive, caring, patient, and thoughtful. At other times, unfortunately, I was a creep. There were times, for example, that I grew so tired of Doreen's being ill that I would lose all patience and criticize her for not being able to handle the pain better. I would tell her that much of it was in her mind and that if only she were stronger the pain wouldn't be as bad. Well, that was all a bunch of baloney, of course. The pain for Doreen was worse than I could ever imagine, and it was real pain from a real disease, not something imaginary.

Other husbands, I have discovered, have equally shameful tales to tell—and good advice for others whose wives suffer from endometriosis.

Kate, 36, founder of a chapter of the Endometriosis Association, has had endometriosis since high school. She married Craig, a math teacher, in 1975. When Kate couldn't get pregnant, Craig recalls, she went to a Boston physician and eventually had a partial hysterectomy. In the years since, Kate has had an ectopic pregnancy, a miscarriage, a ruptured chocolate cyst, danazol treatments, and surgery to remove the endometrial adhesions.

Craig particularly remembers getting a telephone call at school one December and racing home to find Kate in terrible pain. They rushed to the hospital, where Kate was whisked into the operating room for surgery on a ruptured chocolate cyst. Less than two months later, he said, they were trapped in their home by one of the worst blizzards in the city's history when Kate again started having crippling pains. They had to call the police and get permission to drive to the hospital, where Kate was put on pain medication.

"I was painting houses on the side to meet all the bills," Craig recalls. "In those days surgery for endometriosis was not [considered] necessary surgery, so insurance didn't pay for it."

At times, Craig said, their marriage suffered because of the strain. One night Kate became so frustrated with him and with her problems that she simply walked out. "Sure, we had our fights," he said. "Tensions were up."

It was difficult, too, Craig said, for him to come to grips with not having a child.

"At first I was psyched to have kids. I coach soccer, and I wanted a little inside forward, you know? But then I realized I'd better start accepting the fact that, short of a miracle, we wouldn't have kids."

They have, however, learned to live with endometriosis. Since her last surgery Kate has been doing much better. Craig said he has learned over the years that there are many things he can do to help Kate cope with the disease. He's learned as much as he can about endometriosis and the problems it can cause. Sex, for example, can pose special problems for couples coping with endometriosis because intercourse is often so painful as to be impossible. Dealing with such a problem, Craig said, requires awareness and sensitivity on the husband's part.

Craig said he has also tried to be an active participant in meetings of the Endometriosis Association. And he's made it a point to join Kate on her visits to the doctor.

"You go to the meetings as a team," he said. "You gotta make the most of it. I feel like it's Kate and me against the world."

Gene and his wife, Cynthia, were married just a little more than a year ago, though they had known one another for a couple of years. Before he met Cynthia, Gene said, he'd never heard of endometriosis, even though he works full-time as an emergency medical technician in Monona, near Madison, Wisconsin.

For Gene, helping people who are in pain is an everyday thing. It's his job. Yet he still finds himself short of patience sometimes when Cynthia is in pain.

"I deal so much with pain in the street," he said. "And when you come home, you want to unwind. You want to get away from the necessity of having to care for somebody else."

On top of this, Gene added, is a feeling of helplessness when Cynthia is suffering. For him it's the hardest part of dealing with the disease.

"When Cynthia is hurting, I feel bad inside," Gene said. "And there's nothing I can do about it. When someone is in pain in the field, I can stabilize him or her or start an IV. When Cynthia is in pain, I can't do a damn thing."

Gene has learned that there are ways he can, however, help make the pain more bearable. Like Craig, he suggests that husbands whose wives have endometriosis educate themselves about the disease. He suggests that, more than anything else, patience and a willingness to listen are ways to help your wife through the difficult times.

"When someone is hurting, there are times when you can't do anything but be there," Gene said. "Tell her you love her, hold her hand, put a cold compress on her forehead. Show her you care."

Just as Craig and Gene learned, I learned. I learned to listen when Doreen wanted to talk, to take the trouble to rearrange my schedule and go to the doctor with her, to understand when she gently explained that intercourse might be too painful, to be there to hold her when she hurt.

Craig and Gene both said their marriages are stronger for having lived through their struggles with endometriosis. Ours is, too. After all of this, Doreen and I tell ourselves, there surely aren't many obstacles we can't overcome.

And we have decided to adopt a Korean child. Doreen seems to be going through a good time right now, with few pains from the disease. When we talk at night, our conversations are not about endometriosis but about the little black-haired, black-eyed baby that will soon join our family.

■ *Ron Seely is a journalist in Madison, Wisconsin.*

Being Supportive:
Tips for Partners and
Family Members of
Those Who Have Endometriosis

1. Emotional support is very important. All the ways you showed love and support in your home before you ever heard of endometriosis will be even more appreciated now. Try to find new words and actions to show your caring support.
2. Practical support may be especially needed when physical symptoms are dominant. Family members can help in the coping process by taking a larger share of chores and offering more assistance with the daily routine.
3. Maintain a positive attitude. This is crucial, even though difficult at times. Remember that a sense of defeat goes nowhere and does nothing to help.
4. Learn all you can about the medical situation, treatment options, and possible drug side effects. Be involved in medical consultations when possible and be particularly attentive when hospital care is called for.
5. Explore the possibilities of diet, relaxation techniques, and various other lifestyle changes to offer improvement.

Coping with Painful Sex

By Mary Lou Ballweg

"*Since* I had the problem before I married, we became used to having a couple of days each month that I was too sore to make love."

"*Sexually,* both my husband and I have developed a strong personal commitment that enables us to be more patient with each other."

"*Because* of irregular bleeding, we have very little sexual relations. I have to learn to accept myself and my disease and feel that I'm just as attractive and sensual as I was before I was diagnosed."

"*We* tried all kinds of sexual exercises, just touching, music, etc.—but the results were the same. I have lots of problems with painful penetrations . . . like a knife entering you. When he does try to penetrate me, he tries to help me relax, but that helps only a little. I dread going to bed and try to go at a different time than my husband. We don't have sex anymore. I think that even hurts more than penetration."

"*Being* a single young lady and rarely being sexually active, this is a difficult one. . . . I became involved with someone and decided I needed to communicate the difficulties of intercourse due to endometriosis. It seemed understood, but when intercourse became a possibility again, the relationship ended."

"*I* avoid sex entirely."

"*When* it hurts, who wants it?"

"*Experiment* with positions limiting penetration and other sexual activities. Actually, the whole surgery and everything deepened our sexual relationship and friendship, although I was very afraid he wouldn't put up with my disability and would leave me."

"*Sex* was a thought, not an action, so my very understanding husband chews a lot of windowsills . . . humor must be kept or you go crazy!"

Pain with sex is a problem for 59 percent of women with endometriosis and, as is perhaps obvious, that also means it's a problem for their partners and the relationship. Here are a number of tips based on the association's work with thousands of women with endometriosis.

Timing

Determine for yourself when the least problematic or no-problem times are and plan special times of physical intimacy for yourself and your partner at that time. Many women with endo find that the time right after a period and before ovulation is a "good" time for them, and you may find you do not experience pain with sexual activity at that time. Make this a time for you and your partner to make up for the bad times—in fact, together you could make this time so enjoyable and special that you may both find yourselves looking forward to it and planning special events and activities around it.

Sexual Activities

Intercourse. Since deep penetration is most often the cause of pain when endometrial implants are on the uterosacral ligaments or other areas that get stretched, pushed, or pulled with thrusting, positions that control this may make intercourse without pain possible. These positions include the "bridge maneuver" described by Dr. Helen Kaplan Singer in *Illustrated Manual of Sex Therapy*. In this position the man and woman lie side by side or the woman is on top. After sufficient foreplay so that both partners are ready for intercourse (the man erect and the woman lubricated, the equivalent of erection in women), the man enters or the woman guides the man's penis into her and then the couple engage in just enough depth, motion, and rhythm to maintain an erection. At the same time, either partner can stimulate the woman's clitoris with the fingers. "It's a position," says Dr. Andrea Shrednick, a family and sex therapist, "that allows for mutual feelings, mutual satisfaction, touch and closeness, but not the deep penetration that causes pain."

Another method of coping with problems with intercourse might be waiting until the man is nearly ready to ejaculate and limiting actual intercourse to then, with little thrusting. Of course, if even this is painful for the woman, the couple will have to explore other methods of sexual pleasure together.

Couples also can find other positions that are satisfying but do not involve deep penetration. Positions that allow the woman to control the depth of penetration are good because she will know just when it hurts and be able to control for it. Many men enjoy the feeling of being seduced and pleasured that comes from the woman taking a little more action to initiate and "make love" to them.

Sex Is More than Intercourse. Most of us would not like to eat the same meal over and over, even if it was our favorite! Yet, surprisingly, some people think sex equals intercourse. In fact the range of sexual activity is far wider and, once you've experienced it, you'll never go back to the same thing over and over again. If you have not explored these methods before, you'll be amazed at the dimensions your sex life can take on. The endo will perhaps even be a blessing in disguise for having forced you to discover them. Books recommended by a sex therapist that will inform you and spark your imagination are Lonnie Barbach's books *Pleasures, For Each Other: Sharing Sexual Intimacy*, and *For Yourself: The Fulfillment of Female Sexuality*; *Ladies Own Erotica* by the Kensington Ladies Erotica Society; *The New Our Bodies, Ourselves* by the Boston Women's Health Book Collective; and *The Art of Sensuous Loving* by Andrew Stanway.

Intimacy

Even more important than sex is intimacy (of course when they occur together, we can reach true ecstasy!). Intimacy is the personal closeness, sharing, caring for each other, and actions that show true love. Activities that can bring intimacy and pleasure for many couples include massage (which also can help ease the endo pain a bit), hugging and holding each other, kissing, playful physical affection, and cuddling. All of these and sexual activities can be enhanced with music, candles, incense, or sharing a hot bath or shower or special food or drinks and in numerous other ways that will be personal to you and your partner. Many of these are activities you can engage in during the "bad" times with endometriosis to ensure that both of you still feel cared for and loved. During times too painful for sex you may feel better about the situation by remembering this: if your partner were the one in pain, you certainly would be understanding and not insist on having sex. Sometimes a woman is afraid to engage in intimate sharing activities for fear they'll lead to painful sexual activities—these are the times she needs to be clear in communicating with her partner that she is in pain but needs the partner's affection and also wants to show her affection for her partner.

Miscellaneous Tips

Vaginal Lubricants. These can be helpful if a woman experiences vaginal dryness, often a problem during GnRH drug therapy and after removal of the ovaries. (Vaginal lubricants and/or moisturizers currently available include Lubrin, Replens, Creme de la Femme, Astroglide, Gyne-Moistrin, and K-Y Lubricating Jelly.) The lubricant can be used by the man, too—and many men will very much enjoy having you apply it! A cautionary note for those attempting to become pregnant: some vaginal lubricants have been found to destroy sperm (K-Y Jelly or Surgilube) or decrease sperm motility (Lubrin). Glycerin, one of the ingredients of Lubrin, has no effect on sperm, however, according to research reports, so a possible alternative could be glycerin suppositories (available in drugstores) or, according to the editor of *Fertility Review*, a small amount of corn oil.

Sex Therapists. A qualified and carefully selected sex therapist who understands endometriosis can be very helpful. The American Association of Sex Educators, Counselors and Therapists can help you find a sex therapist. For a referral list, send $15 and a self-addressed stamped envelope to 435 N. Michigan Ave., Suite 1717, Chicago, IL 60611.

Communication. Never underestimate the importance of *talking* with each other about your feelings, relationship, work, family concerns, and, most of all, endometriosis and any other problems in your lives. Sexual likes and dislikes also need to be shared. A long-term satisfying sexual relationship is impossible without communication and sharing. All too often unspoken fears and assumptions can ruin a sexual relationship: Is she avoiding sex because she doesn't like me or find me attractive anymore? Has she found someone else? Is she pretending not to feel pain? Fearing this, a man might avoid initiating intercourse, in turn raising some fears and questions in the woman. Loving someone does not mean being able to read his or her mind!

Take Your Partner with You to the Doctor. Assuming you have a competent doctor who understands painful sex as a symptom of endo and is not embarrassed to talk about it and assuming he or she talks to you as a couple, it should help to have the doctor explain why pain occurs with sex in endo. Beware the male doctor who takes a husband off to another room to have a man-to-man talk! And don't assume that a gynecologist automatically knows about painful sex. A recent article in *The Journal of Family Practice* noted that residency programs in gynecology are woefully inadequate in teaching about painful sex.

Treat the Endometriosis. Many members report that hormonal and surgical treatment of the endometriosis removed the pain with sex. However, since the disease is chronic, the pain typically returned when the disease returned. Also, reports on danazol and the GnRH drugs are varied—some women have reported no relief from painful sex; others found reduced pain. It depends on the size and location of implants and numerous other factors. As one association member wrote, "After the second surgery I acquired a very understanding and sensitive boyfriend who helped me deal with my fears of pain during intercourse. I then realized how good sex could be and regret the fact that my ex-husband could not be with me at this time so he could see the problem really *was physical* and not in my head! I've had five surgeries for endo, and intercourse is *always* painless right after surgery, until the endo comes back."

Remember the Most Important Ingredient of All: Gentleness. Be gentle with yourself and your partner. Your partner needs to be gentle and patient with you, and both of you need to be gentle with your relationship. All of us have ego and self-esteem wrapped up in our sexuality. We need to bring as much care and effort to our relationship, if we want it to blossom, as we would to our work or parenting or any other important part of our lives.

11

@/@

Building the Doctor-Patient Relationship

Living with a Chronic Disease: What Do You Want from Your Doctor?

By Mark Flapan, Ph.D.

"*Tell women to interview as many doctors as they can until they feel comfortable with the one they finally choose. I had exams and opinions with five doctors until I found one I trusted and knew would respect my feelings about treatment choices. I have total, complete faith in his skills and knowledge, and believe me, when you are talking about your future ability to bear children and three surgeries in five weeks, you better like and trust him.*

"*Women must learn to make their own treatment decisions and must insist they be given/led to adequate information, not just accept paternalistic decisions made by doctors who have no idea how the patient feels. . . .*"

Linda, Arkansas

"*I am a longtime member of the association and have lived with endo for the past 10 years. . . . I need to share my frustration, which I know isn't unique, but I feel it must be addressed by the association. As most of us are aware, finding an experienced, knowledgeable surgeon presents its own problems. What I find almost incredible, particularly in New York City, is the difficulty in finding other types of physicians and specialists who have the proper interest and capability to help women (and their families) manage their medical condition in between surgeries. My particular problems have required gynecologists, internists, allergists,* urologists, gastrointestinal specialists, etc., most of whom know little or nothing about endo, how it relates to their specialty, the medical options available as treatments, and how to follow up these treatments. What is a side effect of the medication or simply a new and separate, totally uninvolved symptom? Truthfully, I can't even seem to find a gynecologist who is not a fertility specialist with the knowledge to treat my overall needs. . . .

"While I trust my present surgeon, I don't feel that the follow-up, aftercare, and overall medical management are handled properly by these doctors. I also find that their efforts are totally directed to the endo with no interest in this patient's other gynecological needs, such as mammography, weight monitoring, blood pressure, breast exams, chronic yeast infections, etc. How many gynecologists do I need to have?

"The medical community that does show any interest in endo seems to have such differences in opinion regarding monitoring patients on medication that it is frightening. One doctor feels blood tests, [ultrasounds], bone scans, etc. are recommended; another does not. One says every month; another says every three. Dr. A says a medicine can be used only for six months; Dr. B says patients have been treated for 18 months. Wouldn't it be wonderful, and of course, quite idealistic, if teams of doctors were able to treat endo? When I think back over the years of symptoms I have presented to various doctors and how many times I've been told 'It's nothing,' 'It's in your head,' 'You're a hypochondriac,' I explode with anger.

"My greatest comfort and 'sanity preserver' has been maintaining contact with other women who have endo both through your newsletters and my support group. I congratulate you for your efforts in keeping us all in touch with each other and for teaching us to be in touch with ourselves and to try to actively control our own disease by offering us choices. I believe it is of the utmost importance for endo patients to constantly and endlessly keep on sharing their personal experiences with each other.

"One of my greatest fears is for my 14-year-old daughter's future. I hope and pray that my suffering will be something that will never be experienced by her. . . ."

Joan, New York

"I have mixed feelings about the medical profession. We need them, and then again, due to their lack of knowledge, a lot of women have been both mentally and physically scarred."

Julia, Iowa

"It has been an enormous relief and comfort to me to know that there was an Endometriosis Association . . . and the information that you have sent me has been helpful in confirming ideas and in helping me to gain the confidence to 'listen to my body' and to pursue my hunches. Since one rarely gets this from one's doctors—just the reverse—I am overwhelmingly grateful to you. Dreadful to say: as a political theorist my career relies on my ability to think freely to follow my beliefs and instincts in intellectual matters; but the endless denigration, the physical weakness, and the insinuations that one is psychologically troubled *were really robbing me of the confidence necessary to work happily. Your association and the help of two special doctors have started to give that back to me."*

Anabelle, Massachusetts

"Are there any doctors who specialize in this frustrating disease?. . . I feel these doctors have really messed up my life. I don't trust them anymore. . . ."

Betty, British Columbia

"God bless your organization!

"For years I went to my ob-gyn complaining of painful periods and heard 'You'll have to live with it,' 'Get pregnant; it will go away.' (Unfortunately, I wasn't married, so I didn't want a child just to cure me.)

"A couple of years ago I went to work for a health organization that pays for all our medical needs, so I decided I was going to get 'all' my medical problems cleared up. Little did I know that 'they' were related. First I went to my gynecologist since that was my worst problem—painful periods. I was given the same answer—live with it—even though I had stressed the problem of 'painful pelvis.' I was told that the discomfort of my pelvis was not related to gynecology.

"Off to the internist for 'hip pain,' 'painful bowel movements,' and 'constipation.' Barium x-rays and x-rays of my hips and pelvis were done. Nothing out of the ordinary was shown, so I was told to 'eat more fiber.' I gave up until I heard a new 'young' doctor had joined the gyn staff. Since 'she' was a young woman, I thought maybe she had newer ideas.

"She had before her a 'total' health background. She saw in my chart the fact that I had had 'internal' tests and evaluations. She asked questions no other gynecologist had bothered to ask. She asked about bowel and gastric distress; she even asked about painful intercourse. Now why didn't any other doctor ask about intercourse? She said that all these seemingly unrelated symptoms could mean that one more test should be done. She ordered day surgery for that week! A laparoscopy proved her right—endometriosis. . . .

"I consider myself lucky to have found such a compassionate doctor who took the time, then and now, just to listen. . . .My doctor has been a blessing."

Cheryl, Minnesota

"Doctors need to have more information. . . . If they were updated on new findings, and if they were better able to understand the disease and its debilitating effects, then they may be better doctors. One doctor I've seen (who's not on my insurance) has new articles from medical journals on his desk all the time. He corrects me if I have my facts wrong, and he informs me on everything. He also spends a great deal of time in his office with a patient who has lots of questions. He's a wonderfully thorough doctor.

"My other doctor (whom I see because he is on my insurance) is the one who was 'with me' through diagnosis, surgery, and treatment. He has been my doctor for years. After the

laparoscopy, in the postsurgery visit, I was a mess of questions, concerns, and emotions. I wanted information desperately. He neither showed me where to look nor told me much himself. I kept thinking there had to be information on this terrible disease. Even when I asked him about the side effects of the Synarel (holding the patient pamphlet), he said, 'Go and get yourself a medical dictionary and look those words up for yourself. It is not my job to teach you about things you don't need to know.'

"I left his office in tears many times, and his quote will always be in my head. He has said many other hurtful things throughout this ordeal. Unfortunately, I can't change doctors at this time, so I avoid him at all costs. That is not health care to me.

"A bedside manner would be nice, but what I look for now is someone who knows endo and is willing to spend time going over my thoughts or questions. . . ."

Betsy, Colorado

EDITOR'S NOTE: Women with endometriosis face ongoing struggles in their medical relationships, as the accompanying letters and the experiences of almost all of us show, and we thought this article would have much to say to us. (Pronouns have been changed to reflect both male and female doctors by alternating genders from paragraph to paragraph.)

With a chronic, incurable disease, unlike a physical illness for which you go to a doctor, get treated, and are cured, you have a long-term relationship with your doctor. Your doctor becomes a regular, permanent, and important part of your life. She's not just someone you call on occasions when you happen to get sick.

What you want from your doctor now that you have a chronic disease is what you always wanted from your doctor when you were sick—you want him to make it go away. But he can't make it go away because medical research has not yet found a cure for your condition.

It's hard to accept that no doctor has a cure for your illness. Maybe you're still hoping there's some doctor somewhere who has the knowledge, understanding, or treatment to cure you, and you're still hunting for that doctor.

However, if you've lived with your illness for some time, you've probably come to terms with the fact that no cure exists and have settled on a doctor you rely on. You may see her occasionally for a periodic checkup or see her regularly to monitor the effect of some medication. Or you may make special appointments when new symptoms emerge or old symptoms seem to be getting worse.

You Want Something Personal

Although you go to your doctor for him to do something for your body, you want more from him than technically competent physical care. You want something more personal. You want him to listen not just to the beating of your heart but to the *feelings* in your heart. You want him to look at you and see *you* and not just your symptoms. And when he looks at you you want him to see a *person,* not just another case of your disease.

If you keep a stiff upper lip, you want the doctor to recognize that you may be scared to death inside. And if you show your feelings by crying, you don't want her to get upset or think you're a "basket case." You want her to realize you may not hear, understand, or remember what she tells you. This is so because you're nervous when you're with her. Therefore you want her to repeat things when you ask her to, without her getting impatient or annoyed with you or thinking you're stupid.

But most of all, you want to feel the doctor *cares* about you even if he can't cure you. You want to feel, if a serious complication develops, he'll be there for you and will do everything he can to help you.

You want the doctor to show her interest in you by returning phone calls, by not rushing you through appointments, and by listening and responding to your concerns. You want her to explain what's going on in your body in words you can understand. You want her to explain things without upsetting or frightening you, which may not always be possible, because the facts may be frightening. In any case, you want her to put the facts in some hopeful perspective.

You don't want the doctor to try to protect you by being evasive or saying very little. If you feel he's evasive, you get more frightened, wondering what awful thing he's hiding.

Dependency on Your Doctor

You're dependent on your doctor to tell you why you feel the way you do and what your symptoms mean. It's only through her knowledge, her instruments, and her tests that you can find out what's going on inside. Her ability to learn what's going on in your body to learn things you have no way of knowing yourself makes you feel as dependent as a child on her. After all, she's your only hope of ever getting better—you feel your life is no longer in your hands but in hers.

Because of this dependency, everything your doctor says or doesn't say, everything he does or doesn't do, affects you emotionally.

Unrealistic Expectations

One effect of this dependency is that you expect more from your doctor than she can realistically give you. Just as you want her to cure you when no cure exists, you want her to know more about your illness than is medically known.

It's frightening to think that your doctor, on whom you're so dependent for your medical care, doesn't know everything about your disease. How can he help you if he doesn't have an answer to every question? But in reality he can only draw upon available medical knowledge; he can't know more than that. Your doctor, like you, has to wait for medical research to come up with more answers.

Furthermore, you may want more reassurance from the doctor than she can possibly give you. She can't reassure you everything will be all right when she doesn't know everything will be all right—and still keep your trust and confidence.

Moreover, the kind of interest, concern, and caring you want may be unrealistic in a relationship between a doctor and a patient. You would like him to have the kind of concern for you that he would have if it were his own child who was ill or, better yet, if it were his only child who had the illness.

You would like to get an immediate appointment when you call rather than for some time in the future. You would like the doctor to have no other patients before you so you won't have to wait when you arrive. And you would like her to have no other patients after you so you can have all the time you want when you're with her. You would like to be able to reach her on the phone whenever you want but don't want her to answer other patients' calls when she's with you.

You're in Awe of Your Doctor

Your feelings of dependency on your doctor may, on the other hand, lead you to expect too little from him. You may feel overly grateful for anything he does for you. You may feel so intimidated and awestruck by him you're afraid to ask for anything.

You don't want to take too much of her time because she's so busy, so you don't ask all the questions you have or ask her to repeat what you don't understand. You're reluctant to phone her even when something worries you, because you don't want to disturb her. And you wouldn't dare question anything she does in relation to you—after all, who are you to question her judgment? She's the doctor, and you're only the patient.

You don't check out with the doctor things you're doing on your own, like taking vitamins, going on a special diet, or taking some treatment he didn't prescribe.* You're afraid he'll disapprove or think you're foolish, and what would you do then about these extra things you're doing for yourself? As long as you don't tell him, you can continue doing what you're doing, but then you don't get the benefit of his judgment on these matters. All this because you're intimidated by him.

You don't tell the doctor you want to consult another doctor for fear of offending her. You're afraid of doing anything you imagine might annoy, irritate, or anger her. In your mind she's more than your doctor whom you're paying to help you. She's an awesome, imposing authority in whose presence you feel humble and deferential.

---

*Unfortunately, physicians treating women with endometriosis are very often not yet aware of some of the treatments related to rebuilding the immune system, candidiasis, and other approaches that may be helpful.

You Can Feel More Equal

You may have heard that you and your doctor should be partners in your medical treatment, that you should be an informed patient and should even be in charge of your own medical care. But given the nature of the relationship between doctor and patient, you can't be equal partners, let alone in charge of your treatment. Although you and your doctor share the common purpose of your medical care, you and he differ in experience, in the way you look at things, and in the kind of words you use. And no matter how much you have learned about your disease, he's still the medical expert, not you.*

Moreover, you have an illness and are going to your doctor for help, which means you're dependent on her; she's not dependent on you. Of course, she's dependent on having patients to fulfill herself as a doctor as well as to earn a living, but that's different from your dependency on her. You are one of her many patients, while she's your only or main doctor. So in no way can the relationship be equal.

But it's possible to feel more equal than you do. And if you felt more equal, you would be able to ask for the kind of treatment and attention to which you are rightfully entitled. At the same time, you wouldn't expect what may be inappropriate in a relationship between a doctor and a patient, and you wouldn't then feel hurt and angry because these expectations weren't met.

If you didn't expect your doctor to know more than is known about your disease, you wouldn't lose confidence in him if he didn't have an answer for every question. And if you didn't expect him to have some magic treatment, you wouldn't blame him for not caring for your disease or making you better.

While you would continue to expect your doctor to be sensitive to your feelings, you wouldn't expect her to help you with all the emotional reactions evoked by your illness. As it happens, your doctor's training and responsibility are primarily for your physical well-being—not for your emotional and mental state.

If you're feeling particularly upset, frightened, angry, guilty, or depressed by your illness, your doctor can refer you to a mental health professional who can help you with these feelings. A referral for psychological counseling doesn't mean "it's all in your head" or that you're a "mental case."† It simply means you need the kind of help your doctor is not prepared to give you.

---

* Similarly, as accompanying letters and numerous other communications over the years have indicated, it is all too common that women with endometriosis learn much more about their disease than those physicians who have not kept up since they left medical school.

† A referral without any physical care, or even a diagnosis, may, especially with endometriosis, mean the physician does believe the symptoms are in the patient's head.

You and Your Doctor Are Both Human Beings

The more you understand the nature of the relationship between you and your doctor, the more equal and the more like a partner you can feel. Even though you're dependent on your doctor for his special knowledge, he's still a human being like you. He's a human being who went to medical school, and you're thankful for that.

But as a human being your doctor, too, has needs. She needs to feel helpful and of value to you. If your condition gets worse, in spite of everything she does, she feels frustrated, helpless, and inadequate. She wants to be liked, respected, and appreciated by you, just as you want to be thought well of and cared for by her.

Your doctor's manner may be impersonal and aloof for reasons of his own. And he may not think of a relationship with a patient as a potential partnership. But how he is with you is also affected by how you are with him. The more you relate to him as a human being who happens to be your doctor, the more he'll relate to you as a human being who happens to have an illness. Human relationships tend to become reciprocal in this way.

But feeling more equal entails a loss—a loss of a fantasy of having a doctor so knowledgeable and powerful that she can take care of you no matter what. But if, in feeling more equal, you share with your doctor the responsibility for your medical care, then you have a person on your medical team—namely you—who knows better than anyone else how your body feels. And then, in a relationship in which you and your doctor are working together for your physical and emotional well-being, you may not only be more realistic in what you expect from her, but you may also be able to get more of what you need from her.

■ *Reprinted from the* NORD Newsletter, *Vol. VIII, ed. 3, by permission of NORD.*

   Dr. Mark Flapan *has scleroderma and is a founder of the Scleroderma Federation of the Tri-State Area. He is a psychologist in New York City and has a special interest in the emotional effects of chronic illness, both on the ill person and on family members.*

EDITOR'S NOTE: We are grateful to Dr. Flapan and the National Organization for Rare Disorders (NORD) for making this excellent article available.

Standards for
Obstetric-Gynecologic Services

From the American College of Obstetricians and Gynecologists

EDITOR'S NOTE: The American College of Obstetricians and Gynecologists is an international professional organization of ob-gyns that was established, according to one of its publications, "to maintain a cooperating community of physicians to further the goal of the obstetrician-gynecologist." The organization, usually referred to by its initials, ACOG, has more than 29,000 members, most of them physicians in the U.S. and Canada.

The following sections on patients' rights and the rights of the obstetrician-gynecologist are from ACOG's *Standards for Obstetric-Gynecologic Services*, Appendix 4, "Ethical Considerations in the Practice of Obstetrics and Gynecology." Members of the organization are called *Fellows*.

The Patient's Rights in Obstetric-Gynecologic Services

1. To be accorded respect and dignity without reference to age and sex or to marital, socioeconomic, ethnic, national, political, mental, physical, or religious status
2. To be free of exploitation by Fellows for social, sexual, or personal gain
3. To know the truth about her condition and treatment
4. To full disclosure of financial factors involved in her treatment
5. To make decisions regarding her own person, with access to relevant information on which to base such decisions
6. To accept or to refuse treatment
7. To freedom from coercion in such decision-making
8. To high-quality medical care without regard to her status in life
9. To the freedom to choose a physician and obtain additional consultation
10. To know who will participate in her care
11. To be fully informed and to decide whether to participate in or withdraw from medical research without jeopardizing the quality of her care
12. Not to be neglected or discharged without opportunity to find other medical assistance
13. To inviolable privacy except where this right is preempted by law
14. To have an appropriate representative to exercise these rights when the patient herself is unable to do so

The Obstetrician-Gynecologist's Rights in Relation to Patients

1. To refuse care, except in an emergency, to patients with whom no doctor-patient relationship has been established

2. To discharge patients from care, providing adequate opportunity for other care has been extended
3. To refuse to render treatment that is inconsistent with the Fellow's own moral code
4. To retain control of clinical management as long as the physician-patient relationship remains intact
5. To expect honest medically and socially relevant information from patients on which to base care
6. To receive reasonable compensation for services rendered

■ *Reprinted with permission from* American College of Obstetricians and Gynecologists: Standards for Obstetric-Gynecologic Services, *7th ed. (Washington, D.C.: ACOG, 1989): 108–109.*

"As the Pup Worsened, Ignorance Fed Anxiety and Fear": Notes on Medical Communications

By Allan H. Bruckheim, M.D.

EDITOR'S NOTE: Being a good communicator (that means both a good talker and a good listener) is noted again and again in the letters the association receives from women about the traits they look for in an endo specialist. Why communication is so vital when we face a situation in which we are in pain (both physical and emotional), confused, and fearful is explained very well in a column by Dr. Allan H. Bruckheim published in the *Medical Times*. Readers who feel their physician is knowledgeable and helpful but lacks a bit in the communication department may wish to share this column written by another physician. (If you do share it, do so in a kind, positive way—after all, none of us are perfect at our jobs either!)

To teach myself a lesson I thought I already had learned, I couldn't have constructed a better scenario than the events of this past week. I often have speculated on the educational opportunities that could be afforded my residents if I insisted that each be admitted into a hospital in turn and pass through the routines and procedures that all patients experience when hospitalized. Of course, in these days of DRGs* and cost factors, that experience would be far too costly; so, rather than demonstrating the actual negative aspects of this experience, we do a lot of talking about it. Well, that's fine for a hospitalized patient; but how could you construct a scenario in which a physician, with a strong background and reservoir of medical knowledge, could be made to feel the anxieties that can occur during ambulatory care? Since each of us really knows quite a bit about medicine, we find it easy to assimilate the information that is provided to us about our personal condition when we visit the physician.

Last week my daughter's new puppy became deathly ill. Although the situation could be approximated by many experiences that I have had in human medicine, the fact of the matter was that I was pretty much at sea in the complexities of canine pathology and veterinary medicine. As the situation proceeded from bad to grave, and then to the point

---

* DRG is the abbreviation for "diagnosis-related group." This is a designation in a system that classifies patients by age, diagnosis, and surgical procedure, producing different categories used in predicting the use of hospital resources, including length of stay. This system is used by insurance companies to determine how much a hospital should be reimbursed for a claimant's hospitalization.

where the doctor stopped talking about positive outcomes, I found my own ignorance feeding an ever-growing anxiety that developed into debilitating fear. All of this was compounded by the frustration of a caring father who could not deal with his daughter's pain because he lacked the information necessary to provide reassuring explanations.

As reports of the dog's condition became grimmer and grimmer, we sat around the kitchen table, discussing and rehashing the information we had. We did so in an attempt to extract some aspect of logic, some shred of hope, some degree of comprehension to ease the fears provoked by reports of the pup's worsening condition.

While there have been situations such as this with other members of the family, they have never struck home quite as poignantly as this one. My own reserve of knowledge and experience was insufficient to deal with the few facts afforded us by the veterinarian; thus I was unable to construct a comfortable and understandable picture of what was happening and what could happen.

I'm not faulting the veterinarian. His problem was difficult enough, dealing as he was with a new family and a new patient. What I am trying to underline is the fact that in a medical situation, lack of information, lack of instruction, and lack of understanding can, in itself, provoke real pain, anxiety, and anguish. It's so easy to deal with this aspect of care, if only we take those moments necessary to render the advice and explanations that become the most important element during these trying times.

It was an experience that has reaffirmed and strengthened my conviction that patient education is, in fact, an intricate part of health care that deserves a top priority. Incidentally, the pup did survive, and, as of this writing, is doing well. . . .

■ *Dr. Allan H. Bruckheim is clinical associate professor of family medicine at New York Medical College. Dr. Bruckheim also writes a column that appears in many newspapers across the country entitled "Family Doctor" and has authored a book entitled* Answers from the Family Doctor *(Chicago: Tribune Publishing/Contemporary Books, 1994). He has carried information about endometriosis and the association, and many hundreds of women with endometriosis have found us because of his column.*

A Little Help in
Finding Good Doctors

Finding a good doctor for endometriosis is tough. Here are several resources that may be helpful:

- The American Board of Medical Specialties runs an 800-number service (1-800-776-CERT) to verify whether a doctor is listed in a specialty and the year of certification if he or she is certified. While having training in the specialty (such as ob-gyn) does not, of course, guarantee the physician is knowledgeable about endo, it's at least a start. The toll-free line operates 9:00 A.M. to 6:00 P.M. eastern time.

- A resource entitled *Questionable Doctors* lists physicians across the United States who have been disciplined by the state or federal government. Check your local library.

- Disciplinary actions against doctors and dentists as well as malpractice payments must be reported to the United States National Practitioners Data Bank. Established by a 1986 law, the registry does not allow queries by patients, but hospitals have access—in fact, hospitals are legally required to use the registry to check doctors' records.

- The best resources of all are informed members of the association. Be sure to use this wonderful base of experience—join the association if you are not already a member, and attend your local support group meetings and lectures. If no group exists near you, order a contact list. You'll get a list of members in your area who have given us permission to give out their names and phone numbers to other local members. In addition, association literature covers the work of leading experts in the field, including its advisors, top researchers, and innovative clinicians. Taken together, these resources can help you locate an endo specialist. (See the association address and toll-free numbers in "Additional Resources" at the back of the book.)

What You Can Do

"After my own experience and reading the experiences of other women with endometriosis, I strongly believe that educating doctors about endometriosis is essential. These are the professionals we go to with our symptoms and whose correct and early diagnosis is critical for the treatment and management of this disease.

"My suggestion, apart from talking to doctors about the association, is for every woman with endometriosis who can afford the membership fee to take out an association membership in her doctor's name—possibly for both her general practitioner and her gynecologist. I do believe that if they started receiving the newsletter and reading not only the excellent research articles published in it but also the personal experiences of women with endometriosis, this would do much to promote awareness and understanding of this disease. Hopefully the end result would be a lessening of the suffering that we go through before our disease is accurately diagnosed. . . ."

B.Y., Toronto, Ontario

"P.S. When I told my doctor I was giving her a membership in the association for Christmas, she was very pleased."

EDITOR'S NOTE: Readers can also take copies of our popular yellow brochure *What Is Endometriosis?* to their doctors' offices for distribution to other women with endo. Call or write to us (see "Additional Resources")—we'll be happy to send brochures to you for this purpose.

12

~~~~

Endometriosis:
The Patient Perspective

By Mary Lou Ballweg

EDITOR'S NOTE: As we've seen in the preceding chapter, the need to help doctors understand how serious endometriosis can be is great. This article was written to that end. It was originally published in a textbook for physicians, *Infertility and Reproductive Medicine Clinics of North America: Endometriosis,* edited by David L. Olive, M.D. (Philadelphia: W. B. Saunders Co., 1992).

If Endometriosis Is Baffling to Physicians, What Must It Be Like for Those Who Have It?

For decades physicians have called endometriosis an enigmatic disease, a puzzling disease, a frustrating disease to treat. Emery A. Wilson, M.D., editor of the book *Endometriosis,*[1] borrowed a description from Sir Winston Churchill to describe endometriosis: "a riddle wrapped in a mystery inside an enigma." And Robert S. Schenken, M.D., editor of *Endometriosis: Contemporary Concepts in Clinical Management,*[2] writes: "The literature on endometriosis is extensive, but often inadequate or contradictory."

If endometriosis is baffling to doctors who treat it, imagine what it must be like to have it. Recently the Endometriosis Association began conducting focus groups with a professional marketing consultant to learn more about the perceptions of women with endo toward the disease and toward the association. We wanted to learn more about the services women with endometriosis wanted and how the association's services met their needs.

The feelings expressed by the women were striking and resonated with pain, both physical and emotional. Here are some key findings from the consultant's report.

Women were asked to draw their endometriosis as a person. They typically depict it as a sinister male or a devil type of monster. Their drawings show a sadistic and controlling force that enjoys causing pain. The pain and frustration these women feel is apparent as is some degree of acceptance that their endometriosis is here to stay. (Fig. 1)

They also drew the Endometriosis Association as if it were a person. The association was always depicted as a female who was caring, helpful, and empathetic. She is armed with information such as *Overcoming Endometriosis*,[3] the association's book. She is dressed professionally and is smiling in a friendly way, in sharp contrast to the sadistic grins of the disease. She has open arms that are welcoming and big shoulders to cry on. She radiates positive energy. In one extreme she was depicted as a woman on a white horse crusading to the rescue (Fig. 2).

(Some of the letters we receive at headquarters indicate that particularly knowledgeable and skilled physicians are also seen as heroes and deeply appreciated. We give recognition to these specialists in a popular feature in our newsletter entitled "The 'Best Doc' in Town.")

It may come as a surprise to some physicians that the disease affects patients so deeply or that the informational and emotional needs are so great. Because physicians see patients for short amounts of time and these visits are often oriented around specific aspects of the disease, the true chronicity and full scope of the disease may not be apparent. In the first case history presented here, for instance, the young woman, while only 31 years old and

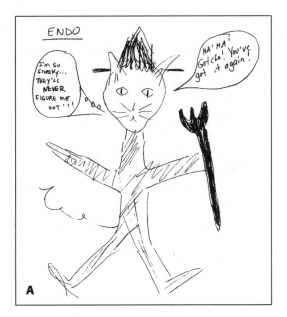

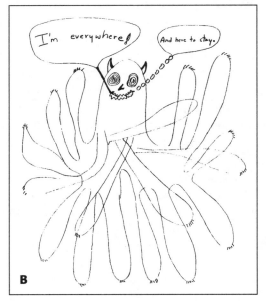

diagnosed via laparoscopy only one and a half years ago, actually has a history and suffering going back to age 11—some 20 years of symptoms and problems, but the physicians treating her are likely to think of her story as starting at diagnosis a year and a half ago.

The number of emotional issues involved in this highly personal disease also contribute to its impact and can make it especially devastating. These issues involve the patient's fertility, sexuality, and ability to work, play, and carry on meaningful personal relationships.

These highly personal issues also mean that the decisions involved in treatments are highly personal, and yet, despite no overwhelming medical evidence to support particular treatments over others at this time, some practitioners do not present a full range of options to patients or allow the patient to be involved in treatment decisions. Adding to the stress, some practitioners are not up to date on the rapidly changing and rapidly evolving specialty of endometriosis and related health concerns. In short, endo can be, from the patient's point of view, a nightmare of misinformation, myths, taboos, lack of diagnosis, and problematic hit-and-miss treatments overlaid on a painful, chronic, stubborn disease.

Let's listen in on some letters from women with endo who can tell the story best in their own words. These are selected from among the hundreds of thousands of stories we've heard since we began the association in 1980. First, the story of Peg is presented.

Dear Endometriosis Association,

I am a first-grade teacher, 31 years old, and was diagnosed through laparoscopy one and a half years ago. I do not have any children, nor have I been married. But I current-

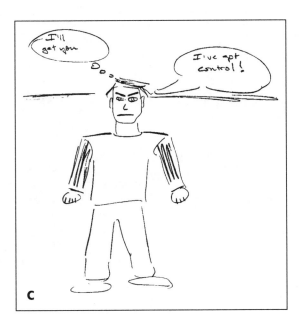

Figure 1 illustrations depicting pain of endometriosis
A (opposite, left), devil
B (opposite, right), devil-type monster
C (left), powerful, sinister male force

ly live with my boyfriend of five years and am looking forward to a day when both of
those things will happen for me. . . .

In the last year and a half I have been reading and learning as much as I possibly
can about endometriosis and management techniques. When I look back at my history, I
now believe that I probably had symptoms of endo since the onset of menstruation, age
11.* Like so many women, I thought that all women experienced the pain and discomfort
I felt.

In the late 1960s and early 1970s people didn't talk about menstruation, at least not
in my circles. It was a hushed subject referred to only as "that time of the month." Like
many endo patients, I never learned what periods were like for other women. I was too

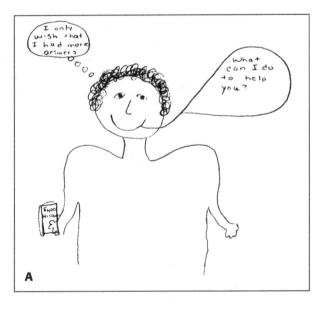

Figure 2 illustrations describing
women's appreciation of the
Endometriosis Association
A (left), maternal, caring symbol
B (opposite, top), active, positive
energy force
C (opposite, bottom), heart symbol

---

*The early onset of symptoms is a common theme in endo stories. Whether these early symptoms are
primary dysmenorrhea or endo, we believe the symptoms should be taken seriously. After all, primary
dysmenorrhea itself is very uncomfortable and disruptive to the youngster's life, and one excellent
multicenter study found primary dysmenorrhea to be a risk factor for endo.[4] As Dr. Robert Franklin stated
in his talk at the association's 10th Anniversary Conference in 1990: "I think those same patients with
primary dysmenorrhea should have a lot of attention paid to them, too. Because . . . they may be having
retrograde flow or they represent a group of patients that look like a lot of prostaglandin is being produced
. . . those same patients often progress on to the early endometriosis, . . . on to more and more bowel
involvement. . . . These are the patients that maybe, with careful watching and medical therapy, we can stop
some of this progression."[5] In the association's large research registry of 3,020 cases, 14.9 percent
experienced their first symptoms before age 15, 25.7 percent at age 15–19, and 19.6 percent at age 20–24.
In other words, an astounding 60 percent of the cases experienced symptoms before age 25.[6]

shy and embarrassed to bring up the subject myself, but I was continually curious why women didn't talk about periods—since they were so incredibly painful and disruptive. The only thing women did say was that they didn't like having periods, periods were a nuisance, and that some women didn't feel well "those days." I assumed all women were sick several days previous to their period, experienced terrible cramps, aching, and nausea to the extent that I did.

The biggest mystery to me was how other women managed the extreme blood flow—no one talked about it. During my teenage years I used to have to run to the bathroom. It seemed like a faucet opened up in my body. This was a giant and embarrassing problem for me, especially since it happened during the sensitive teenage years. Sometimes it happened on dates. How did the other girls manage this? If I had gone to a doctor, I'm sure I would have told him that nothing was wrong. I didn't like what was happening to me, but I didn't know it was not normal.

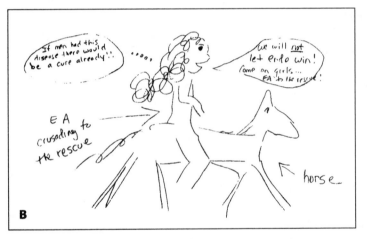

I realize now that people didn't talk about menstruation simply because it was a taboo subject and that probably most of the women around me did not experience as much pain or heavy bleeding as I did—hence many women may have had slightly less reason for the open discussions that would have helped me.

During college years, just by chance I rode my bicycle on a daily basis, exercised using yoga techniques, took lots of naps whenever I wanted, and ate a diet with little or no red meat, little salt, sugars, or dairy products, and very few fast foods—all this because I was on a strict school budget. I ate lots of salads and some fish. My symptoms decreased, and I thought I had simply outgrown terrible periods.

Postgraduation, from the ages of 22 to 26, my symptoms returned even stronger than before. I was less physically active and had moved back home to the luscious and temptingly rich home-cooked foods and occasional fast-food splurges.

By age 26, however, I regained my interest in bicycling and jogging and became extremely fit. I started having severe abdominal pains while climbing tough hills, had an occasional asthma attack[11, 12] which I never had before, and thought it was all because I was exercising too strenuously. I began to slow down physically.

Also at age 26 I got a serious boyfriend, the same one as now, and went to a gynecologist for the first time in my life. I asked for birth control advice. It was then that I first described my periods to any doctor. I still described the pain as though it was a "woman's lot"—after all, I was there for birth control, not pain. To my surprise, the doctor prescribed birth control pills, but not for birth control. He said it would lessen the severe cramping, bloating, and heavy bleeding. It did help me, and he was a wonderfully gentle doctor. I had still not heard of endo, however, or realized that what I was experiencing was anything out of normal.

I went back to school to get a teaching credential and unfortunately had to change my medical plan and doctor. I took birth control pills for five years, occasionally changing the pills . . . after three years of birth control pills I began to experience mild to severe side effects such as breakthrough bleeding, depression, temper tantrums just before my period, and intense migraines that felt like your brain was going to explode. These migraines lasted for one week at a time. . . .

After three years of birth control pills, at age 29, I spent the entire summer in bed with extreme migraines and bleeding every day. I was lucky because as a schoolteacher I had this time off. . . .

I went to my physician twice that summer. I told him everything—bleeding, migraines, and temper tantrums. I was scared he would think I was crazy, but I knew something must be very wrong with me. I could hardly function anymore, my head felt so bad. I had to lie still for hours in the afternoon for weeks at a time. The pain was so severe I thought my brain would burst, and my emotions were out of control. . . .

I asked my physician about it, and I think that's when he did think there was something wrong—in my head. When I asked him if he thought it could be the birth control pills, he said he wasn't sure. He did not honor my request for a glucose tolerance test. He told me that he had known my family for a long time. They were a very good family. He thought that I was just being emotional and had that tendency because I was of Italian descent. He prescribed Valium.*

---

* The medical mismanagement in this letter is obvious—please see other articles in this book for information on proper management. This letter is not that unusual in this regard; it seems some nonspecialists are simply so baffled by endometriosis that they probably should not treat it. Of course, as in this story, there is often no recognition of what it is they're not treating!

[We were shocked, when we first began analyzing data from our research registry, to learn how many women were prescribed tranquilizers for symptoms of endo.][7]

I did not take the Valium or his advice. . . .

Luckily, I earned a new teaching job by the end of summer and was required to have a complete physical and new medical insurance by the district. The district doctor pressed on my abdomen. I was so surprised to find myself screaming in pain. . . . The new doctor listened to everything and immediately set me up with another gynecologist and very good physician.

Before that appointment came, I ran into worse trouble. While my boyfriend and I were visiting friends, the pain erupted. . . . My girlfriend called her gynecologist for me. I talked, rather cried, to him over the phone about how much it hurt. That was the first time I had ever heard the word endometriosis.

"What? This much pain isn't normal, is it? It's a disease? A gynecological disease? That never even occurred to me." I was so surprised. I didn't know anything about endo, but I did know I had tremendous pain. Discovering I had a real condition was a relief. I did not want to hear "You're just an emotional type. Laugh more; you'll be fine." It didn't occur to me at that moment that there wouldn't be a proven cure. At that moment I wasn't worried; I was glad for an explanation. . . .

"Let's Wait and See"

The mistaken notion that all women suffer with their periods, as Peg describes in this first part of her story, is a prevalent belief that greatly hinders diagnosis and treatment of endo. We need all physicians to help educate society that nature does not create an ongoing, monthly bodily function to be painful—pain is a warning sign.

The next section of Peg's letter typifies a number of additional frequent themes in the case histories of women with endometriosis. First, physicians unfamiliar with the chronic problems women with endo tend to experience assume a "Let's wait and see attitude," an attitude that implies that the disease is not that serious. They also fail to realize that by the time a woman comes to them she more than likely has already been experiencing years of pain or life-disrupting problems, or she wouldn't have sought medical attention for symptoms still so routinely considered taboo and embarrassing to talk about. She often also has other symptoms that she does not share at the time of the medical encounter. (In focus groups in New York City some years ago we learned that most of the women present "would rather die first" than tell physicians about pain with sex. One way for a physician to make the statement that he or she is approachable on endo symptoms is to display in the waiting area pamphlets, videotapes, and other materials on endo.)

The physician who would prefer to "wait and see" should probably refer the woman to a specialist in endometriosis. Unfortunately, this usually does not happen. Because the nonspecialist tends to underestimate the important life-disrupting potential of the disease and to be unaware of new treatment modalities that offer the possibility of slowing it down with good management, he or she believes it can be treated by any gynecologist. This, as thousands of case histories show, is a disservice to the woman with endometriosis.

Another all-too-common theme is the "have a baby" answer to endo, regardless of a woman's desire to have a baby or her own and a partner's needs. This presentation of a life choice (and surely the decision to reproduce is perhaps the most profound choice of all in life) as a medical prescription infuriates and insults patients. In addition, as a "treatment" it's scientifically unsound.

Whatever the treatment options, patients appreciate being presented all options and being involved in making the decision, because they affect the patient's life so personally. Patients especially feel they have the right to be involved in decisions involving their sexuality and fertility.

Psychological Denial

Another theme that appears in almost all case histories of women with endo is what we call *denial*, psychological denial that the disease is going to be serious for them or seriously affect their life, that it has returned after treatment, that something involving symptoms that we learned unconsciously were not important could possibly be serious. A delicate balance of denial, hope, and acceptance *is* needed to continue to live life as fully as possible in spite of setbacks with endo and its related health problems. But because of the social milieu surrounding endo, the denial step along the road to psychological acceptance tends to be very prolonged. We see it frequently in women who fail to take steps to learn about the disease, find a specialist, and prepare for a variety of eventualities and instead simply stick their heads in the sand, ostrichlike. Then they come to the association in crisis, often having made poor decisions in the interim. (Sometimes they're under a nonspecialist's care but getting the kind of advice described in the letters reprinted in this article.)

Not only patients engage in denial when it comes to endometriosis, however. It seems hard for doctors also to truly accept that science and medicine do not yet have answers for endometriosis. Even good physicians, who understand that we really don't know the basic scientific facts about endo, still develop the idea that a new surgery or medicine "should do the trick" for a patient. The patient may readily buy into this, at least at first, because she, too, desperately wants a cure. Blind hope, combined with denial, means that the patient (or physician) will even report back great results after a surgery or during a hormonal treatment. One patient relates how her prominent physician wrote on her records, right in front of her, that she was "recovering well" in spite of months of serious bladder and bowel complications following a presacral neurectomy.

The history of endo is replete with individuals who so greatly wanted a cure that they (prematurely, unfortunately) proclaimed one. Danazol was touted as a miracle drug, able to cure, in its early years on the market. Stilbestrol and vitamin B$_6$ were proclaimed the cure in the 1950s. A number of surgeons have been ready to proclaim their particular methods as cures. Hysterectomy and removal of the ovaries have been widely proclaimed as the cure, without any follow-up studies. Recently the association conducted one; unfortunately, for about one-third of the patients hysterectomy and removal of the ovaries did not offer a cure or even relief of symptoms. Forty-four percent of those receiving estrogen replacement therapy experienced a return of symptoms.[8]

Time after time, women write to or call the Endometriosis Association to say their doctors have told them they can't possibly have the disease after surgery because they "got it all out." Women are sometimes afraid to report the return of symptoms, even to a sympathetic physician, for fear of losing the emotional support and rapport sometimes available to a doctor's success stories. One article, emanating from a specialist's hospital, even suggests that women should "develop a new, pain-free point of view." The article presumes that women with endo who have had surgery with the specialist could not possibly still have endo; this at a time when we really do not know what endo is or if implants per se are responsible for the pain. This is simply a more sophisticated version of blaming the victim, implying that she's so used to pain that she continues to feel it despite the disease (defined as implants) being gone or that she imagines or manufactures it.

Given the perplexing nature of endometriosis, treatments should not be presented as cures. No physician or surgeon should feel his ego is on the line in that no one, including yourself, should expect you to cure an incurable disease. Too many, rather than face that basic fact about endo, choose instead to make the patient feel bad about herself or doubt herself. This is putting ego needs ahead of the welfare of the patient.

As difficult as it may be for the patient and the physician, a careful sharing of information about the difficulties of the disease will actually be more helpful in the long run than the ups and downs of unwarranted hope for a complete cure. That kind of up-and-down cycle also tends to keep the patient from doing the things that would most help her find a certain equilibrium and ability to cope with the disease for the long run—that is, "doing her homework," one of the most commonly used phrases in the association, and building her support network, particularly with other women with endometriosis, listening to their stories, mapping out scenarios for different eventualities, and so forth. A woman who has convinced herself that the newest drug on the market, for instance, or getting pregnant will solve all of the problems related to the disease, her husband, and maybe even her work situation will believe she does not need to do the serious homework to deal with the real eventualities.

A personal example might help illustrate this point. After my first serious bout with endo in 1979, during which I had been bedridden, I wanted desperately to believe that all would become just a bad memory for me. My gynecologist warned me, however, that more than likely the disease would be back and would be worse. That was the best bit of advice she could have possibly given me at that point. It allowed me to prepare myself better—save money, firm up relationships, try to find ways to learn more about coping with the disease. Ultimately I found little information, which led to the beginning of the Endometriosis Association, but that's another story. Let's return to the story of Peg.

My physician and gynecologist took me immediately off birth control pills because of the severe headaches I described. My physician wanted me never to take birth control pills again. He said they were too dangerous for me. My new gyn said he suspected that I had endometriosis, just like the gyn on the phone. He said, "Let's just see what happens for a few periods." He told me he wouldn't know for sure except through a laparoscopy, and he wasn't willing to do that yet. He urged me to have a baby. I explained that I was not married, my boyfriend was not ready, and I was just beginning a career and made a very low teacher's salary.

The next four periods off birth control pills were excruciating. Having no severe headaches was fantastic, but bloating, soreness, cramping, two ruptured ovarian cysts, burning, difficulty moving around, and a bladder infection were rough. . . . My doctor continued to urge me to have a baby.

I became blindly optimistic for months. "I'll be OK," I said. "I don't think anything will happen to me. I've been a 'good kid.' What's a little pain—I feel fine today. There's probably a way they treat this disease. They'll look at me someday and say I don't need treatment. They'll treat me, and I'll respond."

I was ignoring the fact that several times in the last four months I had debated whether or not to go to the emergency room.

(I've learned now that there is a better way to view the disease: to accept it and manage its symptoms—a year and a half later.)

After four months I couldn't stand it anymore. I was barely hobbling around, wondering how much worse I needed to get before my doctor decided I did have endo and that we needed to treat it. I finally begged him to do something. We scheduled a laparoscopy. I went to a very kind doctor who seconded his opinion, only she said she would have done it sooner and would do an emergency laparoscopy right now if I was her patient.

Two days before my scheduled laparoscopy, I almost collapsed in my classroom and was rushed to the hospital for an emergency laparoscopy. My gynecologist found and cauterized several implants in my cul-de-sac, on my broad ligaments, and in a few other places. None were spotted on my ovaries. . . . He said my fertility was not yet jeopar-

dized and again urged me to have a baby. He suggested that if I did not have my first baby within two years I probably would be forfeiting my fertility. Nothing had changed between my boyfriend and me, so this was very disturbing.

One month after my laparoscopy I was put back on Ovcon 35 for pain management and to reduce ovarian cysts. The pain in my abdomen was happily gone, but the severe headaches came back. I was returning to the once-a-month temper tantrums. I asked my doctor if he thought it could be the pill, but he warned me that I couldn't go off them. Which would I rather have? Severe pelvic pain, reduced fertility, or monthly headaches? I really didn't know what to do.

For several months I just continued, with on-again, off-again side effects. Then, one year after the laparoscopy, I felt the endo come back. Deep in my heart I realized there was no denying the disease this time. Everything I had read was true, and now I'd have to face it head-on. . . .

My gynecologist said it couldn't be endo because he had gotten all he could see a year ago. I knew he was wrong. He sent me to my physician thinking I had irritable bowel syndrome and migraine headaches not related to the pill.

My physician wasn't sure about the endo coming back; he did think I had irritable bowel syndrome, and he wanted me off birth control pills immediately because of the headaches. He performed magnetic resonance imaging and found a birth defect called a venous angioma. For five days I sweated to find out what my venous angioma was. Finally I learned it was a nontumorous, benign knot of blood vessels that did not need to come out but just be watched. He took me immediately off birth control pills and said I may never go on them again. My gynecologist reluctantly agreed; he was worried about the endo. The pills caused the headache, not the venous angioma, but the physician thought those terrible headaches were warning signs of impending stroke.

That was a month and a half ago. I am now 31. Without receiving hormonal treatment for endo I suddenly feel the full force of how it has affected my body. . . . I feel enormous, constant pain.

The first month off the pill was the most difficult simply because I was not prepared for the kind of pain it was. It interrupted every activity of my life. I still went to work every day except when I caught a terrible flu. I sat with heating pads at home, cleaning and cooking meals much less. My boyfriend had to serve me many meals at first. It got so bad that Easter weekend I wasn't sure anymore if my abdomen was actually experiencing something else—like appendicitis. The emergency staff thought I might have an intestinal flu or ovarian cyst. My abdomen was so sore that touching it caused extreme pain. They gave me 75 cc of Demerol which barely helped the pain but helped me sleep better.

Since that time I spent many weekends devoted to reading and studying the disease. . . . I was afraid I would have to quit work and go on disability. I couldn't even walk three blocks to the store without coming home in wrenching pain.

My gynecologist has offered to give me 200 mg of danazol daily. But I have read about the side effects. . . . So far I have said a powerful no.

It looks like I have been accepted into a Stanford research study about the effects of gonadotropin-releasing hormone [GnRH] on bone metabolism. . . .

I don't really believe I think there is an end-all cure. I guess I'll believe it when I experience it. But I feel like I'm on the right road. I have just begun visualization and believe acupuncture may help me the most.

I hope that you will have the time to read my story. It is not over yet. It will be interesting to see what happens. My gynecologist thinks I will have a hysterectomy by the time I reach age 35. My Stanford gynecologist thinks that GnRH will bring me into complete remission or cure, and my acupuncturist thinks that he can possibly bring me to a complete cure because he's read about so many cases.

Sincerely,
Peg, California

"I Found a Doctor Who Was Always Ready to Listen"

Dear Mary Lou:

I am a new member of the association. As a new member, I requested a lot of reading material, which I just recently received. I pored over the information just as soon as I received it. I can barely put my feelings down on paper. I am 29 years old, I had a total hysterectomy three years ago, and I have no children. I was originally diagnosed with the disease at age 17, after an emergency surgery was performed. I had a cyst the size of a baseball, which had ruptured. Obviously, every woman with this disease has a different story. The articles that I read last evening brought tears to my eyes. . . .

The one thing that really hit home was the mental state this disease and its treatment can cause. After nine years of treatment, which included two conservative surgeries and countless minor surgeries, I was a mental wreck. I am very fortunate, as I found a doctor who was always ready to listen to my ideas and feelings. However, the thing I would like to stress is that each woman has to make decisions based on her own life and course of the disease. I made my own decision to have a hysterectomy. The mental anguish I went through to reach that decision was one of the hardest things I have ever done in my life. Now, thanks to you, I realize there are other women with similar feelings.

After having discovered your association, I started to develop a goal in my mind. My goal is that if I could help one 17-year-old from going through what I went through, then my disease would have benefited someone.

Sincerely,
Debbie, Indiana

Not Taking the Early Symptoms Seriously
Leads to Medical and Patient Confusion

To: Endometriosis Association

As a kid I had always had really painful periods. My father carried me to emergency rooms monthly for pain medications. In the early 1970s a female physician invented Ponstel, and I thought I had "died and gone to heaven."*

Six months after my second birth (which was incredibly painful and only 13 months after my first horrible one), I started having vertigo, ear ringing, and left-sided chest pain. The onslaught of physicians started, at least 15, and a trip to the L. Clinic. After three years I decided they were right—I was just depressed and stressed out (despite newly developed asthma and hair loss).

I started working out for one hour daily. I gained some muscle mass, could breathe easier, and felt less mentally miserable. Within 18 months my high started to diminish, I was tired, and the pain was creeping down my left side and into my left leg. I worked out harder, I started getting monthly upper respiratory infections, nosebleeds, and a continuously decreased white count. My left [side] pain started to burn and pull. I increased my consumption of Ponstel, and oddly, it helped. In January 1989, I began having a very difficult time standing up straight without falling. The medical community said Ménière's disease.†

In the spring it occurred to me that I was taking Ponstel at least 15 days a month. By May my left side burned almost continuously. I started warming up longer, thinking I had pulled a ligament in my left side.

Finally, while on annual training in New York, I hit rock bottom. After a military physician said I had pelvic inflammatory disease, I took a taxi to a local ER and was told that it was adenomyosis.

---

* The writer is referring to Dr. Penny Budoff's work in finding that nonsteroidal anti-inflammatories counteracted the symptoms of primary dysmenorrhea. Dr. Budoff's story is fascinating and highly recommended reading.[9] It's clear that traditional gynecological training on primary dysmenorrhea (that it's rooted in psychogenic causes) has caused great harm to girls and women with endometriosis as well as to those with primary dysmenorrhea.

† Women with endo often report other health problems, some of which, we have learned over the years of listening to patients and studying them in our research program, are very common in endo. While it's not entirely clear what problems were occurring for this particular woman, one of the common problems is thyroid disease. British research has identified increased incidence of thyroid autoimmune problems in women with endo.[10] Others are allergies, asthma, a history of mononucleosis, fibromyalgia, lupus, and other known or suspected autoimmune diseases.[11–15] An in-depth personal and family history can elicit these diagnostically helpful patterns. Have a young person check with older family members for medical histories, because young people often are unaware of family medical histories.

I consulted Mary Jo at the Maine Chapter of the Endometriosis Association; she provided me with a Boston endo specialist.

In late September 1989 I had an exploratory laparoscopy. After a diagnosis of endometriosis, the disease was lasered. It was located on the left side, predominantly in the back and on the uterosacral ligament. . . .

At this writing the vertigo is totally gone. The ear ringing persists, but it has been suggested that the Ponstel (antiprostaglandins can cause ringing) causes this. The left-sided pain is greatly diminished, but I still have some during ovulation and menstruation. Unable to take the pill and testosterone, I am seeking the services of an acupuncturist and chiropractor. Both seem to be helping a little.

The chronicity of illness is devastating, especially if no one is able to tell you that what you feel indeed does exist. It is incredibly miserable when you start to believe that they are right and you are wrong. It affects every waking moment, and you think, Oh, no, this can't be happening—not again. Your family tries to help, but they, too, can't bear it. With the diagnosis, at least you can wake up and say, "I hurt, but there's a reason. I'm not nuts." After five years of hell I am just beginning to see a light at the end of the darkest medical tunnel, filled with self-doubt and frustration. For me it is only the beginning of knowing. I'm not sure if the disease or the medical community has caused me more despair.

God bless,
Linda, Maine

Lack of Validation Lowers Self-Esteem

The following letter touches on a number of common themes in the endo patient's perspective. First we sometimes hear from women from families in which primary dysmenorrhea and endometriosis are endemic that they were told to expect problems or came to expect them because of the experiences of female relatives around them. These mothers and other older female relatives, unfortunately, are passing along the medical advice they received in their earlier decades, that the pain was normal, or they'd have to learn to live with it, and if they couldn't, they had some psychological flaw. The Endometriosis Association has been following families with endometriosis for some years now.[11] We find the lack of diagnosis in preceding generations a major problem.

Second, the way endo and related health problems tend to begin in the girl's puberty, when she is so young and still very much in the process of developing her sense of self, often has devastating consequences for her self-esteem. This is, unfortunately, all too often reinforced by society. Friends, family, and medical personnel, rather than listening to her problems and offering help, are all too likely to reinforce the taboos surrounding her symptoms and to suggest that her problems are psychogenic. Her physical pain is then enveloped with emotional pain, confusion, the sense that she is a bad girl with a problem that shows she is inadequate as a person. This is later enhanced by the feeling she is inadequate as a woman if she develops pain with sex and infertility.

As one nurse wrote the association, "Too many physicians make their female patients think their problems are psychological when they aren't—which becomes almost a self-fulfilling prophecy. . . . It would spare many women's self-esteem if their doctors would admit they don't know what's wrong rather than suggesting psychological causes for physical symptoms." Unfortunately, low self-esteem robs a person of a vital ingredient needed to pursue health. Low self-esteem was identified as a profound factor in women's health choices by a scientific advisory panel representing 25 medical specialties and professional organizations at a meeting convened by the Society for the Advancement of Women's Health Research in Washington, D.C., in spring 1991. The panel identified the following as a topic of concern: "The acknowledgment that the low self-esteem of many women, occurring as a result of the socialization process that begins during childhood and adolescence and continues into maturity, profoundly affects choices throughout a woman's life."[16] Certainly those who treat endometriosis could help change this. I believe deep-seated attitudes about women's bodies and reproductive functions, especially menstruation, underlie much of the low status and low self-esteem inculcated in our girls and teens.

It Affects Every Waking Moment. . . .

Dear Members,

I started my periods when I was nine years old. I had always matured faster than the other kids. I can only remember having two or three periods that were pain-free at first. I can remember sitting at my desk in the fifth grade with a terrible ache in my lower back. My parents never told me much about my periods except that it was the "woman's curse." The pain steadily got worse over the years. I went from regular physicians to several gynecologists.

At 13 I went on the pill until I was 17 years old. I was pain-free for about two years after starting the pill. Then, just as before, the pain got steadily worse. So I finally went off the pill because of migraines and leg cramps.

From there I took danazol for six months. It did not work. As soon as I start my period I will be having another laparoscopy. He is going to laser all of it off that he can, cut the nerve to the uterus, uterine suspension, and anything else he can do in outpatient surgery. I am having trouble starting my periods back. It has been 10 weeks since I went off the danazol. I have been very sick in these 10 weeks. I started Provera yesterday to start my period. These make me even sicker. But I keep looking forward to after the surgery, when hopefully I will be better, even if just for a little while.

Sometimes the depression and the "poor little me" syndrome still sets in, but not as bad as before or as often. I hope that I don't have to end up with a total hysterectomy, but if it comes to that I will accept it. I will do anything it takes to stop the pain. People just don't understand that. You can't believe some of the responses I've gotten from friends and family on the subject of a hysterectomy. They really think I should endure anything to keep being a "full woman." People should be more informed. But for now I have hope, and for once in my life I feel I have a chance at a normal future. It feels wonderful!

Thanks,

Shari, Tennessee

From the patient's perspective, endo is almost indescribable: it's taboo, it's embarrassing, it's frightening, it's sneaky, it's sadistic. Endometriosis, and the treatment the sufferer receives from others because of it, leads women to a deep feeling of having been betrayed by their own body and also by others in society whom they thought were there to help, including doctors.

"It"—this disease, described in our focus group as a sinister devil-type of monster that enjoys causing pain—has the power to destroy your dreams, your dreams of a loving relationship with your husband or partner, your dreams of having children, your work goals, your dreams of a healthy body, your plans for building a financially secure and happy life. "It" hurls you into a world of vulnerability, and just when you're feeling most vulnerable and afraid, it hurls you into a world where your vulnerability and powerlessness are emphasized. You are a young woman, maybe only a teenager, and must find a way to navigate the power relationships of patient-doctor (often made worse by our society's male-female power imbalances) at a time when you're confused and afraid, the bureaucracies of hospitals and insurance companies, the harsh realities of trying to support yourself financially when you're sick.

We invite you to attend a support group meeting of the Endometriosis Association. Anyone who takes the time to listen to and talk with many women with endo about their actual experiences with the disease soon learns that while some lucky individuals may appear relatively unaffected by it, too many others have suffered years of pain and emotional stress, have been unable to work or carry on normal activities at times, and have experienced financial and relationship problems because of the disease. Listening to the stories, you just might find yourself inspired, as I have been over the years, by the courage of many of these young women and decide to join in partnership with us to find answers to this mysterious disease.

Notes

1. E. Wilson, *Endometriosis* (New York: Alan R. Liss, 1987): 1.
2. R. Schenken, *Endometriosis: Contemporary Concepts in Clinical Management* (Philadelphia: J. B. Lippincott, 1989): Preface.
3. M. L. Ballweg, *Overcoming Endometriosis: New Help from the Endometriosis Association* (New York: Congdon & Weed, 1987).
4. D. W. Cramer, E. Wilson, and R. J. Stillman, "The Relation of Endometriosis to Menstrual Characteristics, Smoking and Exercise," *JAMA* 255 (1986): 1904.

5. Endometriosis Association. *Endometriosis: The Experts Speak.* 10th Anniversary Conference Cassette Tapes (Milwaukee, 1990).

6. "Research Recap: Four Studies from the Association's Research Registry Program," *Endometriosis Association Newsletter* 10, no. 2 (1989).

7. "Data Bank Results Are In!" *Endometriosis Association Newsletter* 4, no. 5 (1983).

8. K. Lamb, L. Breitkopf, K. Hamilton, et al., "Does Total Hysterectomy Offer a Cure for Endometriosis?" *Endometriosis Association Newsletter* 12, no. 3 (1991).

9. P. Budoff, *No More Menstrual Cramps and Other Good News* (New York: G. P. Putnam's Sons, 1980).

10. M. G. Brush, "Increased Incidence of Thyroid Autoimmune Problems in Women with Endometriosis," *Endometriosis: A Collection of Papers Written by GP's, Researchers, Specialists and Sufferers About Endometriosis,* compiled by the Coventry Branch of the Endometriosis Society (March 1987).

11. K. Lamb, R. Hoffman, and T. Nichols, "Family Trait Analysis: A Case-Control Study of 43 Women with Endometriosis and Their Best Friends," *American Journal of Obstetrics and Gynecology* 154, no. 3 (1986): 596–601.

12. K. Lamb and T. Nichols, "Endometriosis: A Comparison of Associated Disease Histories," *American Journal of Preventive Medicine* 2, no. 6 (1986): 324–29.

13. T. Nichols, K. Lamb, and J. Arkins, "The Association of Atopic Diseases with Endometriosis," *Annals of Allergy* 59, no. 11 (November 1987).

14. K. Thorson, *Fibromyalgia Network* 11, no. 18 (October 1990).

15. "Two-Fold Risk of Endometriosis in Hospitalized Patients with Lupus," *American Journal of Obstetrics and Gynecology* 153, no. 179 (1985).

16. M. Bass and J. Howes, "Towards a Women's Health Research Agenda: Findings of the Scientific Advisory Meeting," convened by the Society for the Advancement of Women's Health Research, Washington, D.C., 1991.

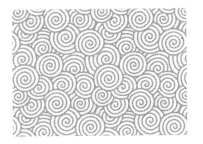

PART IV

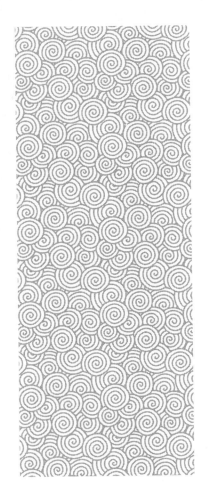

New Research Directions

13

@/@

Endometriosis: A New Picture of the Disease Is Emerging

Statement for Scientific Advisory Meeting III:
Women's Health and the Environment
Sponsored by the Society for the Advancement of Women's Health Research

By Mary Lou Ballweg

"*I joined the association because I knew that there must be answers somewhere to our many questions about endo. Like so many other women, I had to learn the hard way that physicians do not have those answers. I had to learn that the basic science for this disease has not yet been done and that until it is done my treatment decisions, like those of every other woman with endo, would be made in a sea of uncertainty. . . .*

"*Somebody said that every generation stands on the shoulders of the generation before. I think of my mother's generation, who endured this painful disease for the most part unaided. Because the Endometriosis Association allows us to act together, pooling the experiences of many thousands of women, we stand on their shoulders, and we can see further than our mothers could.*

"*I think of young women who have just been diagnosed, of teenagers who suffer from severe dysmenorrhea without knowing that their illness has a name, and of little girls who are even now approaching puberty, unaware of what it may bring. These are the next generation of women with endo who will stand on our shoulders. They look to us, asking us to find the answers.*

"*As I see it, we have a choice. We can sit and hope that someone else finds the answers. Or we can take the suffering and frustrations of this disease and use them to get more research done.*"

Barbara, Ontario

"*What* women need to keep in mind with all the advances in medical technology is how much more we could be getting done now if there were more hands doing the work. We could make tremendous strides. Back when the EA started, we were just trying to get in the door, but now that the actual research is happening, we could do so much together.

"*If your daughter has endometriosis, what do you want to be able to give her—a support group or a cure?*"

Sue, Wisconsin

"*I* am very interested in this disease, having had experience within my family. I am a twin, age 58. My twin sister and I had endometriosis. I had a hysterectomy at age 42 and my sister at age 47. My daughter has endometriosis. She had one ovary and fallopian tube removed five years ago. She had been on danazol, had a remission for three years, and now is back on danazol. Knowing the emotional, physical, and mental stress we each have gone through, it means so much to know serious research is being done. . . .*"

Vada, Virginia

"*M*edical science has done all it can for me at this point in time. My concern is now with my young niece who is fast approaching puberty. I do not wish her to suffer the living nightmare of pain, agony, and despair of endometriosis. . . .*"

Lena, North Carolina

"*M*aybe my daughter will not have to suffer the same way her grandmother and aunt did.*"

Kristen, Manitoba

"*O*ur lives have been made difficult by endometriosis (if not painful), and therefore we would be more than happy to contribute to research that could lessen the suffering of others. . . .*"

Denise, Ohio

EDITOR'S NOTE: In June 1992 I was asked to present the association's research on dioxin and endometriosis at a meeting sponsored by the Society for the Advancement of Women's Health Research in Washington, D.C. Following are excerpts from that statement. Information on our dioxin research is incorporated into the chapter that follows.

Endometriosis is a puzzling disease affecting an estimated five million women in the United States and millions more worldwide. It is a nightmare of misinformation, myths, taboos, misdiagnosis, and problematic hit-and-miss treatments overlaid on a painful, chronic, stubborn disease.

Women with the disease have been much maligned—supposedly they were white, stressed-out, perfectionistic, upper-socioeconomic-level women who brought the disease on themselves by postponing childbearing.[1] Only when the Endometriosis Association began in 1980 and systematically gathered data were we able to disprove all these myths. With the largest Research Registry on endometriosis in the world (established with our leading medical advisors and housed at the Medical College of Wisconsin), the association has categorically disproved these myths. Endometriosis is, in fact, an equal-opportunity disease affecting all races, personalities, and socioeconomic groups, as well as all ages of females from as young as 10 or 11 to as old as women in their 60s and 70s.[3]

Future generations of feminists and sociologists will, we are certain, study endometriosis as a touchstone for the sexism in our society. Why is it that in the 20th-century, post–World War II era in which there had been so many unprecedented changes the first place physicians looked to lay blame for what seems to be a huge increase in the numbers of women with endometriosis was at the women themselves? Women with endometriosis are routinely told the problem is all in their heads or due to stress or, if the disease has been confirmed, it's still their fault for not having a baby early enough.[2] (These doctors are forgetting that the age of menarche, the first period, is now 10 to 12 years old and are not aware that the symptoms begin before age 20 for 41 percent of those with endometriosis.[3]) The terrible impact on young women can be seen in the fact that there has been a 250 percent increase in hysterectomies for females aged 15 to 24 between 1965 and 1984 due to endometriosis; a 186 percent increase in the same years for women aged 25 to 34.[4] (This is based on data from the U.S. National Center for Health Statistics and analysis by Dr. Gary Berger, medical director of Chapel Hill Fertility Center, Chapel Hill, North Carolina. Dr. Berger is board-certified in epidemiology, preventive medicine, and ob-gyn.)

Black women with symptoms of endometriosis are frequently diagnosed with pelvic inflammatory disease (PID)—based on a racist assumption that black women are sexually promiscuous and therefore are more likely to have a sexually transmitted disease. In one study 40 percent of the black women diagnosed with PID actually had endometriosis.[5] We believe that centuries-old taboos about menstruation, female sexuality, and infertility combined with a lack of science have created a situation in which doctors and others have felt all manner of societal prejudice can be heaped on this disease.

Endometriosis now affects an estimated five and a half million girls and women in the United States and Canada. But before 1921 there were only 20 reports on it in the world literature.[6] Rather than blame women, as some in the medical establishment have done without any scientific proof, the Endometriosis Association has been systematically studying all aspects of the health and experience of women with endometriosis, listening to the stories of hundreds of thousands of women with the disease, and publishing reports based on our studies in medical journals. *It appears that what we call endometriosis is just the tip of the iceberg for a whole range of health problems that have underlying them hormonal/immune dysregulation. The type of endometriosis that I am describing is the most severe form of the disease, tends to occur in families with endometriosis and a host of related health problems, and tends to cause numerous health, work, financial, marital, and social problems.*[7]

In the new picture of the disease that is emerging, one sees not only the traditional symptoms of endometriosis—chronic pelvic pain, pain with sex, gastrointestinal and bladder problems, infertility, and others—but also high rates of atopic (allergic) diseases in the individuals and their families including allergies, food intolerances, asthma, eczema, and sometimes debilitating sensitivities to environmental chemicals such as perfumes, cigarette smoke, cleaning agents, and others;[8, 9] a tendency to infections and mononucleosis;[3, 9] problems with *Candida albicans*,[9–11] mitral valve prolapse,[12, 13] fibromyalgia, and chronic fatigue immune dysfunction syndrome;[14] and a greater risk for autoimmune disorders including lupus[15] and Hashimoto's thyroiditis.[16]

The Research Registry

In 1980, when the association began, it didn't take long to figure out that the reason there was so much misinformation on endo was that serious ongoing study of women with endometriosis across patient population groups had never been undertaken. We set out to find answers. We developed a questionnaire and distributed it to every woman with endometriosis willing to fill it out. By the fall of 1980 we had received more than 300 completed questionnaires, and with the help of Dr. Karen Lamb we started working with the Medical College of Wisconsin to computerize and analyze our data.

From that process we were able to develop, for the first time in history, solid information on large numbers of women with endo. The registry grew over time to 3,020 cases.

Most of the association's literature and information has been rooted in our research registry, as well as our informal information gathering. In addition to developing our own huge body of lay information on the disease, we began the serious endeavor of scientific research using the registry. Dr. Lamb, for many years assistant professor of preventive medicine at the Medical College of Wisconsin and director of the association Research Registry, was instrumental in this. Five of the research studies produced by her and others working with her were published in medical journals. One of the published articles is simply a description of the data registry. The other four studies touch on various subjects Dr. Lamb and research team members have studied over the years and are summarized here. Another study was published in the association's newsletter and is included in the hysterectomy portion of Chapter 2; data from the registry is included in Chapter 16.

• "Tampon Use in Women with Endometriosis," *Journal of Community Health* 10, no. 4 (winter 1985). Karen Lamb, R.N., Ph.D., and Nancy Berg, B.A. The study found that women with endometriosis were no more likely to use tampons than women without endometriosis, so at least in this study, no link between endometriosis and tampons was found.

• "Family Trait Analysis: A Case Control Study of 43 Women with Endometriosis and Their Best Friends," *American Journal of Obstetrics and Gynecology* 154, no. 3 (March

Because of our attention to the whole woman and our long-standing research program, we at the Endometriosis Association have recently been able to make possible a major research breakthrough linking endometriosis to environmental toxins—especially dioxin. (See the next article.)

Breakthroughs in women's health are possible if one *listens* to women with the health problems being studied. Because we've been listening to *all* the health problems of women with endometriosis for so many years, because we had documented that immune dysregulation clearly was part of the endometriosis picture, because we have always had a research program, and because we had the funds available to support a colony of research monkeys at least briefly, we were able to realize the significance of endometriosis being the cause of death in the dioxin-exposed colony (described in the next article). If we had not had that

---

1986). Karen Lamb, R.N., Ph.D., Raymond G. Hoffmann, Ph.D., and Thomas R. Nichols, M.S. This study found an increased risk for endometriosis in families of women with endometriosis, and the risk appears to follow the mother's side of the family. As one reviewer of three family studies wrote: "First-degree relatives of patients with endometriosis are at significantly increased risk of developing endometriosis . . . and more likely to have severe endometriosis than are women who do not have an affected first-degree relative."

- "Endometriosis: A Comparison of Associated Disease Histories," *American Journal of Preventive Medicine* 2, no. 6 (June 1986). Karen Lamb, R.N., Ph.D., and Thomas R. Nichols, M.S. This study found a strong family tendency (in the families of women with endometriosis *and* in the women) to allergic problems. "Vaginal yeast infections, mononucleosis, eczema, hay fever and food sensitivities occurred among women with endometriosis more frequently than should be expected from rates determined from a comparable group of females."

- "The Association of Atopic Diseases with Endometriosis," *Annals of Allergy* 59, no. 11 (November 1987). Thomas R. Nichols, M.S., Biostatistical Consultant, Dept. of Biostatistics & Epidemiology, Cleveland Clinic Foundation; Karen Lamb, R.N., Ph.D.; and John A. Arkins, M.D., Department of Medicine, Allergy-Immunology Section, Medical College of Wisconsin. (Atopic: allergic reaction, specifically one with strong familial tendencies.) This study expanded on and corroborated the previous study. Eighty-one women with demonstrable endometriosis reported a higher incidence of allergy-related symptoms, especially food intolerances, hay fever, and yeast infections, than 81 matched controls.

The implications of the last two studies are broad. They point strongly toward the probable importance of the immune system in the development and/or maintenance of endometriosis in families with the disease. They also point the way to possible new diagnostic, treatment, and even preventative approaches to the disease. A noninvasive immunologic test may one day be feasible. The study findings could lend validity to the exploration of alternative avenues of treatment. It may be that modulation of the immune system and/or allergy management techniques will benefit women with endometriosis.

background, the colony would have been dispersed completely, and the valuable information they held would have remained unknown. I shudder to think how many more decades it would have been before we discovered the link to organochlorine toxins.

We believe there may be other breakthroughs linking environmental toxins and health, and I believe that women will need to be in the forefront making those breakthroughs. If one looks closely at the most confusing health problems of modern women—breast and ovarian cancer, osteoporosis, the autoimmune diseases that afflict primarily women, endometriosis and its related diseases—one finds a rather constant theme of hormonal/immunological dysregulation.[17] Why are women in modern society plagued by these diseases? There isn't going to be enough money to fund all of the research needs of women, or of men for that matter, if we continue to look at our health needs in a piecemeal fashion, disease by disease. And the specter of women's health groups fighting each other for a piece of the limited funding pie is too gruesome to fathom. Do we pit grandmothers with osteoporosis against their teen granddaughters with severe endometriosis? Women in their thirties and forties with breast cancer against women with autoimmune diseases? Who could possibly be the Solomon wise enough to make these decisions?

Instead, let's work smarter . . . let's look for the synergy, the ways that smart research might pay off in many ways for many women. Basic research that addresses the hormonal and immunological differences in women compared to men could go a long way to helping provide desperately needed answers for all of these problems.

We believe the most critical research needs facing us at this time include addressing these questions:

- Why are women in the modern world plagued by diseases of hormonal/immunological dysregulation?
- How can we characterize the critical interplay between the endocrine and immune systems in women?
- How do the endocrine and immune systems communicate with each other?
- What regulates their delicate balance so that fertility occurs, so that a mother and her embryo are protected and the embryo not rejected immunologically?
- How do compounds like dioxin act to create their hormonal and immunological effects?
- How do dioxin and other organochlorine compounds affect the embryo, fetus, newborn—all stages of life profoundly more susceptible to immunological and hormonal damage than adults are?

Notes

1. N. H. Lauersen and C. DeSwaan, *The Endometriosis Answer Book: New Hope, New Help* (New York: Rawson Associates, 1988).
2. L. Halstead, P. Pepping, L. Haile, and W. P. Dmowski, "Women's Experiences with Endometriosis: Delay and Disbelief." *Abstracts, Third World Congress on Endometriosis* (Brussels, June 1992).

3. Data from Endometriosis Association Research Registry, partially published in *Endometriosis Association Newsletter* 10, no. 2 (1989).

4. *Hysterectomies in the United States, 1965–84.* Vital and Health Statistics, U.S. Department of Health and Human Services, Public Health Service, Centers for Disease Control, National Center for Health Statistics, series 13, no. 92 (1987).

5. D. L. Chatman, "Endometriosis in the Black Woman," *American Journal of Obstetrics and Gynecology* 125, no. 7 (1976): 596–601.

6. J. Older, "Leeches and Laudanum: Grandmother and You: Historical Highlights," *Endometriosis* (New York: Scribner's, 1984).

7. K. Lamb, R. G. Hoffman, and T. R. Nichols, "Family Trait Analysis: A Case-Control Study of 43 Women with Endometriosis and Their Best Friends," *American Journal of Obstetrics and Gynecology* 154, no. 3 (March 1986): 596–601.

8. T. R. Nichols, K. Lamb, and J. A. Arkins, "The Association of Atopic Diseases With Endometriosis," *Annals of Allergy* 59, no. 11 (November 1987).

9. K. Lamb and T. R. Nichols, "Endometriosis: A Comparison of Associated Disease Histories," *American Journal of Preventive Medicine* 2, no. 6 (1986).

10. M. L. Ballweg, "The Endometriosis-Candidiasis Link," *Overcoming Endometriosis: New Help from the Endometriosis Association* (New York: Congdon & Weed, Inc., 1987): 198–219.

11. "Research News: Candida—Chronic Fatigue Link," *Endometriosis Association Newsletter* 10, no. 4 (1989).

12. M. L. Ballweg, "A Heart Defect in Endometriosis: Another Clue to a Bigger Picture?" *Overcoming Endometriosis,* 228–31.

13. N. Fletcher, "Mitral Valve Prolapse," *Endometriosis Association Newsletter* 13, no. 2 (1992).

14. M. L. Ballweg, "Fibromyalgia/Endometriosis Link? . . ." *Endometriosis Association Newsletter* 12, no. 3 (1991).

15. D. A. Grimes, S. A. LeBolt, K. R. T. Grimes, and P. A. Wingo, "Two-Fold Risk of Endometriosis in Hospitalized Patients with Lupus," *American Journal of Obstetrics and Gynecology* 153, no. 179 (1985).

16. M. G. Brush, Department of Gynaecology, St. Thomas Hospital Medical School, London, "Increased Incidence of Thyroid Autoimmune Problems in Women with Endometriosis," *Endometriosis: A Collection of Papers Written by GPs, Researchers, Specialists and Sufferers About Endometriosis,* compiled by the Coventry Branch of the Endometriosis Society (March 1987).

17. M. L. Ballweg, "Testimony for Research Funding," presented to the Office of Research on Women's Health, National Institutes of Health, June 12, 1991; reprinted in *Endometriosis Association Newsletter* 12, no. 4 (1992).

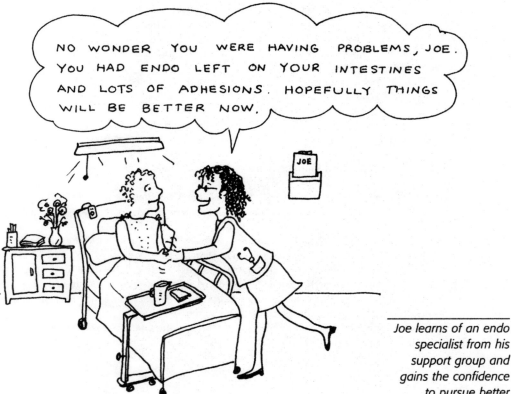

Joe learns of an endo specialist from his support group and gains the confidence to pursue better treatment.

14

∾∾

Endometriosis and Environmental Toxins

By Mary Lou Ballweg

EDITOR'S NOTE: The dramatic news that endometriosis in monkeys could be caused by exposure to dioxin was first published in the association newsletter in the summer of 1992.

At the workshop "Basic Pathophysiology of Endometriosis" held in Washington in September 1991, a research paper was handed around that marked a surprising finding. It described a very high rate of endometriosis in rhesus monkeys that have been studied by the U.S. Air Force and National Aeronautics and Space Administration over many years to learn about the effects of radiation.[1]

The endometriosis developed spontaneously in 53 percent of the monkeys in the study group during a 17-year period after radiation exposure. In the control group of monkeys that received no radiation, the incidence of spontaneous endometriosis (endo that developed on its own, not due to endometrium transplanted for research purposes) was 26 percent.

The authors note: "Endometriosis in our monkey colony was conclusively linked to whole-body-penetrating energies of ionizing radiation. Women receiving whole-body, or in particular, abdominal, exposure to penetrating doses of protons or x-rays should possibly be considered to be at higher risk of developing endometriosis than unexposed women."

The radiation study brought to mind another study our medical advisor Dr. Paul Dmowski had mentioned in the past on PCBs causing endo in monkeys. I began a fascinating detective effort to track down information about those monkeys once and for all. I learned that this very interesting study involving PCB-induced endo in rhesus and cynomolgus monkeys was reported by now-retired Ottawa physician James Campbell to the Ontario Association of Pathologists in October 1985. The report—entitled "Is Simian

Endometriosis an Effect of Immunotoxicity?"—had received little attention.[2] "Simian" refers to monkeys or apes. The study was carried out by the Canadian federal government to determine the effects of PCBs in food. The endometriosis finding was a surprise to the researchers.

In the abstract for his presentation Dr. Campbell wrote: "The endometriosis in these rhesus monkeys was much more productive of inflammatory reaction than the otherwise similar process in humans. . . ." The abstract notes that spontaneous endometriosis is regarded as rare in monkeys and apes. In another presentation on the findings in 1988, Dr. Campbell also noted that the animals experienced marked impairment of reproduction.[3]

PCBs are pollutants that were discharged as waste water by industrial plants until they were banned. They are long-lasting, accumulate in water and soil and in animal and human fat, and are secreted in breast milk. The Great Lakes basin is the most PCB-contaminated area of North America; Great Lakes fish are particularly contaminated.

Is it possible, based on the PCB study, to speculate that the disease of endometriosis might have been a mild, mostly tolerable disease in the past (except presumably for a few unlucky souls) that has become severe and distinctly intolerable with the additional effects of modern pollutants in our bodies? Perhaps these studies will help explain why there seems to be an epidemic of endometriosis worldwide in this century.

From Dr. Campbell I learned that there was another colony of rhesus monkeys in which two animals had died of endometriosis. This colony had been part of a toxicology study to evaluate long-term effects of TCDD (2,3,7,8-tetrachlorodibenzo-p-dioxin), another environmental pollutant. Groups of eight animals received either 25 parts per trillion (ppt; high dose) or 5 ppt dioxin (low dose); control monkeys received no dioxin.

TCDD (2,3,7,8-tetrachlorodibenzo-p-dioxin) is the most toxic of a group of chemicals widely prevalent in the environment from herbicides, industrial wastes, and other sources. Dioxin is known to cause immune suppression (based on animal research), cancer, and birth defects. In addition, it has the ability to act like a hormone in the body.

Dioxin acts with the same mechanism of toxicity as PCBs do according to Dr. Bob Bowman, a researcher involved in the TCDD study. Although the study was originally begun to study the impact of TCDD on reproduction, it was difficult, according to the researcher, because the animals exposed to the chemical had a lot of problems producing viable offspring.

In both the Ottawa study and the TCDD study, reproduction by the animals was markedly impaired. Sixty of the PCB-treated monkeys achieved only 26 pregnancies, with nine stillbirths, four deaths within 1 to 11 days after delivery, and three miscarriages. Sixteen control monkeys achieved nine live births, with two stillbirths.

Removal of the ovaries was carried out in some of the animals to control the disease but was not always successful, lending further support to the EA study showing that removal of the ovaries does not always cure the disease. (For more on this, see "Does Hysterectomy and Removal of the Ovaries Offer a Cure for Endometriosis?" in Chapter 2.)

Obviously these studies are of extreme importance, providing clues about endo that might not have been found for decades since no one thus far has suspected a link to environmental pollutants and radiation. Also in the TCDD study, endometriosis did not show up until *many* years after the exposure, making it easy to overlook the link.

At the time I learned of these animals, the original research team had disbanded except for Dr. Bowman, who had been studying the behavioral effects of dioxin in the offspring. And EPA funding for the colony had run out. Our efforts to secure further funding failed. The university where the monkeys are housed began selling them but had not yet shipped them. I called an emergency board meeting of the Endometriosis Association, and we decided to fund the colony for two months and carry out laparoscopies on the entire colony to determine if endometriosis was present in those still alive.

We asked our medical advisor Dr. Dan Martin, a leading endo surgeon, to carry out laparoscopies on the monkeys. He was assisted by our vice president of research Sherry Rier and advisor Paul Dmowski, M.D., Ph.D. At the end of a long day of laparoscopies—when the researchers broke the code to determine which animals were dioxin-exposed and which were not*—they were astounded by the highly statistically significant results.

Seventy-nine percent of the animals exposed to dioxin had developed endometriosis. Moreover, the disease increased in severity in direct proportion to the amount of dioxin exposure (the more dioxin the animal had received, the more severe the disease). Control monkeys tended to have no disease or minimal disease; exposed monkeys moderate or severe, depending on the amount of dioxin exposure. *The dose-dependent relationship was highly statistically significant (p<0.001) using the American Fertility Society and revised American Fertility Society classifications.*†[4]

The Endometriosis Association decided to raise the money to maintain the colony for at least three years (beginning in 1992), when the monkeys would probably be in menopause. Our members, primarily women with endometriosis, have generously contributed more than $230,000 thus far for this research. Our goal was to learn as much as possible from the colony. We alerted the research community and requested proposals for further research.

This is a tremendous breakthrough for a disease in which decades of research had not led to any clear understanding of causes of the disease and in which researchers have never been able to cause spontaneous development of the disease. (All the animals studied previously have required researchers to transplant endometrium, the lining of the uterus, into the animal's abdomen. However, there is no guarantee that transplanting endometrium results in a situation in which the immunological factors that perhaps lead to the dis-

---

*For the sake of objectivity, the animals are given a number code so that researchers will not know which were part of the dioxin group and which were controls during the surgeries.

†The American Fertility Society is now called the American Society for Reproductive Medicine.

ease are re-created in the animal model, meaning that the conclusions drawn from models with transplanted endometrium could be misleading.) So, besides pointing the direction to a possible cause of the disease, this dioxin work also provides a much-needed animal model for studying the disease. (In Brussels, at the Third World Congress on Endometriosis, it was pointed out that endometriosis develops in cycling, menstruating women and should be studied in a cycling, menstruating animal.)

Obviously this work also raises numerous questions and takes us into the completely new area of toxicology. While dioxin is known to cause changes in the immune system, what those changes may be related to endometriosis is still being studied. Sherry Rier, Ph.D, has continued her immune studies related to endometriosis and the dioxin colony, now as the Tracy H. Dickinson Research Chair of the Endometriosis Association. This program was established at Dartmouth Medical School in fall 1994. (See the next article.)

Work with the dioxin colony will continue as long as funding is available and as long as scientifically valid work can be done with the aging rhesus colony. The original dioxin findings were published in *Fundamental and Applied Toxicology* in November 1993. Adding to the probable significance of our work, a German study has been published finding that women with endometriosis and antithyroidal antibodies had higher levels of PCBs in their blood.[5]* (Interested researchers may contact association headquarters—see "Additional Resources"—for a translation of the study.)

Our work has also been presented at the Society for Gynecologic Investigation (1993), the American Association of Immunology (1993), the Estrogens in the Environment conference (1994), the EPA (1994), and at the National Institutes of Health Endometriosis 2000 conference (1995). (The last conference came about because of testimony I gave at a U.S. Senate hearing on hysterectomies called by Senator Barbara Mikulski. After the hearing, Senator Mikulski's staff asked what needed to happen next for women with endometriosis. When I said we needed a forum for bringing together toxicologists and endocrinologists so we could make sense out of the new dioxin work, a process that might take 10 to 15 years without a special push, Mikulski's office wrote legislation appropriating funds for the conference!)

Fortunately, the research community has responded with significant interest to the dioxin work (in part because research funds were available). As of this writing, more than 15 studies have been initiated because of the association's dioxin work. Here's a sampling:

- The National Institute of Environmental Health Sciences is carrying out a study to determine blood levels in women with endometriosis of dioxin, furans (another pollutant closely related to dioxin), and PCBs.

Antithyroidal antibodies means antibodies, immune cells, that react against one's own thyroid, an autoimmune disease. A writer is preparing an article on thyroid problems in women with endometriosis for an association newsletter.

- The Environmental Protection Agency (EPA) is carrying out a study to determine if dioxin causes endometriosislike changes in rats with transplanted endometrium.
- A study of natural killer cell activity is being expanded by scientists Christopher Coe and Sherry Rier. (Natural killer cells are immune cells that attack tumor cells and virally infected cells.)
- A study of antiphospholipid antibodies is being carried out on serum from the animals by Paul Wooley, an expert on the role of these antibodies in autoimmune diseases such as lupus.

The dioxin breakthrough was also covered by leading scientific publications. *Science* magazine, in an article entitled "Dioxin Tied to Endometriosis" by Ann Gibbons that appeared in the November 26, 1993, issue, introduced the subject in this way:

> More than 5 million women in the U.S. have endometriosis, and nobody knows why. The disease, in which tissue from the uterus mysteriously migrates to the abdomen, ovaries, bowels or bladder, often causes internal bleeding, severe pelvic pain, infertility, and other problems. Researchers have speculated that the disease might be caused by menstrual blood that flows backwards or by a developmental disorder that causes tissue to form where it should not, but proof hasn't been forthcoming. Now a study has fingered a new suspect, one with a decidedly unsavory reputation: dioxin.
>
> In human beings, this environmental toxin causes cancer and birth defects, among a host of other ills, and in a colony of female rhesus monkeys researchers have found that it can also play a key role in endometriosis. . . . "This is the first big piece of evidence that environmental toxins may be involved in the pathogenesis of endometriosis," says David Olive, chief of reproductive endocrinology and infertility at the Yale University School of Medicine. "It opens up a whole new area of research."

Scientific American; Science News; Chemical and Engineering News; Environmental Health Perspectives: Journal of the National Institute of Environmental Health Sciences, and others also carried stories. The fact that these respected scientific publications made space for the story indicates the importance of this research. Association members can be proud of these accomplishments—they would not have happened without us.

Notes
1. J. W. Fanton and J. G. Golden, "Radiation-Induced Endometriosis in *Macaca Mulatta*," *Radiation Research* 126 (1991): 141–46.
2. J. S. Campbell, J. Wong, L. Tryphonas, D. L. Arnold, E. Nera, B. Cross, and E. LaBossiere, "Is Simian Endometriosis an Effect of Immunotoxicity?" Presented at the Ontario Association of Pathologists Forty-Eighth Annual Meeting (London, Ontario, October 1985).

3. J. Campbell, "Is Reproductive Wastage and Failure Related to Environmental Pollution? Considerations of Human Data and Findings from a Rhesus Model," Symposium, "Toxicological Pathology: Quo Vadis?" (Ottawa, September 1988).

4. S. E. Rier, D. C. Martin, R. E. Bowman, W. P. Dmowski, and J. L. Becker, "Endometriosis in Rhesus Monkeys (*Macaca mulatta*) Following Chronic Exposure to 2,3,7,8-Tetrachlorodibenzo-p-Dioxin," *Fundamental and Applied Toxicology* 21, no. 4 (1993): 433–41.

5. I. Gerhard and B. Runnebaum, "Grenzen der Hormonsubstitution bei Schadstoffbelastung und Fertilitätsstörungen," *Zentralblatt für Gynäkologie* 114 (1992): 593–602.

Immunological Findings in Rhesus Monkeys Exposed to Dioxin

By Sherry Rier, Ph.D.

Although it is not known what factors are responsible for the development and progression of endometriosis, recent studies suggest that endometriosis is associated with immune dysfunction.[1,2] It is known that endometrial tissue is found within the peritoneal cavity of most women; however, only a percentage of women develop endometriosis. Immune cells within the peritoneal cavity may play an important role in the establishment and maintenance of endometriosis. These cells may normally destroy endometrial cells or discourage their growth within the peritoneal environment. Substances produced by cells of the immune system (cytokines) may also participate in endometriosis by influencing the ability of endometrial cells to grow and flourish where they do not belong. In this regard, we have shown that peritoneal leukocytes and endometrial cells from patients with endometriosis aberrantly produce the cytokine interleukin-6 which may result in unregulated growth of endometrial cells.[3,4]

Some studies suggest that endometriosis is associated with changes in systemic immunity, that there may be differences in how the immune cells that circulate throughout the body function in women with endometriosis.[1] Cytokines are important in regulating the function of immune cells both within the peritoneal cavity and throughout the body. Thus, one approach that scientists have used to study alterations in immunity which accompany different diseases is to study cytokines. If either too much or too little is produced, disease can result. To evaluate how immune cells in the blood in general circulation function in rhesus monkeys both with and without endometriosis, we have examined the ability of these cells to produce interleukin-6 and another cytokine called tumor necrosis factor.[5,6] Recently we have also studied the types of circulating immune cells and their ability to produce several other cytokines (including interferons, and other interleukins) important in immune function.

In studies funded by the Endometriosis Association, differences were found in the ability of the immune cells to produce interleukin-6 and tumor necrosis factor alpha. Cells from monkeys that had either mild or severe endometriosis could easily be stimulated to produce tumor necrosis factor, while cells from monkeys with no disease could not.

In contrast, animals with disease were able to produce less interleukin-6 than normal monkeys. In fact, less interleukin-6 was produced in severe disease than in those with mild endo. Cells from monkeys with *no* disease could produce substantially more interleukin-6 than monkeys with disease (either mild or severe).

Interestingly, cytokines are also produced by other cells, including uterine endometrial cells (the cells that are abnormally implanted in the peritoneum of endometriosis patients). It is also known that hormones such as estrogen influence the production of cytokines. A newly emerging idea is that the immune system influences the endocrine (hormonal) system and vice versa—that hormones can influence immunity.

Studies are in progress to further define differences that exist in the immune system of monkeys with endometriosis compared to those that are healthy. It is our hope that continued work will unravel the mystery of how the immune system and endocrine system may function differently in women with endometriosis. This will provide clues to what causes the development of disease and lead to possible prevention or therapy directed at the underlying cause of endo.

Notes

1. J. A. Hill, "Immunologic Factors in Endometriosis-Associated Reproductive Failure," *Infertility and Reproductive Medicine Clinics of North America: Endometriosis* 3 (1992): 583–96.
2. W. P. Dmowski, D. Braun, and H. Gebel, "The Immune System in Endometriosis," *Modern Approaches to Endometriosis*, E. J. Thomas and J. A. Rock, eds. (Boston: Kluwer Academic, 1992): 97–111.
3. S. E. Rier, A. K. Parsons, and J. L. Becker, "Altered Interleukin-6 Production by Peritoneal Leukocytes from Patients with Endometriosis," *Fertility and Sterility* 61 (1994): 294–99.
4. S. E. Rier, P. N. Zarmakoupis, X. Hu, and J. Becker, "Dysregulation of Interleukin-6 Responses in Ectopic Endometrial Stromal Cells: Correlation with Decreased Soluble Receptor Levels in Peritoneal Fluid of Women with Endometriosis," *Journal of Clinical Endocrinology and Metabolism* 80 (1995): 1431–37.
5. S. E. Rier, B. L. Spangelo, D. C. Martin, R. E. Bowman, and J. L. Becker, "Production of Interleukin-6 and Tumor Necrosis Factor-Alpha by Peripheral Blood Mononuclear Cells from Rhesus Monkeys with Endometriosis," *Journal of Immunology* 150 (1992): 49A.
6. S. E. Rier, D. C. Martin, R. E. Bowman, and J. L. Becker, "Immunoresponsiveness in Endometriosis: Implications of Estrogenic Toxicants," *Environmental Health Prospectives* 103 (1995).

■ *Sherry Rier, Ph.D., formerly the association's vice president of research, now holds the Tracy H. Dickinson Research Chair of the Endometriosis Association and heads the association research program established at Dartmouth Medical School in November 1994.*

Dioxins, PCBs, and Endometriosis—What Do We Need to Know to Protect Ourselves?

By Mary Lou Ballweg

Since our news of the startling findings of endometriosis in a research monkey colony exposed to dioxin, an environmental pollutant, many women with endometriosis have expressed concern about dioxin exposure. How are we exposed to dioxin? What are the dangers? Can we protect ourselves from it and how? This article is meant to start to answer those questions.

We will also cover the same questions for PCBs since some monkeys in a research colony studied by the Canadian federal government reportedly developed severe endometriosis and impaired fertility following PCB exposure. Also, a German study has found higher levels of PCBs in women with endometriosis and antithyroidal antibodies.

Organochlorines

It is unfortunately entirely possible that other chemicals in addition to dioxin and PCBs could be related to development of endometriosis. Dioxin and PCBs are part of a large group of chemical compounds called *organochlorines*. Organochlorines are made on purpose or by accident (as a by-product of other processes) by combining chlorine with

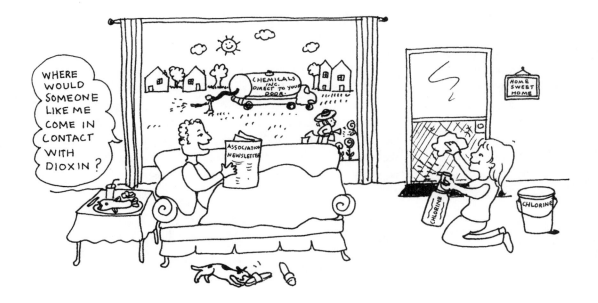

organic substances, usually petrochemicals. Organochlorines began being manufactured and used widely in the 1940s. They were the result of wartime experiments to create more lethal chemical weapons.

Organochlorines are now found everywhere on earth according to a publication by Greenpeace, the international environmental organization. At least 177 of them have been found in human tissues and fluids in the United States and Canada, including in fat, mother's milk, blood, semen, and breath. They are responsible, researchers believe, for the declining sperm counts of men over recent decades. They are passed from one generation to the next through the placenta in pregnancy and in breast milk.

Organochlorines are almost completely foreign to nature according to Greenpeace, although some dioxins may be produced in nature in small quantities. Synthetic, human-made organochlorine compounds are extremely resistant to breakdown and can take hundreds of years to break down completely. Meanwhile, these synthetic organochlorines are taken up and are stored in the fatty tissue of animals and humans. The concentration in fatty tissues increases with time even at low levels of exposure. This process is called *bioaccumulation.*

To make matters worse, another process, called *biomagnification*, occurs. As plants and small animals are eaten by larger animals, the amount of toxins consumed by each higher organism increases. For instance, bottom animals and plants in a lake with contaminated sediment are eaten by small fish, which are eaten by bigger fish, which are eaten by seabirds and humans. Humans who eat animal products at the top of the food chain can thus consume significant concentrations of toxins. (Vegetarians consume significantly less, since they're eating at the bottom of the food chain—plants.)

Only a few of the organochlorines have been banned (including PCBs and DDT, but not dioxin),* but even those that have been are still widely prevalent in the environment. This is due partly to the compounds' long life as well as to continued use and dissemination of the compounds illegally or by wind, water, and products from countries where the compounds are still legal. The book *Whitewash: Exposing the Health and Environmental Dangers of Women's Sanitary Products and Disposable Diapers—and What You Can Do About It*, by Liz Armstrong and Adrienne Scott (Toronto: HarperCollins, 1992), notes that "hypocritically, we still manufacture DDT in North America for export to other countries."

Greenpeace, which notes that there are 11,000 organochlorines now in commerce, calls for a complete ban on organochlorines in its 1991 report "The Product is the Poison: The Case for a Chlorine Phase-Out." The International Joint Commission, a U.S.–Canadi-

---

*New regulations for dioxin are being considered by the United States Environmental Protection Agency (EPA), which released a 2,000-page report on dioxin in fall 1994. Much as the tobacco industry did, the industries involved in dioxin pollution are paying selected scientists and lobbyists handsomely to fight regulation of the toxin and to try to discredit the studies showing dioxin is harmful, including the association's studies. Readers, we need your continued support.

an organization established in 1909 to oversee binational concerns related to the Great Lakes, has also stated that "the use of chlorine and its compounds should be avoided in the manufacturing process."

Greenpeace notes that enough is known about the persistence and toxicity of organochlorines as a class to justify a ban but that only a tiny portion of the compounds have been subjected to even preliminary hazard assessments. A similar problem was noted at a Medical College of Wisconsin conference, "Health Implications of Great Lakes Pollution." Speakers noted that while more than 70,000 chemicals are in use in industry today, toxicological data exists for only 5,000 to 6,000 of these chemicals, and the data on even these is incomplete.

"Hindsight is always 20/20," the saying goes, but even still it's hard to imagine why so many chemicals were and still are allowed to be produced and disseminated widely in the environment without prior testing to assure safety for humans, animals, and plant life. This widespread dissemination means that every person and animal in the industrialized world (and many in the third world also, since water, wind, and products have spread the contaminants worldwide) has what scientists call a "background" of contaminants they carry in their bodies, from the embryo stage on. Because of this background load, the only way to know what any particular chemical does is to study it under controlled laboratory conditions without exposure to other chemicals. In addition, because the chemicals have bodywide impact and scientists do not yet understand what these impacts are, especially in the incredibly complex immune, reproductive, and nervous systems, they must study the chemicals in animal models.

Hormonal and Immunological Effects

In fact it is only a recent realization that these compounds *have* profound immunological and reproductive impacts. In prior decades the focus of research and governmental regulation was almost exclusively on cancer. Now scientists are learning that many very toxic immune and reproductive consequences occur with exposure to levels of pollutants far below the level known to cause cancer. Dioxin, for example, can induce hormonal reactions at exposures a hundred times smaller than the exposures associated with cancer, according to animal research cited by the United States Environmental Protection Agency (EPA).

Scientists studying animals in and around the Great Lakes were among the first to notice these effects. The Great Lakes are about average in their level of pollution compared with other lakes, according to the recent "Health Implications of Great Lakes Pollution" conference. But because less than 1 percent of the water in the Great Lakes flows out of them into the ocean each year, "the effects of organochlorine contamination thus show up more quickly in the Great Lakes than in other aquatic ecosystems," according to Greenpeace. Thus, what's happening in the Great Lakes may serve as an early warning.

The Great Lakes also have been studied more extensively because of their importance to so many states and provinces. The lakes contain 95 percent of the fresh surface water of the United States. Twenty percent of the U.S. population and 50 percent of the Canadian population lives in the Great Lakes basin, the area that drains into the Great Lakes, according to an EPA publication.

The World Wildlife Fund has noted: "Since the mid-1950s, problems with the endocrine systems of birds, fish, and mammals in the Great Lakes have been reported. . . . In each instance, high concentrations of organochlorine chemicals were found in these animals or other individuals in the same populations. . . . More recent research documents similar problems. Researchers from Guelph University can no longer find an adult salmonid [a family of salmon] in the Great Lakes that does not have an enlarged thyroid, nor can Canadian Wildlife Service researchers find a herring gull without an enlarged thyroid."

The International Joint Commission notes in a recent publication that "scientists noticed in the 1960s and 1970s that almost entire populations of cormorants, herons, and gulls living on the lakes started to die." And studies of children of mothers who ate Great Lakes fish showed they were born sooner, weighed less, and had smaller heads than the infants from the same community whose mothers did not eat Great Lakes fish. The infants showed significant behavioral problems, including jerky, unbalanced movement, increased startle reflexes, and decreased interest in new stimuli. In tests at seven months and four years of age these children had difficulty learning because of impairments in short-term memory and other mental functions.

Recently a group of scientists gathered at Wingspread in Racine, Wisconsin, for a conference, "Endocrine Disrupters in the Environment." They issued a consensus statement after assessing the current knowledge on endocrine (hormonal) effects of polluting compounds:

Many wildlife populations are already affected by these compounds. The impacts include thyroid dysfunction in birds and fish; decreased fertility in birds, fish, shellfish, and mammals; decreased hatching success in birds, fish, and turtles; gross birth deformities in birds, fish, and turtles; metabolic abnormalities in birds, fish, and mammals; behavioral abnormalities in birds; demasculinization and feminization of male fish, birds, and mammals; defeminization and masculinization of female fish and birds; and compromised immune systems in birds and mammals. . . .

The mechanisms by which these compounds have their impact vary, but they share the general properties of (1) mimicking the effects of natural hormones by recognizing their binding sites; (2) antagonizing the effect of these hormones by blocking their interaction with their physiological binding sites; (3) reacting directly and indirectly with the hormone in question; (4) altering the natural pattern of synthesis of hormones; or (5) altering hormone receptor levels.

Twenty-three compounds or groups of compounds were cited by the scientists as having known ability to disrupt the endocrine system. Thus far, however, the precise impact of this disruption in humans is not known. If the dioxin and PCB links to endometriosis are borne out by further study, it may be the first human disease definitely linked to hormonal/immunological disruption due to pollutants.

At the conference the scientists used DES exposure as a model of what they expect may happen in humans. Based on the animal studies, they expect the effects, like DES, will be worse in the offspring exposed to the toxin in the mother's uterus than in the parent exposed as an adult. And, like DES, the manifestations of the exposure may not occur until sexual maturity, making it very difficult to trace the source. As the first generation to be conceived after the introduction of these chemicals, are the baby boomers the first generation to show these effects?

The gap between exposure and observable signs of disease makes it harder to be sure what is happening, at least in humans. (In the dioxin monkey colony the monkeys were fed the dioxin in their chow as young adults, and the evidence of endometriosis was noted 10 years after exposure started. Similarly, in the PCB monkey colony, endometriosis was not noted until years after the chemical exposure.) "Because functional deficits are not visible at birth and may not be fully manifested until adulthood, they are often missed by physicians, parents, and the regulatory community, and the causal agent is never identified," the Wingspread scientists wrote.

They also pointed out that the scientific and public health communities are generally unaware of the presence of hormonally active environmental chemicals. (It was noted at the Medical College of Wisconsin conference that only two medical schools in the United States even offer a course in environmental medicine, meaning physicians are woefully uninformed on these matters.) The Wingspread scientists call for broadening the testing of products beyond simply looking for cancer and specifically studying hormonal effects in animals.

Dioxins

Let's move on to specifics on dioxins and PCBs. Dioxins comprise a group of 75 related compounds, with TCDD (2,3,7,8-tetrachlorodibenzo-p-dioxin) being the most toxic. In fact TCDD has been called the most toxic chemical ever produced by humans.

TCDD is the dioxin involved in the rhesus monkey colony the association saved. In the monkeys this potent chemical caused development of endometriosis in very minute quantities—5 ppt (parts per trillion) and 25 ppt. To imagine how infinitesimal this is, imagine a trillion (1,000,000,000,000) drops of water and only 5 drops of dioxin in that trillion drops of water. Or, as a researcher involved with the dioxin experiments for the last 15 years described it, that's like spitting into an Olympic-size swimming pool.

TCDD, according to a confidential American Paper Institute report released by Greenpeace, is present in trace amounts in the whole range of chlorine-bleached paper products: sanitary napkins and tampons, toilet paper and facial tissues, disposable diapers, paper plates and towels, coffee filters and cigarette papers. Perhaps worse, hundreds of organochlorines are released in the bleaching process as the products are manufactured, compounds that then find their way into water and air (one million metric tons of chlorinated organic materials enter United States and Canadian waterways every year!).

But saddest of all, as the authors of *Whitewash* so eloquently point out, the bleaching process and "whiter-than-white" results are completely unnecessary, especially in women's sanitary supplies. The authors suggest that the sanitary supply industry bleaches the pulp used in the products to contribute to the illusion that the products are sterile (which they are not). They suggest that women in North America launch a campaign to force the industry to stop chlorine bleaching of these products. Such a campaign was successful in six weeks in England for sanitary napkins (but not tampons, which are probably more critical, since they're worn internally and the vagina is apparently quite an absorbent organ).

The most important source of dioxin for the average person, according to Linda Birnbaum, Ph.D., director, EPA Environmental Toxicology Division, is, alas, our food because of pesticide contamination and bioaccumulation in animals. Dioxin is also created by the burning of toxic waste and municipal garbage in incinerators, leaded gas in vehicles, certain wood preservatives, and the manufacturing and use of certain products—pesticides, solvents, and organochlorine chemicals.

PCBs

PCBs (polychlorinated biphenyls) are compounds that were used widely as electrical insulators and were used formerly in carbonless paper, specialty inks, and paints and as additives in plastics manufacturing. Industrial waste water from these manufacturing processes and from municipal sewage treatment plants that process these wastes were sources of PCB contamination of water and soil.

The FDA allowed defined levels in dairy products, poultry, eggs, animal feeds, and other food products—5 ppm (parts per million) were allowed in poultry and the edible portion of fish, for example. Even these standards covered only foods shipped between states, not foods shipped within states unless the state adopted the standard. A Wisconsin Department of Natural Resources paper from 1974 assures readers that "the Food and Drug Administration Standards are established with a wide margin of safety well below the level of toxicity to humans." The very same paper, however, notes that levels of PCB at only 2 ppm in fish in the diet of mink led to reproductive failure. The FDA currently allows 2 ppm of PCBs in fish.

PCBs last a very long time. They are basically a life sentence, as one speaker at the conference "Health Implications of Great Lakes Pollution" stated. Once you have them in your body, they'll essentially be in your body for the rest of your life. Even worse, like other organochlorines that are stored in our body fat, they are passed along to our children when we are pregnant with them and breast-feed. Work by Wayland Swain, Ph.D., Michigan, showed that it may take six generations before PCBs are cleared from our bodies even with no further exposure. This work was calculated on the basis of the first mother in the six generations having the average level of PCBs in her breast milk currently found in Michigan mothers who consumed PCB-contaminated fish. The study also assumed that each mother had her baby at age 20 when some PCBs would have passed out of her body but not as much as would have later (again assuming no further exposure).

PCBs have been banned in both the United States (since 1979) and Canada (since 1980) but are still widely prevalent in the environment. The load of PCBs in beluga whales in the St. Lawrence River leading into the Great Lakes is so great, for example, that their bodies are declared hazardous waste when they die.

The most serious exposure to PCBs for many people generally would be in contaminated fish. In Wisconsin, the Department of Health and Social Services advised pregnant women not to eat Lake Michigan fish (Lake Michigan is heavily contaminated with PCBs) beginning in the mid-1970s, and others were advised not to eat fish from PCB-contaminated lakes more than once a week. Next people were told to avoid certain sizes and species of fish (the larger, older fish at the higher end of the food chain). Today, with greatly increased understanding of the dangers, the Michigan Medical Society has advised that children and anyone who ever plans to have children, male or female, should eat no Great Lakes fish!

Contact your local governmental health units to attempt to learn what contamination levels may occur in your area and what precautions to take. At the "Health Implications of Great Lakes Pollution" conference, speakers suggested low-fat ocean fish were generally safer than freshwater fish and that the smaller fish such as cod and halibut were less contaminated than larger specialty fish.

Anyone attempting to limit the PCBs to which they and their families are exposed should take the fish warnings very seriously. At the "Health Implications" conference, it was pointed out that *one* fish meal of contaminated fish could result in as much PCB in your body as drinking the water from Lake Michigan and breathing the air in the area for 119 years! In addition, remember that the FDA-allowed levels may be too high to avoid the hormonal/immunological effects discussed in this article. The amount of TCDD (dioxin) currently allowed in fish is 50 ppt! Severe endo occurred in the monkey colony at 25 ppt.

In addition to endometriosis, there may be other pressing reasons to eliminate exposure to PCBs as much as possible. A preliminary study has suggested that PCBs and pesticides may be involved in breast cancer, which has increased in prevalence from one woman in 20 in the United States developing it in 1940 to one woman in 9 today. The study found elevated levels of PCBs and pesticide residues in fat samples from women with cancer compared with those who had benign breast disease. [The study, "Pesticides and Polychlorinated Biphenyl Residues in Human Breast Lipids and Their Relation to Breast Cancer," appeared in *Archives of Environmental Health* 47, no. 2 (March/April 1992).] Possibly this finding, if confirmed, will make sense out of past observations that high-fat diets seem linked to breast cancer and that women who breast-feed have a lower incidence of breast cancer—can we speculate that perhaps this could be because toxic chemicals bioaccumulate in fat tissues such as the breast and because breast-feeding results in dumping some of the toxic chemical load into the infant? In the dioxin monkey colony the monkeys lost up to 20 percent of their body burden of dioxin in pregnancy and breast-feeding, with breast-feeding being the greatest source.

All this information on environmental pollutants and their health consequences can certainly feel overwhelming. But perhaps we can take heart in knowing that information is the first step toward taking action. And action is what's needed, both individually and socially. There are many steps you can take to reduce your exposure to these toxins. See "Avoiding Dioxin and PCBs—What You Can Do." And remember, *together* we can make a difference. If indeed toxic pollutants are a part of the endometriosis story, *only* working together will make it possible for us to overcome this nightmare.

Avoiding Dioxins and PCBs—
What You Can Do

By Mary Lou Ballweg

Although dioxins, PCBs, and other organochlorines are very prevalent in the modern world, there are some clear steps you can take to avoid at least some of the exposure. Here are some suggestions:

1. Avoid contaminated fish (see the preceding article, "Dioxins, PCBs, and Endometriosis . . .").
2. Consider eating lower on the food chain—more vegetables and grains; fewer animal products. The more animal products you consume, the more pollutants you will encounter since pollutants accumulate in the fatty tissues.
3. Trim away the fat from meats and fish you do eat, and remove the dark stripe down the back of fish fillets. Cook foods in ways that allow the fat to drain away from what's eaten (meat on racks, for instance) and don't use the fat for gravies, etc.
4. Even better, go organic. Organic growers guarantee their foods have been grown without toxic chemicals and hormones added to the feed. Even tasty organic poultry and meats are now available in natural food stores. If organic food is too expensive, consider using it at least before conception and during the most critical first six to eight weeks of pregnancy.
5. Check on the pollutants in your water supply with local authorities or by having testing done. (If the water supply comes from the Great Lakes, you can skip this step and go straight to getting a water purifier!) Excellent water purifiers now exist that can remove PCBs, lead, mercury, chlorine, and other contaminants and will cost less over time than buying bottled water. If you use bottled water, check that the bottler is a member of the International Bottled Water Association (IBWA), which requires members to meet certain standards. At the very least, use pure water during pregnancy.
6. Substitute cloth products for bleached paper ones that have dioxin residues: hankies for facial tissues, cloth towels for paper towels, cloth napkins for paper ones. Switch to unbleached coffee filters. Bathroom tissue manufactured in a dioxin-free process is available from some specialty and health stores and from the Seventh Generation catalog. (Seventh Generation Catalog Request, Colchester, VT 05446-1672.)
7. Switch to menstrual products that do not have dioxin residues in them. See the following article, "Dioxin Danger in Tampons . . ." for sources. And before you throw out that last box of napkins or tampons, call the 800 number with the product and tell the company why you're switching.

8. Find safe substitutes for chlorine bleaches and cleaning products used in your home (and workplace too if possible).

9. Recycle paper and use recycled paper. Encourage recycling and using recycled paper at your workplace. Use both sides of the paper. As many as 1,000 organochlorines are released with paper bleaching. (The association uses recycled paper in its newsletter.)

10. If you're among the fortunate who are able to invest, consider "green" investing. Quite a number of "alternative" funds are available that screen companies for both traditional financial criteria and their environmental record. A helpful resource, *You, Your Money, and the World*, is available from Co-op America, 1612 K St. N.W., Suite 600, Washington, DC 20006, 1-800-584-7336.

11. Write to paper companies and ask them to do something important for their future and ours—plan to phase out chlorine bleaching and plan for less toxic manufacturing processes. The book *Whitewash* has much background information that will help you with this step. It is available from Women and Environments Education and Development (WEED) Foundation, 736 Bathurst St., Toronto, ON, Canada M5S 2R4, (416) 516-2600. WEED has begun a campaign to eliminate organochlorines in sanitary products.

12. And now for a really tough one—what about breast-feeding? One wonders if there are testing services available as there are for water. If indeed one's breast milk is contaminated, would it make sense to pump it and dispose of it (as hazardous waste presumably)? The true tragedy of toxic pollution is clear in an issue like breast-feeding—pollution could rob us of the ability to have children and to engage in something as beautiful and powerful as breast-feeding! Ideas, anyone?

Dioxin Danger in Tampons—How to Obtain Safe Sanitary Supplies

By Mary Lou Ballweg and Karen Gould

With the discovery that dioxin is linked to endometriosis, we may all be wondering how we can avoid it and other toxins that may damage our health. One problem area that we may not have considered is the use of tampons and sanitary napkins. Most women assume these products are sterile (they are not) and also that governmental regulations protect them. Unfortunately, there is very little regulation of sanitary protection products—manufacturers are not even required to inform consumers of the ingredients used in the products, for instance.

Because of chlorine bleaching of the pulp used in the products, dioxin traces are left behind. The *Wall Street Journal* reported in June 1992 that a congressional panel had accused the Food and Drug Administration (FDA), the U.S. federal agency charged with ensuring that drugs and medical devices are safe, of ignoring a possible danger to women from tampons that may contain dioxin. The congressional panel uncovered an FDA document that noted that the risk of dioxin in tampons "can be quite high." However, according to the article, the FDA deleted a statement about these possibly significant risks from an agency report without a full investigation.

In addition to the danger to our health from dioxin traces in sanitary products made from chlorine-bleached pulp and paper, the process of manufacturing these products adds pollutants to our environment. And dioxin and related compounds aren't even the whole story. An article entitled "The Truth About Tampons" in the November/December 1990 issue of *Garbage Magazine, The Practical Journal for the Environment* cites a 1981 FDA study that found boron, aluminum, copper, waxes, surfactants (chemicals to improve absorbency), alcohols, acids, nitrogen compounds, and hydrocarbons occurred in tampons. In addition to the health hazards, especially for chemically sensitive women, as many with endo are, these contaminants contribute to pollution. (Sanitary napkins and tampons *never* belong down the toilet, according to the article—they contribute to plumbing problems, they must be strained out of sewage systems and sent to a landfill, and all too many of them end up being flushed straight into waterways, including the ocean.)

Surprisingly, quite a number of companies are offering alternative sanitary products. Realizing that women with endo, who perhaps use more of these products than anyone, now have yet another reason for using the healthiest products available, we're listing sources here.

Three categories of products are available: pads, tampons, and rubber cups. Each has advantages and disadvantages; pads and tampons offer a range of choices.

Pads are available in both disposable and washable cloth varieties. The disposable pads are chlorine-free and usually cotton-sheathed. They are convenient but of course still add to the load in our landfills. Also, they may still contain irritants that can bother extremely chemically sensitive women.

Reusable cloth pads come in many varieties. Most are cotton flannel or fleece. They sport a wide variety of prints and colors (some are vegetable-dyed). Securing options include belts, Velcro, and wings that fasten. For the especially chemically sensitive, organic untreated cotton reduces problems that might arise from pesticides used to cultivate most cotton and dyes used to produce cloth in the pad. Some of the pads and their cases are very pretty—just seeing them can start to change one's perspective on periods! One company offers a beautiful young woman's beginner kit.

The issue of care of reusable pads is addressed in the book *Whitewash: Exposing the Health and Environmental Dangers of Women's Sanitary Products and Disposable Diapers*:

"For many women, the big concern is how they'll care for reusable pads after years of just throwing the disposables away," says Lynn Burrows, founder of the reusable sanitary product company, Women's Choice. "'What will I do with these messy things?' they ask. The answer is simple: Soak them in a bucket of cold water, which dissolves the blood and prevents permanent staining, then run them through the regular laundry. These pads wash up very easily, and they dry well, too."

Women working away from home have other concerns. "They wonder if reusable pads are appropriate, but it's just a matter of being prepared if you're out of the house for several hours. Store the used ones in an airtight bag until you get home; *then* toss them in a bucket of cold water," Lynn Burrows advises.

Tampons are also available in disposable and reusable varieties. The disposable tampons are 100 percent cotton without chlorine bleaching. Natural sea sponges can also be used as tampons. Sponges have serious disadvantages. They may be contaminated with sand, fungi, or ocean pollutants. They also need to be rinsed out promptly and thoroughly after use. For further discussion and instructions about the use of sea sponges, consult *The New Our Bodies, Ourselves*, p. 250 (by Boston Women's Health Book Collective, Touchstone, 1992).

A rubber cup called *The Keeper* is a third type of alternative. It's a small reusable rubber cup advertised to last at least 10 years. The rubber might be an irritant for the chemically sensitive.

With so many choices available, some combination of products that best suits your needs should address the issue of convenience. Once they switch, many women report that they are more comfortable.

Alternative menstrual protection products are available primarily through mail order, although many health food and ecology stores carry some of these items. Today's Choice, a line of chlorine-free pads and panty liners, and Natracare tampons are often available in these stores.

Chlorine-Free Disposable Pads and Tampons

Seventh Generation, 49 Hercules Dr., Colchester, VT 05446-1672, 800-456-1177: Chlorine-free pads and liners.

Body Elements Terressentials Catalog, 3320 N. 3rd St., Arlington, VA 22201-1712, (703) 525-0585: *Natracare* 100 percent cotton, chlorine-free tampons.

Washable Cloth Pads

Body Elements Terressentials Catalog (see disposables): Moon Wrap pads with wings in cotton flannel, floral, and organic cotton, Moon Pouch for transporting, Moon Bowl for soaking.

GladRags, PO Box 12751, Portland, OR 97212, (503) 282-0436: Flannel pads in colors or organic cotton fit inside a cotton liner that attaches around the crotch of panties.

Menstrual Health Foundation, 104 Petaluma Ave., Sebastopol, CA 95472, (707) 829-3154: The Menstrual Health Foundation is a nonprofit women's organization that promotes "products, programs and publications for menstrual well-being and empowerment," including 100 percent organic cotton knit reusable menstrual pads. The foundation notes its pads "provide a healthy alternative to current commercial disposable products which are bleached with chlorine and create toxic dioxins, harmful to humans and the environment."

Many Moons, #14-130 Dallas Rd., Victoria, BC V8V 1A3, Canada, (604) 382-1588: Flannel pads attach with belts or wings, in prints, colors, or organic unbleached cotton, carrying bag, soaking pot.

Modern Women's Choice, PO Box 245, Gabriola, BC V0R 1X0, Canada, (604) 247-8433: Cotton fleece pads with nylon backing, Velcro attachment, wings, and Velcro-added panties, purse carrier.

The Natural Baby Co., Inc., 816 Silvia St., 800 B-S, Trenton, NJ 08628-3299, (609) 771-9233: Flannel pads in white, floral, or untreated cotton with Velcro fasteners and waterproof purse bag.

The Natural Choice, 1365 Rufina Circle, Santa Fe, NM 87501, 800-621-2591: Organic cotton pads.

Rubber Cup

The Keeper, Box 20023, Cincinnati, OH 45220.

■ *Karen Gould, Austin, Texas, is a consultant in medieval and renaissance manuscripts and freelance writer who suffers from chronic fatigue and multiple chemical sensitivities.*

15

෨෨

Is Your Home a Health Hazard?

By Lyse M. Tremblay

"*Shortly after moving into a new apartment complex in Texas, my husband and I became very ill, exhibiting symptoms of neurotoxicity. We later discovered that the symptoms were caused by urea-formaldehyde foam insulation installed in the walls of the apartment (which gives off toxic formaldehyde gas) and organophosphate pesticide sprayed within the apartment.*

"*As a result of the toxic chemical exposure, my immune system was damaged, and I developed many allergies to many foods and chemicals. Now, whenever I eat a food to which I am allergic or expose myself to cigarette smoke/perfume/petrochemicals, I become fatigued, dizzy, disoriented, and achy, and pressure develops in my forehead/face that if severe enough can affect the muscles in my face, making it difficult for me to make facial expressions, speak, or smile.*

"*However, by controlling the environment in my home (not allowing cigarette smoking or pesticide/herbicide use and not using scented products, cleaners containing solvents, etc.) and watching my dust closely, my allergy reactions have improved. Since I am so sensitive to perfume and cigarette smoke and it is difficult to avoid these in public, I have not worked outside of the home since the chemical exposure four years ago.*

"*My husband and I own and manage a wholesale tool distributorship business we operate out of our home. I am able to perform all of the office duties associated with the business—accounting, ordering and receiving merchandise, answering the phone, secretarial, etc. I do not mind what I am presently doing, and it keeps me busy, but I miss teaching, and I really miss being financially independent! . . .*

"*I had been seeing my allergist for nearly a year and the headaches were finally improving when I began to experience the strange symptoms I now think are partially due to endo and partially due to interstitial cystitis. (Sometimes I feel like a 'basket case.') I think the endo/cystitis symptoms are also attributable to the immune system damage from the chemical exposure I had four years ago. Believe it or not, I was quite healthy before that. . . .*"

G., South Dakota

"*I developed severe endometriosis after being exposed to a pesticide with dioxin while work-ing in a plant store. . . . With increasing frequency, toxic chemicals are invading the home, school, and workplace. Most often they are components of construction materials (particu-larly carpeting), petrochemical pollutants, pesticides, and synthetic fragrances.*

"*Although the cancer connection to chemical exposure has long been suspected, a grow-ing number of experts attribute the alarming increase in cases of allergies, asthma, auto-immune disorders, and neurological conditions (including depression, hyperactivity, and insomnia) to chemical contamination. The national impact of related health care and dis-ability costs as well as lost productivity are important factors to consider.*

"*The effects of chemical contamination are long term and can be devastating, creating disease as well as contaminating the air and groundwater. My hope is that when the effects of toxic chemicals on humans and the environment are more fully understood, our society will demand safe alternatives and stronger regulation. . . . I hope you will pass on to your readership the importance of using nontoxic products and also putting pressure on industry to eliminate toxic chemicals from their products.*"

Linda, California

"*I have just finished reading your most recent mailing regarding the link between endometriosis and dioxins. It left me with a cold, terrified feeling. Unnecessary chemicals, toxins, pollution—I'm not surprised to find that we are polluting ourselves sick. I have endo (laparotomy in 1991 with cautery and removal of implants in my umbilicus, cul-de-sac, ovary, etc.). It was in remission until a few months ago. Now I can actually palpate a tender mass near my umbilicus. . . . I have two children. My daughter is 15 months old. I breast-fed her for six months because she had an anaphylactic reaction to milk. Allergies are the result of a mixed-up immune system. She is doing OK now but cannot eat any dairy products, eggs, nuts, or fish. She has the characteristic dark circles under her eyes. Fortunately there are soy milk formulas available. It is my understanding that she is among a growing number of children with severe allergies.*

"*Questions galore fill my mind. Why are dioxins produced? How can anyone discharge these substances into our water/soil/air with a clear conscience? How do we stop this in-sanity? Recently I heard a woman speak about her experience living near Love Canal. She described her children—both mentally retarded. The daughter had been born with a variety of deformities, including a double row of teeth. How many tragedies have to occur before we stop polluting and dabbling in toxic chemicals? Should we really be spraying poisons on our yards—spaces that are supposed to be safe for our families? . . .*

"*I am dumbfounded at what risks we take for minor conveniences and silly little 'gains.' Dazzling white paper products, weed-free, thick, green lawns, and blemish-free fruit are not worth it if we end up with cancer, endometriosis, or a baby with birth defects. What kind of existence can our children expect to have? I do believe that if people understood the implica-*

tions they would think twice. When it comes right down to it, protecting the environment means protecting ourselves and our children.

"I wish the association the best of luck with its research and, especially, with confronting government and business about the toxins that are ending up in our food, water, and air. Please give us guidance as to what we can do at the consumer and patient level. United voices will get results! Perhaps printing a sample letter that could be sent to producers of offending products and to government officials would be an effective way to get ourselves heard. . . . Together we make a difference!"

Patty, Ontario

It is now acknowledged by the U.S. Environmental Protection Agency (EPA) and the Canada Mortgage and Housing Corporation (CMHC) that houses contain substances that may be hazardous to our health. In fact the air inside the home may be more seriously polluted than the outdoor air in the largest and most industrialized cities. In view of the fact that approximately 90 percent of our time is spent indoors, the risks to our health from indoor air pollution for many of us may be greater than the risks from outdoor air pollution.

Most houses contain a number of pollutant sources, and while exposure to one pollutant source may not in itself be a problem, exposure to a number of them can present a serious risk. These pollutants can enter our bodies in one of three ways: (1) through our food or water, (2) through materials and furnishings we touch, and (3) through the air we breathe. Although houses are mostly responsible for pollutants absorbed as a result of the air we breathe, these will be in addition to the rest of the pollutant load that our bodies have absorbed, thereby increasing our total load.

Naturally, not everyone will be affected in the same way by exposure to pollutants. Factors such as heredity, diet, lifestyle, age, and preexisting medical conditions all affect our particular susceptibility.

Who Is Most at Risk

CMHC separates people into three categories ranging from those most at risk to those least at risk. Most at risk are individuals who are hypersensitive to a number of agents and who react adversely to extremely low levels of exposure. This condition is commonly described as *environmental allergy, environmental hypersensitivity,* or *environmental illness.* According to a report on housing for the environmentally hypersensitive prepared for the Research Division of CMHC, the symptoms reported by those affected ranged from central nervous system problems such as tension, fatigue, headaches, depression, and inability to concentrate to problems with other physical systems such as gastrointestinal, respiratory, musculoskeletal, genitourinary, EENT (eyes, ears, nose, and throat), skin, and cardiovascular. The symptoms were often severe enough to interfere with a person's ability to function normally. Biochemical individuality (heredity or mother's health and nutritional state during pregnancy), total body burden (biological stress including illness, psychological state, and all forms of irritants and toxic contaminants), and nutritional state were noted as factors that may predispose a person to hypersensitivity.

The onset of environmental hypersensitivity was reported as being triggered by the following:

- serious injury or severe stress
- serious illness often requiring surgery or prolonged drug therapy
- chronic exposure to low-level contamination such as molds or formaldehyde in homes and buildings, industrial emissions at work or in a polluted neighborhood, or chemicals in the food and water
- acute exposure to toxic agents during industrial accidents or pesticide applications

The report also notes that the chemical sensitivities of hypersensitive individuals were almost always associated with parallel sensitivities to biological contaminants such as molds and dust as well as to food allergies. Hypersensitive individuals tested positive in conventional allergy tests as well as clinical ecology tests. It was also reported, however, that a reduced exposure or total avoidance of the environmental irritants or incitants reduced the food allergy sensitivities to some extent and that all the participants reported an improvement in their health following a change of habitat that excluded chemical exposure to even minute levels of contaminants but included clean air, clean water, and clean food.

It is interesting to note the similarities between this group and most sufferers of endometriosis. In addition, the profile of the respondents who had made modifications to their homes to improve their health indicated that 83 percent were female, 93 percent were over the age of 30, 76 percent became ill in adult life, 93 percent had been sick for more than six years, and 27 percent were currently disabled. In light of the research on dioxins and endometriosis, the similarities may be more than just coincidental.

The second group at risk are the people with known health problems such as respiratory or cardiovascular diseases, allergies, chemical sensitivities, or chronic illnesses, or those who spend a large amount of time in the home such as women, children, the elderly, or the infirm. For this group the home needs to be altered to lessen the effects of any known irritant and avert risk.

The third group consists of people who have no known reaction to low levels of contaminants and are in relatively good health. The issue for them would be to improve comfort and prevent potential health problems from occurring. Prevention for this last group is indeed very important because just as some health effects may be experienced soon after a single pollutant exposure, other effects may not occur until years later. Some people can become sensitized to biological and chemical pollutants as a result of a high exposure level or a long and repeated exposure level.

It is therefore important to deal with the issue of indoor air pollution even if physical symptoms are not noticeable and particularly important to take corrective action if you have a known health problem or are hypersensitive.

Pollutants, Health Effects, Sources, and Solutions (Compiled from EPA and CMHC sources)

Biological Contaminants

Substance: Molds, mildew, dust mites, pollen, animal dander and cat saliva, bacteria, and viruses.

Health Effects: Eye, nose, throat irritation; shortness of breath; dizziness, lethargy, fever, digestive problems, asthma, humidifier fever, influenza, infectious diseases, sensitization to substances, allergic reactions, hypersensitivity pneumonitis, allergic rhinitis.

Sources: High (above 60 to 70 percent) humidity levels; leaky house components or pipes causing water accumulation; humidifier, air conditioner, or refrigerator trays or drainage pans; condensation on interior surfaces; rotting house structures (e.g., windows, floors and framing); damp or moist house furnishings (e.g., carpets, furniture, wall coverings, mattresses, paper, clothing); potted plants (soil can support fungal growth); cold, uninsulated, or unventilated places (e.g., cold cellars, crawl spaces, basements); drains; dirty filters; indoor storage of firewood; damp and dirty surfaces; house dust (e.g., furnishings, mattresses, carpets, ducts, exposed surfaces); pollen (e.g., indoor plants, nearby outdoor plants); pets.

Solutions: Reduce humidity level in house with dehumidifier or air conditioners; ventilate to prevent moisture buildup in kitchens, bathrooms, basements, and attics; minimize the use of humidifiers and clean them regularly, keep drain pans clean; repair household leaks and remove rotting, damp, or water-damaged materials; clean regularly and vacuum, preferably with a central vacuum system vented outdoors; avoid dust-accumulating furnishings (e.g., upholstered furniture, drapes, carpets); use allergen-proof mattress encasements; use electrostatic or high-efficiency filters in air-handling units, and clean or replace them frequently; cover soil on potted plants and do not overwater them; confine pets to one area of the house or eliminate them entirely.

Chemical Contaminants

Substance: Combustion gases and respirable particles (carbon monoxide and nitrogen dioxide).

Health Effects: Carbon monoxide—in low concentrations: fatigue in healthy people and chest pains in people with heart disease; at higher concentrations: impaired vision and coordination, headaches, dizziness, confusion, nausea, flulike symptoms; at very high concentrations: fatal. Nitrogen dioxide—eye, nose, and throat irritation, potential impaired lung function, and increased respiratory infections in young children. Respirable particles same as nitrogen dioxide with the addition of bronchitis and lung cancer.

Sources: Unvented kerosene or gas stoves, and heaters, woodstoves, fireplaces, leaking or backdrafting chimneys and furnaces, automobile exhaust, tobacco smoke.

Solutions: Vent furnaces, gas stoves, and space heaters to outdoors; replace gas devices with electric devices; select properly sized woodstoves with tightly fitting doors that are certified to meet EPA emission standards; have trained professionals inspect, clean, and tune up central heating system annually; do not idle car in the garage; do not smoke in the home or, if smoking cannot be avoided, increase ventilation where smoking takes place and use exhaust fans.

Substance: Pesticides, insecticides, termicides, fungicides, rodenticides, and disinfectants.

Health Effects: Irritation to eyes, nose, and throat; damage to central nervous system and kidneys; increased risk of cancer.

Sources: Pesticide use, pesticide residue in homes from previous pesticide use, products on lawns and gardens that drift or are tracked inside, mothballs, stored pesticide containers, household surfaces that collect and then release pesticides.

Solutions: Use alternative pest control methods; do not store pesticide containers inside the home; store clothes with moth repellent in separate ventilated areas; use pesticides only when absolutely necessary and with care.

Substance: Organic gases (volatile organic compounds, or VOCs) and formaldehyde.

Health Effects: Eye, nose, and throat irritation; headaches; loss of coordination; nausea; damage to liver, kidney, central nervous system; cancer or suspected cancer; skin rashes; severe allergic reactions; fatigue; wheezing and coughing.

Sources: Paint, paint strippers, varnishes, furniture oils, caulkings, glues, adhesives, wood preservatives, aerosol sprays, cleaners and disinfectants, moth repellents, air fresheners, stored fuel and automotive products, dry-cleaned clothing, hobby supplies, drywall compound, soft plastics, pressed wood products, urea-formaldehyde foam insulation, permanent press fabrics in clothes, furnishings, furniture, and draperies, carpets and underpads, wall coverings or floor coverings made of vinyl, plastic, or other synthetics, upholstered furniture containing synthetic foam, personal care products (perfumes, cosmetics, and toiletries).

Solutions: Substitute unscented, nontoxic products; avoid cleaning agents containing chlorine and other organic solvents; store supplies outside or in closet equipped with exhaust fan; use low-toxicity, low-odor paints, varnishes, oils, caulkings, and other building materials; air out dry-cleaned clothes; do not use room deodorizers, mothballs, or fabric softeners; replace pressed wood products with low-toxicity products or seal pressed wood products with appropriate sealers; increase ventilation to one air change every three hours and maintain moderate temperature and humidity so as to discourage the release of formaldehyde; use low-toxicity, natural, nondyed, nonfireproofed, nonmothproofed, nonallergenic furnishings and materials. (*All natural* does not necessarily mean nonallergenic.) Controversy exists over the use of plants as significant absorbers of formaldehyde and other gases (natural air cleaners); do not rely on them exclusively.

Substance: Lead.
Health Effects: Affects practically all body systems; can cause convulsions, coma, and death at high levels; at low levels, it can have health effects on the central nervous system, kidneys, and blood cells. It can also impair mental and physical development.
Sources: Lead-based paint, contaminated soil or dust, lead-based water pipes, lead-based dinnerware.
Solutions: Do not disturb lead-based paint in good condition; do not sand or burn lead-painted surfaces; seek expert help in removing lead paint; do not bring lead dust into the home; have house water pipes tested for lead contamination; test dinnerware for lead contamination.

Substance: Asbestos.
Health Effects: Long-term risk of chest or abdominal cancers and lung diseases. Smokers have increased risk.
Sources: Deteriorating, damaged, or disturbed insulation, fireproofing, acoustical materials, and floor tiles.
Solutions: Leave undamaged asbestos materials alone. If material is damaged, consult expert asbestos removal contractors.

Substance: Radon.
Health Effects: Lung cancer. Smokers are at higher risk.
Sources: Earth and rock beneath the home may produce gas that seeps in through openings in the foundations; well water in radon area; radon-laden building materials.
Solutions: Have home tested for radon exposure.

Once a thorough evaluation of your home has been made and the sources have been identified, you need to develop a plan of action. It is important to identify the true source so that money is not spent needlessly fixing something that is not the major problem. The basic strategies of any action plan are:

1. Eliminate the source whenever possible.
2. Separate the source from the rest of the house if you can't eliminate it. This is done by sealing in the source or by air-sealing the house to prevent the entry of the outdoor contaminants or by creating one safe, clean oasis within the house.
3. Ventilate to evacuate pollutants and bring in fresh, clean air (filters may be needed depending on the quality of outside air). Ventilation does not replace the elimina-

tion of the offending sources, but it is necessary to provide clean air at an affordable cost. This applies to both newer, tightly sealed houses and older homes.

The action plan can be phased in over a period of time (start with the least costly and more effective solutions first) or done all at once, depending on the needs of the individuals and the resources available. It may involve minor renovations or modifications, major alterations, or even relocation to another home or the construction of a new custom home.

In conclusion, there are many factors in our environment that are difficult to control, but the elimination of pollutants in our home is not one of them. This is something we can choose to do something about, assuming we have the knowledge to make informed choices. CMHC reminds us that, regardless of our health needs, clean indoor air can provide the basis for a nurturing environment. It can improve the quality of our health and our sense of well-being. It is therefore deserving of our attention and our resources.

Bibliography
1. Breecher, Maury M., and Shirley Linde. *Healthy Homes in a Toxic World*. New York: John Wiley and Sons, 1992.
2. "The Clean Air Guide, CMHC," CMHC NHA 6695 (1993).
3. CMHC, "Healthy Housing: A Guide to a Sustainable Future," CMHC NHA 6725 (1993).
4. EPA and CPSC, "The Inside Story: A Guide to Indoor Air Quality," EPA 402-k-93-007 (September 1993).
5. "Housing for the Environmentally Hypersensitive," prepared for CMHC Research Division, CMHC PE 0090 (July 1990).
6. Leclair, Kim, and David Rosseau. *Environmental by Design*. Washington (USA) and British Columbia (Canada): Hartley and Marks, 1992.
7. Pearson, David. *The Natural House Book*. New York: Simon and Schuster, 1989.

Other Resources
EPA and CMHC have a number of other publications available. Local offices can provide information.
Rosseau, David, W. J. Rea, and Jean Enwright. *Your Home, Your Health and Well-Being*. Berkeley: Ten Speed Press, 1988.
Bower, John. *Healthy House*. New York: Carol Communications, 1989.
Ashford, N., and C. Miller. *Chemical Exposures: Low Levels and High Stakes*. New York: Van Nostrand Reinhold, 1991.
Dadd, Debra Lynn. *Non-Toxic, Natural and Earthwise*. Los Angeles: Jeremy P. Tarcher Inc., 1990.
Venolia, Carol. *Healing Environments*. Berkeley: Celestial Arts, 1988.

Newsletters
Environmental Building News, RR 1 Box 161, Brattleboro, VT 05301.
Environmental Resource Guide, American Institute of Architects, 9 Jay Gould Court, PO Box 753, Waldorf, MD 20604.
The Environmental Review, Citizens for a Better Environment, 647 W. Virginia St., #305, Milwaukee, WI 53204.

Directories

Home Grown Green, Richard Kimbell, 105 Franklin, Roseville, CA 95678.

Chemical Injury Information Network, Cynthia Wilson, (406) 547-2255, PO Box 301, White Sulphur Springs, MT 59645.

National Green Pages, Co-op America, 1850 M Street NW, Suite 700, Washington DC 20036.

Tackling Toxics in Everyday Products: A Directory of Organizations, by Nancy Lilienthal, Michele Ascione, Adam Flint. Inform Inc., 381 Park Ave. So., New York, NY 10016-8806.

Environmental Health and Toxicology: A Selected Bibliography of Printed Information Sources, U.S. Department of Health and Human Services, Centers for Disease Control, National Center for Environmental Health, Information Resources Management Group, Atlanta, GA 30333.

■ *Lyse M. Tremblay, Longueuil, Québec, is a consulting architect (architectural and M.B.A. degrees from McGill University) specializing in healthy buildings. She has served on town planning committees, written articles for health magazines and healthy building publications, and spoken on the subject to self-help groups and on television. Having endo, asthma, and multiple allergies herself, she has personal experience with problem buildings.*

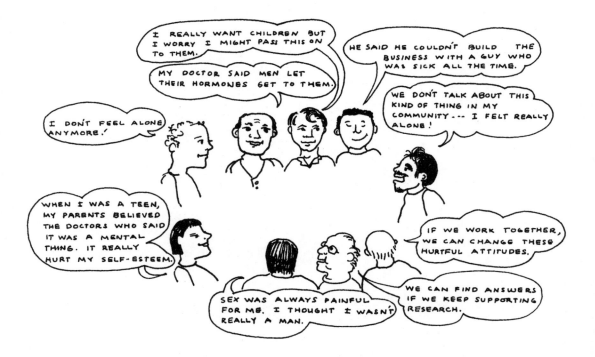

16

◉◉

The Puzzle of Endometriosis

By Mary Lou Ballweg

Endometriosis remains an enigma to the practicing gynecologist.[1]

Endometriosis provides a unique clinical and scientific challenge.[2]

The literature on endometriosis is extensive, but often inadequate or contradictory.[3]

. . . a riddle wrapped in a mystery inside an enigma.[4]

Most people enjoy a puzzle—be it a jigsaw puzzle, a three-dimensional maze, a magician's sleight of hand, a Rubik's Cube, a mystery or detective novel or movie—as a pastime. Real-life puzzles are not so much fun. No one tells us the answer at the end. People living with the puzzle have no easy way to explain for themselves and everyone around them what is happening to them. And if we must interact professionally with people afflicted by an illness that is a puzzle, the puzzle can deprive us of meeting some basic human needs—to be successful, to understand the things around us, to be able to help those who come to us for help, to be able to make a difference.

Endometriosis has certainly earned a reputation as perhaps the most puzzling entity in gynecology. And with an estimated 5.5 million women in the United States and Canada with the disease and probably millions more worldwide, there is an overwhelming need to solve the puzzle. Not that people have not been trying. In the past quarter century more than 5,000 articles have been published on endometriosis (although scientific rigor has been applied only recently according to one authority).[5]

With so much energy going into this endeavor, why do we seem only a little closer to solving the puzzle of this disease? Just as with other puzzles in our lives, it may be useful to step back, reframe the problem, question assumptions and premises, and ask new questions. Answers could be staring us right in the face.

Endometriosis may resemble those trick pictures in which you can see two pictures, but once you visualize one it is difficult to see the other until you force yourself not to see the first picture. You have to create a blank slate in your mind. If we view endometriosis only as a gynecologic disease tied to endometrial implants, we may miss other, even obvious, ways of seeing the disease.

Just What Is Endometriosis? Oh, sure, it's endometrial implants that somehow appear in ectopic locations. But is it? The fact that endometrial implants can be found in more than 40 percent of women; that symptoms may or may not be associated with these implants; that extent of implants does not correlate with symptoms; that removal or atrophy of the implants does not necessarily improve symptoms or cure the disease; that the classification schemes, tied to extent of implants, tell us little about symptoms or prognosis; that some women undergo repeated laparoscopies for symptoms that any experienced clinician would wager are endometriosis and no implants are found (later laparoscopies sometimes find implants, sometimes not)—all lead to the conclusion that implants may not be the quintessential element, the sine qua non, of the disease.[6–14]

A consortium of European leaders on endometriosis has already defined the disease as more than the mere presence of implants. "Endometriosis is a disease affecting many women during their reproductive life. However, the mere presence of what is defined as endometriosis histologically cannot be equated per se to the presence of a disease. Endometriosis as a disease should be defined as 'the presence of ectopic endometrium, in association with evidence of cellular activity in the lesions and of progression, such as the formation of adhesions, or by its interference with normal physiological processes.'"[15]

While lauding the excellent scientific work being done at the cellular level to determine the activity of the implant and its similarities to and differences from endometrium, it seems time also to look beyond the endometrial implant. If the puzzle of endometriosis is a systemic immunological, biochemical, or metabolic one, implants could come to be seen as peripheral to the root of the problem, as sequelae that perhaps must be treated in addition to addressing the underlying disorder.

To continue to equate endometriosis strictly and solely with implants could lead to erroneous conclusions. Some researchers already are concluding that since so many women can be found to have ectopic endometrial tissue endometriosis is not a disease or that endometriosis (defined as implants) does not cause pain, that women with implants and pain have psychological reasons for their pain since other women with implants have no pain.[16–19] Others, while agreeing that endometriosis causes pain, suggest that pain that continues after thorough surgery (directed at implants) must be from something other than endometriosis.[20] All are blocks in our thinking based on defining endometriosis as implants when all evidence suggests something more is involved. Continuing to equate endometriosis strictly with implants could also mean we harness ourselves to treatments that might be directed only at the tip of the iceberg.

No doubt looking beyond the implant is hard—after all, the definition of endometriosis as ectopic endometrium has been taught since the 1920s. It's human nature to hang on

Table 1. Symptomatology Of Endometriosis
(From EA Research Registry)

From 3,020 case histories from the Endometriosis Association Research Registry. Registry is composed of medical histories (500+ variables) from patients from all states and provinces.

	Number	*Percent of Total*
Dysmenorrhea and/or pain throughout the menstrual cycle	2,904	96.2
Dyspareunia (Painful sexual intercourse)	1,801	59.6
Infertility	1,340	44.4
Heavy or irregular bleeding	1,971	65.3
Nausea, stomach upset at time of menses	1,744	57.7
Diarrhea, painful bowel movements, or other intestinal upsets w/menses	2,385	79.0
Dizziness, headaches w/menses or pain	1,782	59.0
Fatigue, exhaustion, low energy	2,478	82.1
Low-grade fever	889	29.4
Low resistance to infection	1,182	39.1
No symptoms	80	2.6

Note: 45% detailed other symptoms, including muscular aches and emotional fluctuations (10.2%).

tenaciously to what we think we "know." But in a case like endometriosis, where so little is really known, it's dangerous to hang on to old ideas to the exclusion of new. We dare not laugh at new ideas, though at first glance they may seem outlandish, because we truly do not know where the answers will come from. Remember the lessons of the past—in the Middle Ages, for instance, it was outright heresy to suggest that there might be any cause for disease other than God's will. And later, when Louis Pasteur proposed that "invisible enemies" might be causing disease, he was considered crazy. After discovering the bacteria that cause several diseases and also the method of vaccinating with inoculations to protect against these diseases, he became a hero. But before that the doctors of his time would not listen to him since he was not a physician and because his ideas were so revolutionary.[21]

Beyond Implants: What Is Endometriosis Associated with Besides Implants? What Else Does This Disease Do? So, if we need to look beyond the implant, where do we look next? As with all puzzles, we may need to go back to the source—the disease itself, which all can agree lies somewhere in the patient. If we look at patients closely, listen to them carefully, listen without shutting out symptoms that do not fit our preconceptions, we will find we hear over and over again systemic complaints, complaints that go far beyond the pelvis.

The Endometriosis Association Research Registry, housed at the Medical College of Wisconsin, consists of over 3,000 case histories of women with confirmed endometriosis. The registry was begun in 1980 by the women who started the Endometriosis Association to help answer, scientifically, the many questions we had about the disease. Common symptoms reported by women in the registry include "fatigue, exhaustion, low energy" experienced by 82 percent; bowel problems by 79 percent; and a wide range of bodywide symptoms such as muscular aches. A smaller group also report low resistance to infections (39 percent) and low-grade fever (29 percent).[22]

In a selected group of these women, those with family histories of endometriosis, we also find a propensity to atopic diseases, including allergies, eczema, and asthma.[23–25] There is also a tendency to infections, and sometimes sore throats, and problems with fungal infections, especially those caused by *Candida albicans*.[26] These symptoms, repeated in the histories of women with endometriosis that pour into headquarters and the more-than-150 chapters and support groups of the Endometriosis Association, point to particular types of immune problems. *Candida albicans*, for example, is kept in check by cell-mediated immunity, which has been speculated to be faulty in women with endometriosis. These symptoms, including the nongynecological ones, may offer important clues to the nature of endometriosis.

Dysmenorrhea is the single most frequent symptom reported by women with endometriosis. Over 96 percent of the women in the association registry report it.[22, 27] In addition, primary dysmenorrhea seems to precede (or occur simultaneously with) endometriosis in the majority of cases.

Physicians must ask patients about dysmenorrhea since so many believe menstrual pain and menses-associated problems are normal and do not report it. At the Endometriosis Association we often hear a woman say she first developed symptoms of endometriosis at such-and-such an age—when questioned about cramps and illness with her period, or bowel problems with her period, or pain with or after sex, she will often say she just has the "usual cramps and things everyone gets."

Granted, many women do experience primary dysmenorrhea in the modern world—however, that does not mean it is normal or healthy or has always been the case. There may be factors in our modern world—environmental, dietary, or others—causing these problems. The Endometriosis Association's recent work with a dioxin-induced endometriosis animal model has brought to light the powerful impact of pollutants on hormones, for example.[28, 29]

Despite being the most frequent and usually the earliest symptom reported in endometriosis, dysmenorrhea has not been studied much, although one multicenter study found primary dysmenorrhea to be a risk factor for endometriosis.[30] Clearly, studies delin-

Table 2. Does Anyone Else Among Your Blood Relatives Have Endometriosis? (From EA Research Registry)

	Number	Percent
Yes	671	25.6
No	1,597	60.9
Don't know	353	13.5
Total	2,621	100.0

Missing data = 34 (1.3%)

Table 3. Do You Have Other Health Problems in Addition to Endometriosis?

	Number	Percent
Yes	1,360	56.9
No	1,032	43.1
Total	2,392	100.0

Missing data = 263 (9.9%)

Table 4. A Comparison of Medical Histories of Women with Demonstrable Endometriosis and Their Control Group[25]

	% Cases	% Controls
Food intolerances	31.8	18.2
Hay fever	36.4	21.6
Nonspecific yeast infections	52.3	29.5

eating the relationship of primary dysmenorrhea to endometriosis are needed. Where does one end and the other begin, or are they on a continuum? What is the natural course of primary dysmenorrhea? Why does primary dysmenorrhea occur in families as does endometriosis? What is the relation of this symptom and others seen in endometriosis (such as allergies) that may also be related to prostaglandin synthesis and fatty acid metabolism?

Table 5. Pain Profile Relative to Menstrual Cycle and Patients' Characterization of Severity Levels (From EA Research Registry)

	Number	Percent
No pain relative to menses	80	2.7
At time of menses only	384	12.9
At ovulation only	39	1.3
Throughout the menstrual cycle	2,481	83.1
Total	2,984	100.0
Missing data = 36 (1.2%)		
Mild	92	3.2
Mild to moderate	234	8.1
Moderate	310	10.8
Moderate to severe	1,145	39.7
Severe	546	18.9
Varies, mild to severe	558	19.3
Total	2,885	100.0
No pain = 78 (2.7%) No response = 57 (1.9%)		

Physicians have paid more attention to some symptoms associated with endometriosis than others; strangely, the symptoms they attend to most are not the most prevalent ones. In an Australian study, for example, women who reported period pain, heavy bleeding, back pain, and bowel pain had longer diagnosis delays than those who did not report these symptoms. Women who reported period pain, the most common symptom of endometriosis, had a diagnosis delay of 4.9 years compared to 2.3 years for those who did not report period pain.[31]

Moreover, the symptoms girls and women often find most disruptive to their lives are sometimes not the ones physicians address. Patients tend to think in terms of the impact of the symptoms on their lives—some symptoms may not even matter to them, while others may be destroying their self-image, their relationships with family or a sexual partner, or their ability to work or study. The teenager with life-disruptive dysmenorrhea and her family may care much more about that symptom than her future fertility but find that her

Table 6. Have You Ever Been Unable to Carry Out Your Normal Work and Activities?

	Number	Percent
Yes	2,241	74.8
No	755	25.2
Total	2,996	100.0

Missing data = 24 (0.8%)

physician, while concerned about her future fertility, considers the pain not worth follow-up investigation. (If we were diagnosing and treating the 15-year-old with endometriosis and incapacitating pain, perhaps she might not be infertile at 25!)

Pain is the most commonly reported symptom, yet one recent textbook on endometriosis does not even have an index heading for pain.[32] As a British physician recently noted: ". . . there is a definite gulf between the patient and the gynaecologist. The patient actually goes to see the doctor because she has got something that is seriously interfering with her life, which is pain. The gynaecologist, however, is more interested in what is causing the pain and not so much in the interference with her life. If he does not find what is causing the pain he tends to give up at that point, and that produces intense resentment on the patient's part, who after all is not interested particularly in endometriosis—she just wants her pain dealt with. I think pain is poorly taught at medical school, with the result that the histories taken by doctors do not cover the detailed components of pain that may actually lead to a much greater understanding not only of the cause, but of how to relieve it."[33]

Looking at the timing of symptom onset might also help us unravel the puzzle of endometriosis. For instance, over 40 percent of women in our registry, 42 percent in an Australian Endometriosis Association study, and 35 percent in a British Endometriosis Society study report experiencing their first symptoms of endometriosis by age 19. But only 2 to 6 percent were diagnosed before age 20; also, 83, 79, and 71 percent, respectively, reported their first symptoms before age 30, but only 52 to 56 percent were diagnosed before age 30.[31, 34] Because of the delay between onset and diagnosis, many clues may be lost by the time diagnosis occurs. Clearly, if we are to solve the puzzle of endometriosis, we will have to try tracking the clues while they are still warm (if not hot). We may even need to look at youngsters before puberty. In families with endometriosis it is common to hear the same stories over and over of allergies, asthma, low resistance to infections, and problems with *Candida albicans* long before puberty.

**Table 7. Age Endometriosis Symptoms First Presented
(From EA Research Registry)**

	Number	Percent
Under 15 years of age	431	14.9
Age 15–19	746	25.7
Age 20–24	567	19.6
Age 25–29	675	23.3
Age 30–34	363	12.5
Age 35–39	117	4.0
Total	2,899	100.0

No symptoms = 56 (1.9%)
No response = 65 (2.2%)

What about infertility? In our registry 44 percent of the women report infertility. The history of medical interest in endometriosis in recent decades is that infertility specialists were the first to be concerned about the disease. But the relationship between endometriosis and infertility has been questioned widely in recent years.[35] In our registry the patients who report no symptoms (3 percent) invariably are infertility patients.[22]

Selection bias may be inflating the significance that infertility has in endometriosis, since infertility patients are far more likely to be investigated for endometriosis.[36] This selection bias also means that we may be closing our eyes to other symptoms that may offer important clues to the nature of the disease. Women with endometriosis who have bladder symptoms, for instance, are sometimes told they have urinary tract infections or receive a diagnosis of interstitial cystitis.[37] Women with endometriosis with bowel symptoms are sometimes "diagnosed" with irritable bowel syndrome or spastic colon.[38]

Other Health Problems of Women with Endometriosis. The full range of frequently reported health problems in women with endometriosis provides valuable clues. But too often, as specialists, there is a tendency to look only at the pelvic symptoms or at those traditionally associated with endometriosis. The reported association with lupus; atopic diseases; thyroid disease, especially Hashimoto's thyroiditis (an autoimmune disease); mitral valve prolapse; problems with *Candida albicans*; and a susceptibility to chronic fatigue immune dysfunction syndrome (CFIDS) or fibromyalgia are clues that much more is going on, at least in the most problematic form of endometriosis.[25, 39–44] The Endometriosis Association and the nonprofit groups serving those with related problems (including CFIDS, fibromyalgia, interstitial cystitis, and candidiasis) have noted the overlapping nature of these problems. (A report appearing in the association newsletter on fibromyalgia, following the observation by a member that so many of the women in the Fibromyalgia Network with confirmed fibromyalgia had a history of endometriosis, resulted in more than 600 letters from association members to the network, for example.)

The following letters, samples from the hundreds of thousands the Endometriosis Association has received, show the difficulties encountered because of the currently fragmented way of looking at the disease and provide examples of the related health problems noted in our research registry.

Dear Endo Assoc.

I have undergone three laparoscopies in 10 months (each with a new doctor familiar with previous treatment) due to extensive endo. In each case I was gripped with pain to a point of having to have surgery.

I also was very put off by my struggle with feeling so ill only to have gynecologists dissuade me from believing there was an underlying problem in need of further investigation. Finally, after a third surgery and Lupron treatment for severe endo . . . as well as a negative colonoscopy (due to my irritable bowel concerns), done by an internist who allowed the gynecologist's diagnosis to completely dictate his evaluation, I broke through to an internist specializing in rheumatic diseases. Prior to any lab work, I fit into a description of fibromyalgia. After specialized blood work . . . I have been diagnosed with systemic lupus erythematosus (SLE).

Ablating endo implants is, in my case, a frustrating experience in treating the tip of the iceberg. One specialty doesn't know or want to know about the other, and the patient becomes a victim of a medical evaluation system that has more blind spots than truly exist. All the answers are not in, but better and extensive evaluation may do a patient more justice. You can bet I have the last paragraph of p. 205 highlighted in my book [Overcoming Endometriosis].[45] What if endometriosis is a symptom of immune system problems rather than a disease itself? How do we educate the medical profession to evaluate the whole patient? . . .

Deborah, California

Dear Mrs. Ballweg:

Over the past five years I have been diagnosed with fibromyalgia, chronic fatigue immunodeficiency syndrome, mitral valve prolapse, candidiasis, and endometriosis . . . The latest diagnosis of fibromyalgia came from an autoimmune and connective tissue specialist at the Mayo Clinic in Jacksonville, Florida. . . .

While my overall health has improved greatly from the above treatments [for the various conditions] in terms of a reduction of abdominal pain, extreme fatigue, vaginal itching, low-grade fevers, joint and muscle pain, etc., I am still unable to locate a physician who will assist me in pulling each of the diagnosed illnesses together and work with me in treating them collectively. Based on my own experiences and research, I am confident that the illnesses and symptoms are all related, but I am very frustrated by the lack of interest and knowledge each doctor exhibits in regard to my entire medical history. Each doctor who has helped me wants to concentrate on only one aspect of my symptoms (his own area of expertise), and as a result I feel treatment and improvement are limited. . . .

Margaret, Florida

Dear Mary Lou:

The article in the newsletter on fibromyalgia sounded hauntingly familiar. For the past six months I have taken between 1,400 and 2,400 milligrams of ibuprofen per day to keep symptoms similar to what was described under control. The fatigue I have felt the past two years has been overwhelming, but I kept telling myself it was "all in my head. . . ." I finally got the courage to go back to my gynecologist for a physical. . . . I expected him to say, "Everything is fine; come back in a year." But he ended up biopsying a vaginal lesion he thought was endometriosis. The pathology report stated "chronic inflammation." As I reviewed my pathology report from my hysterectomy, a frequently used term was chronic inflammation. It seemed to describe everything they removed. . . .

I was sent back to my family practice doctor for possible lupus or arthritis testing. Some of the other symptoms I frequently experience are aching joints, low-grade fever, general achiness, and sensations of numbness in fingers, toes, and lips. A blood count showed signs of—you guessed it—"chronic inflammation." I started thinking of myself as a walking "chronic inflammation." No wonder my body was so tired all the time—it was chronically inflamed. I pictured little white cells constantly coursing through my system looking for something to attack and, finding nothing, attacking those very cells they were supposed to protect. Needless to say, my allergies have been almost overwhelming over the past few years, and I have frequently been on Hismanal to control sinus problems as well as rashes. . . .

The changes I experienced on the ibuprofen have been dramatic. For the first time in years I feel alive again. I have energy to do things I haven't done for years. I have discontinued the Hismanal, except for a few weeks of hay fever in the summer. I have decreased my estrogen (Ogen) replacement therapy by half. . . .

Susan, Utah

Dear Madam,

On vacation I returned to my parents' home in London, England, where, despite having just had a laparoscopy, which had diagnosed and cauterized my mild endo, I continued to have severe stomach pains, feelings of cystitis and yeast infection, and constant exhaustion—the symptoms that had, finally, led to the laparoscopy. After seeing my local general practitioner and being told that it was an "unspecific virus" that was troubling me (since all tests were negative), I finally found help. . . .

The help came, first, from a doctor I was referred to for back trouble who said that he thought that I might have food allergies . . . he referred me to an allergy doctor, who decided that I had acute candidiasis and food allergies (for which I'm still being tested). After only three days on the diet many of my symptoms improved, and by the end of the week I felt, for the first time in several years, alive, free of pain of all sorts, and full of energy.

It's amazing: the past year has been an enormous struggle to get control over endless cystitis and yeast infections and to get help for the dreadful stomach pains I had for most of my menstrual cycle (they became unbearable one week before and during my period), for the back pains, the migraines, and the sudden fevers. . . .

As it is, the year has been a living nightmare, a constant battle simply to get through each day awake and not give in to the fury, depression, and helplessness provoked by the doctors as much as by my symptoms. . . .

On my mother's side of the family (my grandmother, my mother's twin) there is a history of severe allergies, and my sisters and I used to have allergic reactions to bubble bath, petrol, etc., when we were small (swollen faces, rashes, nausea). . . .

Anabelle, Massachusetts

To Endometriosis Association

I am a DES daughter. My mom died at the age of 37 of ovarian cancer. I have been treated for a yeast infection since I was eight years old. Many doctors would even accuse me of poor hygiene as to why I suffered from this recurring problem. I had painful periods, but my stepmother told me that was normal. At the age of 20 I suffered with a virus that the doctors never could explain. They thought I had mononucleosis, but the test was negative. I was married and became pregnant and had a healthy baby boy. At age 29 I was found to have Hashimoto's disease. I had a large tumor on my thyroid gland. . . .

At age 30 I developed a soreness around my upper abdomen. The doctor told me it was probably a pulled muscle. Then I had a severe attack of pain, diarrhea, and fever, and they rushed me to the hospital thinking it was my appendix. It wasn't. For the next six months I was sent from doctor to doctor thinking it was Crohn's disease. I lost 20 pounds and felt miserable. . . . I have pain constantly in my upper abdomen, fatigue, slight fever at times, and twice a month I lie in bed for two or three days in severe pain. The pain in my back has become so severe that I am unable to walk.

Just yesterday I went to a gynecologist at B. Hospital in New York. He seemed puzzled by my medical history and didn't offer any help. He said either I take the pill or have a hysterectomy, as I am high risk for ovarian cancer. Recently they did find an ovarian cyst, but he told me it was nothing to worry about. I left his office in tears from frustration, but also the exam was so painful. . . .

If only you knew what joy it brought me to read your book and newsletters. I have felt so very, very alone with all of this. People close to me don't understand the pain and also feel endo is not a "big deal." . . . I am on welfare now, as I have been unable to work. . . .

I have been disabled with this for the past two years, and I'd like very much to find a way to become functional again. . . .

Lisa, New York

Gaps in Other Fields Affect Our Understanding of Endometriosis. The gaps in other fields also converge on endometriosis to create more holes in our knowledge. For instance, endometriosis is a disease that clearly involves the female hormones and also appears to involve the immune system. But the interlinking of hormones and the immune system is still a big mystery. As long ago as 1985, *Science* magazine published an article on the interactions between the gonadal steroids and the immune system, but the precise nature of this link is still a puzzle.[46, 47]

The finding that certain pollutants can cause endometriosis in rhesus monkeys may help us understand this link.[28, 29, 48–53] The toxicology literature is filled with examples of how pollutants such as dioxin appear to act as hormones in the body and at the same time disturb immune response. There are at least 23 chemical families of pollutants, like dioxins and PCBs, that have known ability to disrupt the endocrine system, according to a consensus statement issued by scientists gathered at a conference, "Endocrine Disrupters in the Environment," held July 1991.[53]

Another example of how gaps in other fields impinge on our ability to understand endometriosis is the lack of understanding of how immune abnormalities, particularly subtle ones, relate to clinical problems. The first report on the dioxin-induced endometriosis monkey colony indicated that despite altered T cell ratios there was no clinical evidence of immune deficit in the monkeys.[54] Endometriosis had not yet been found in the monkeys—two were to die over the next few years, and two others were experiencing pain with their menses, and it was difficult for these researchers in immunology to understand the implications of the alterations they found. But the conclusion that there was no clinical evidence of immune deficit, despite their failure to look for such evidence, is the kind of statement that contributes to confusion. Similar statements have been made about women with endometriosis.[55]

Why So Many Myths and Misconceptions? Medical mysteries are not the only puzzles about endometriosis. There are also sociological ones (which have contributed to keeping endometriosis a medical mystery). One member of the Endometriosis Association recently wrote that her physician said endometriosis is a disease of "overeducated women who wait too long to get pregnant," that she was "too educated for her own good," and that "you don't see Miss [Hispanic name], the 15-year-old migrant field worker, having any problems getting pregnant." Her physician's comments are a perfect example of the way

Table 8. What Would You Have Liked to Have in Making Treatment Choices? (From the EA Research Registry)

	Number	Percent
More information	539	35.8
Someone to talk over options	63	4.2
Both of above	174	11.5
To talk to others with similar symptoms	106	7.0
Honesty from doctor, more information, someone to talk over options	143	9.5
Better and earlier medical attention	91	6.0
Other needs	392	26.0
Total	1,508	100.0

Note: Although about half expressed no difficulty in making treatment choices, fully 61 percent (519) needed more than they received in the medical encounter.

myths work—drawing on common biases and prejudices in society to explain puzzles society has not yet resolved.

It appears to be human nature to make up answers when none are forthcoming because it so frustrates us not to have answers. This occurs particularly in the area of taboo subjects, such as the symptoms of endometriosis. The myths take on a life of their own because they pick up the nonconscious ideologies at the heart of society—the unspoken things that everyone just "knows" and does not question. When the nonconscious becomes conscious, spoken, discussed, investigated, true science and change can take place.

We like to believe that medical science is beyond myth and taboo, especially as we approach the 21st century, but just as often deeply seated taboo or myth colors science. An example of how mythmaking and taboos taint science is the story behind the myth that black women do not get endometriosis. A leading gynecologist, involved internationally in training gynecologists, confided to me soon after we began the Endometriosis Association in 1980 that gynecologists would almost automatically diagnose a black woman with symptoms of endometriosis as having pelvic inflammatory disease. The underlying reason was an assumption that black women were sexually promiscuous, a contributing factor in contracting PID. Statistical analyses then showed that black women had a lot of PID but not endometriosis, further perpetuating the myth that black women did not get endometriosis but did get PID. Except that the numbers, now in the guise of science and separated from their human element, could not so easily be accused of racism! And the numbers, based on racism, reinforced the scientific "truth" that black women did not get endometriosis.

Myths and taboos also make it harder for the physician to do his or her job. Because of the myths and taboos, women and girls are reluctant to share all of their symptoms with the physician, or they delay seeking help. Because they are not sharing a complete picture of their symptoms with their physicians, they make it harder for the physicians to diagnose endometriosis. (Physicians can help patients know they are approachable on endometriosis symptoms by displaying pamphlets, videotapes, and other patient education items in their waiting rooms.)

But why have physicians themselves perpetuated misconceptions about the disease, especially the one that symptoms, particularly dysmenorrhea and pain with sex, are in a woman's head? A study at one endometriosis center found that although women complained of classic symptoms of endometriosis, physicians and other caregivers tended to diagnose their complaints as normal menstrual events. The majority of the women were led to believe they were overreacting to the pain and their symptoms were psychological in origin.[56, 57]

Few of us today really believe endometriosis is an imaginary disease, but somehow unconscious taboos and subtle training that teach that women are not reliable reporters about their bodies take over in actual encounters with patients.[58] Remember that well-known study in which women and men presented with the same symptoms and the men were referred for medical work-up and the women, in much greater proportion, were referred for psychological counseling?[59]

We have all had the experience of thinking we understand something—say divorce or heart attack or the loss of a loved one—but when we went through it ourselves realized we really had not. Add to this natural experience the fact that men do not have the organs and cycle that women do, even without a perplexing disease to complicate the picture, and that it is easier to think a girl or woman is exaggerating or that a problem does not exist than to constantly remember that she is describing something men cannot easily relate to unless they are very empathetic and willing to put themselves in another's shoes. Male conditioning teaches boys and men *not* to put themselves in female shoes, unfortunately.

This tendency of human nature to define reality as one's own reality, as well as the tendency to disbelieve the experience of women's reality, especially when it comes to reporting pain and problems with their reproductive organs, has tended to distort care. For example, the whole category of mental disorders called *somatization disorders,* affecting primarily women according to the psychiatric literature, is based on physical symptoms of primarily female disorders (the differential diagnoses include lupus and multiple sclerosis, and should include endometriosis). Why are we not surprised to find obvious symptoms of endometriosis on the list of diagnostic criteria for somatization disorder?!

Obviously it is a disgrace that such clear symptoms of endometriosis are listed as a "mental" disorder, and we call on endometriosis specialists to work to have this changed. The following letter shows some of the distortions in care (and unnecessary costs to the medical system) that result from the myths and taboos surrounding endometriosis.

> *To whom it may concern:*
>
> *I am 28 years old, married for eight years with no children. . . . My story is typical. I've been sick with stomach problems for 12 years, but my doctor kept telling me that there's nothing physically wrong with me. She sent me for all kinds of tests and specialists, but everything came back negative. I was sent to psychiatrists [who] told me to get a job and stop feeling sorry for myself. They said I was a nervous type of person, which they felt caused my stomach problems. For years I really thought it was all in my head, but that didn't make me feel any better. My family believed the doctors, so I had no one to talk to. . . .*
>
> *My doctor was getting fed up with me going to her and complaining all the time, and she even told me so. After about nine years of feeling sick and crazy, my doctor sent me to a gynecologist.*
>
> Teresa, Ontario

EDITOR'S NOTE: Teresa was diagnosed with endometriosis on her ovaries, appendix, bowel, and cul-de-sac.

As dangerous as the idea that these symptoms are part of a mental disorder if complained about is the idea that they are a normal part of being female. To be female is to suffer?

So, if it seems that endometriosis has gathered numerous myths and misconceptions around it, in part because of the taboo nature of many of its symptoms, the next obvious sociological mystery is why these symptoms are taboo. Even normal menstruation and female sexual issues are taboo, although they are life elements at the very heart of survival of the human race. It is the nature of taboos to be about the subjects most feared or most involved with the power relationships in a society. Certainly sexuality and reproduction are powerful forces. And the exclusively female nature of menstruation and female sexuality have made them easy targets for myth and taboo in a world that for the last several thousand years has been patriarchal. (Many millennia before that appear to have been predominantly matriarchal.)

A number of modern books have delved, some with sociologically and anthropologically careful science, into the mystery of the taboos surrounding menstruation and female sexuality. Physicians who work in gynecology and fertility will find these volumes of great interest and helpful in their work. Worth mentioning are *The Curse: A Cultural History of Menstruation* and *The Woman in the Body: A Cultural Analysis of Reproduction.*[60, 61]

Why Is Endometriosis Not Seen as a Serious Disease? Finally, there is another sociological myth that perhaps contains seeds of answers to the other puzzles and questions we have addressed. That is, why is endometriosis not seen as a serious disease? How can the same disease that is considered "all in their heads" or "just cramps" by some end up in hysterectomy and surgical castration for hundreds of thousands of women?[62] The only answer to such a contradiction is that the disease and women are not taken seriously. Only if women, their bodies, and their life needs are not taken seriously can one so easily dismiss their complaints. And only if it does not matter (in a society in which women are devalued) whether women have their sexual organs can one so simply remove their female organs if the complaints continue. Whereas most men would react violently to the idea of castration, it is so commonplace in this society for women that few even question the great disparity in the number of women who have had their reproductive organs removed versus the number of men. Are our industrialized societies really that much more civilized about this issue than the African countries that so routinely and crudely carry out female genital mutilation?[63]

Of course, several factors complicate the picture of why it might be difficult to see the disease as serious. First, the cyclicity of the symptoms, at least at the beginning, may make it harder to quantify the loss. Second, there's the invisible nature of the illness (although many other invisible illnesses are taken seriously.)[64] Third, women may hide the symptoms because they are taboo or they may feel, with shame, that the symptoms reflect poorly on their femininity. Finally, there is the selection bias mentioned earlier, which means that only certain symptoms have been looked at rather than the whole picture of the disease.

Another indication that female status is the problem is the frequent unwillingness, in the woman and her family or in the physician, to help the girl or woman suffering from endometriosis. The following two letters describe situations in which the girl or woman cannot get a pelvic exam until she is sexually active. What clearer statement could there be that women's bodies, especially their sexual organs, belong to males?! Can anyone imagine an illness in which a boy or man would be expected to live with severe pain in his sexual organs until he was no longer a virgin? The very idea is ludicrous. It is always easier to see the blind spots in a culture other than our own, especially if more exaggerated, so we are including an excerpt from a letter from an Algerian woman that articulates the same issue:

Dear Sir or Madam:

I am a young girl suffering. . . . I attempted many treatments, mostly hormonal treatments based on Duphaston and danazol. All were inefficient, since I am still suffering, and the disease grows more and more serious as I get older.

Just at the very beginning before undertaking any treatment, doctors found big enlarged ovaries full of cysts in the ultrasonographic examination. Concerning my periods. . . . these are very painful and full of big clots. . . .

If I am addressing you, it is just because you are my only hope which keeps me alive. I am seriously ready to serve for any medical test for new treatments. . . . there is the problem of virginity; all doctors refuse to practice a gynecological examination, which is very vital for me, for fear that they would rupture my hymen. . . . *[emphasis added]*

S., Algeria

To whom it may concern,

My name is Lorie. I am married, and I have an eight-year-old son. I'm 24 years old. The baby and the marriage came young, but I wouldn't trade that for the world. It sounds as if I should be content and happy, doesn't it? I would be except for one major problem. I have severe endometriosis.

It all started when I was 10 years old and started menstruating. My "time of the month" was a very excruciating week of pain. The doctor said I just had difficult periods. I would scream for hours, and if I got out of bed I would faint.

At 13 I made love for the first time, so the doctor could now do a pelvic exam *[emphasis added]. I was in his office every month because of my pain. He said I had ovarian cysts, which were normal for a girl that age, and gave me codeine to help with the pain. . . .*

I turned 16 in August, had my baby in September, got married the following June, life was great. Then came my period in November. . . . The pain was every bit as terrible as before, but more so. I went to my gynecologist, and he found a large cyst on my right ovary and said I needed surgery. He removed a softball-size cyst, and I was released four days later. . . . in February I was back in the hospital having a cyst removed from each ovary and part of my right ovary removed.

In March I found out I was pregnant and started feeling great. In the last week of June I began having severe cramps and bleeding. I lost my baby and had a D & C.

In September I switched gynecologists, and after he removed three grapefruit-sized cysts, one from each ovary and one from my intestine, he told me I had endometriosis. I was put on Danocrine but didn't get any better.

In February, I had a hysterectomy and oophorectomy. I was only 17, and I was heartbroken. The doctor said that my problems were over.

I was OK for a while, for about a year and a half. Then the pain was back. I decided to go to a doctor in B., and he did a laparoscopy. I had adhesions, and they were removed. I was put on Premarin. He saw no endometrial lesions. I was constantly in pain, and nothing was being done. I suffered a nervous breakdown three months later.

I suffered with the pain until August 1990. I was in such severe pain I felt I would die. My doctor in B. couldn't see me for six weeks, so I went to a gynecologist here. He did a laparoscopy and found a large cyst on my small intestine. I was sent to a general surgeon who, because I had no money to pay, refused to do the surgery to remove the cyst. I found another surgeon who did emergency surgery and told me I still had endometriosis. . . .

[My doctor] told me that less than 1 in 100 women still have endometriosis after a hysterectomy and I am that less than one.* I was continued on the Premarin and was also put on Provera. Two months ago the pain got worse, and I was back at the doctor. I was told I may have a cyst on the intestine. I am having trouble urinating and was told I possibly have the disease on my bladder and was referred to a urologist. The Premarin and Provera were discontinued pending what he says. I had to wait seven weeks to see him.

I saw the urologist this Monday after several weeks of pain, urinating every half hour, sometimes in my pants, and not sleeping enough to say so. He performed a cystoscopy and said my bladder is capable of holding only 130 cubic centimeters of urine and that amount causes pain. . . . My kidneys are now causing pain, but he didn't do anything yet. . . . I won't go back to him until October 24th, and I don't know if I can take it until then. I'm tired. I hurt. And after 14 years I want some relief.

Through the years I've had lasting and loving support from a lot of friends and my family. I have people who ask how much it takes mentally to deal with this and have been told I'm an extremely strong person. Well, I don't feel strong anymore. I want this over and don't know how. We have no money to pay for all these medical bills and medication and are on the verge of bankruptcy. . . .

In all these years I feel as if I haven't gotten any better or been helped to understand why this is happening to me. I pray every night for my health back. My husband keeps telling me he thinks I'm going to die because he knows they can't keep taking out my organs one at a time. I can't make him understand any differently because I am also confused. I'm too young to live my life like this. I want energy and just a day without pain. I want a doctor who'll understand my fears and who'll help me feel better without waiting months and possibly getting worse in that time. I want to make love to my husband without pain, and I want my sex drive back. I want this to end, and I want a life because this isn't living. This is endometriosis, and it really is hell . . .

Lorie, Vermont

Ultimately, perhaps the last sociological puzzle (why the disease has not been seen as serious) is not so mysterious after all—it is related directly to the status of women in society. The bigger mystery is what it will take to change it. As noted by the authors of *The Curse: A Cultural History of Menstruation,* "It is impossible to escape the conclusion that menstrual politics has dominated social and economic relations between the sexes since the beginning of time."[66]

---

*Hysterectomy and removal of the ovaries have been widely proclaimed as the cure, with little long-term follow-up study. Recently the association conducted one; unfortunately, for about one-third of the patients, hysterectomy and removal of the ovaries did not offer a cure or even relief of symptoms. Forty-four percent of those receiving estrogen replacement therapy experienced a return of symptoms.[65]

But if we apply ourselves to reframing the questions related to endometriosis (and indirectly to some of the most important things involved in life), we may be able to solve the puzzle. After all, if there were five million young men with endometriosis in the United States, young men whose dreams were in danger of being destroyed by a disease, whose ability to function sexually were at risk, whose fertility were at risk, whose ability to build a satisfying work life and carry out the normal activities of living were at risk, and who even would face the threat of castration—if this were happening to young men, no one would dare say it was not serious. Men would have banded together long ago, research institutes would have been devoted to it, and by now it would be not only curable but also preventable. The puzzle would be solved. Can we afford to do anything less for women and girls?

Notes

1. D. L. Olive, *Infertility and Reproductive Medicine Clinics of North America: Endometriosis* (Philadelphia: W. B. Saunders Company, 1992), 3:3, xi.
2. E. Thomas and J. Rock, *Modern Approaches to Endometriosis* (Lancaster, England: Kluwer Academic Publishers, 1991), ix.
3. R. Schenken, *Endometriosis: Contemporary Concepts in Clinical Management* (Philadelphia, J. B. Lippincott, 1989), ix.
4. E. Wilson, *Endometriosis* (New York: Alan R. Liss, 1987), 1.
5. D. L. Olive, ed, "Future Directions for Endometriosis Research," *Infertility and Reproductive Medicine Clinics of North America: Endometriosis* 3, no. 3 (1992): 763.
6. J. M. R. Rawson, "Prevalence of Endometriosis in Asymptomatic Women," *Journal of Reproductive Medicine* 36 (1991): 513.
7. D. E. Pittaway, "Diagnosis of Endometriosis," *Infertility and Reproductive Medicine Clinics of North America: Endometriosis* 3, no. 3 (1992): 619.
8. D. B. Redwine, "Treatment of Endometriosis-Associated Pain," *Infertility and Reproductive Medicine Clinics of North America: Endometriosis* 3, no. 3 (1992): 701–06, 708–13.
9. M. Nisolle-Pochet, F. Casanas-Roux, and J. Donnez, "Histologic Study of Ovarian Endometriosis After Hormonal Therapy," *Fertility and Sterility* 49 (1988): 423–26.
10. I. A. Brosens, "The Endometriotic Implant," *Modern Approaches to Endometriosis*, 30.
11. D. L. Olive and A. F. Haney; "Associated Infertility; A Critical Review of Therapeutic Approaches," *Obstetrical and Gynecological Survey* 41 (1986): 538.
12. M. W. Vernon, J. S. Beard, K. Graves, et al., "Classification of Endometriotic Implants by Morphologic Appearance and Capacity to Synthesize Prostaglandin F," *Fertility and Sterility* 46 (1986): 801.
13. D. B. Redwine, "Age-Related Evolution in Color Appearance of Endometriosis," *Fertility and Sterility* 48 (1987): 1061–63.
14. A. A. Murphy, W. R. Green, D. Bobbie, Z. C. dela Cruz, and J. A. Rock, "Unsuspected Endometriosis Documented by Scanning Electron Microscopy in Visually Normal Peritoneum," *Fertility and Sterility* 46 (1986): 522.

15. A. Audebert et al., "Endometriosis 1991: A Discussion Document," *Human Reproduction* 7 (1992): 432–35.
16. J. M . R. Rawson, "Prevalence of Endometriosis in Asymptomatic Women," 515.
17. E. J. Thomas and J. A. Rock, "The Future," *Modern Approaches to Endometriosis,* 291.
18. R. C. Reiter, R. L. Shakerin, J. C. Gambone, and A. K. Milburn, "Correlation Between Sexual Abuse and Somatization in Women with Somatic and Nonsomatic Chronic Pelvic Pain," *American Journal of Obstetrics and Gynecology* 165 (1991): 104–09.
19. I. Gottesfeld, "Chronic Pelvic Pain: Stalking a Clinical Enigma," *Today's Woman* (October 1991).
20. D. B. Redwine, "Conservative Laparoscopic Excision of Endometriosis by Sharp Dissection: Life Table Analysis of Reoperation and Persistent or Recurrent Disease," *Fertility and Sterility* 56 (1991): 634.
21. M. L. Ballweg, *Overcoming Endometriosis: New Help from the Endometriosis Association* (New York: Congdon & Weed, 1987), 221.
22. Endometriosis Association Research Registry, "Characteristics of Women with Endometriosis," *Endometriosis Association Newsletter* 10, no. 2 (1989): 2.
23. K. Lamb, R. G. Hoffmann, and T. R. Nichols, "Family Trait Analysis: A Case Control Study of 43 Women with Endometriosis and Their Best Friends," *American Journal of Obstetrics and Gynecology* 154 (1986): 596–601.
24. K. Lamb and T. R. Nichols, "Endometriosis: A Comparison of Associated Disease Histories," *American Journal of Preventive Medicine* 2 (1986): 324–29.
25. T. R. Nichols, K. Lamb, and J. A. Arkins, "The Association of Atopic Diseases with Endometriosis," *Annals of Allergy* 59 (1987): 360–63.
26. M. L. Ballweg, *Overcoming Endometriosis,* 198–219.
27. M. L. Ballweg, "Data Bank Results Are In! from Endometriosis Association Research Registry," *Endometriosis Association Newsletter* (May 1983): 1.
28. M. L. Ballweg, "Research News—Endometriosis Linked to Radiation and Environmental Pollutants in Research Studies," *Endometriosis Association Newsletter* 13, no. 2 (1992): 1–2.
29. M. L. Ballweg, "Research News—Exciting Findings in Dioxin Monkey Colony," *Endometriosis Association Newsletter* 13, no. 3 (1992): 1–2.
30. D. W. Cramer, E. Wilson, R. J. Stillman, et al., "The Relation of Endometriosis to Menstrual Characteristics, Smoking, and Exercise," *Journal of the American Medical Association* 255 (1986): 1904.
31. R. Wood, "The Pathway to Diagnosis of Women with Endometriosis," Endometriosis Association (Victoria), Melbourne, Australia, presented at Third World Congress on Endometriosis (Brussels, June 1992).
32. D. B. Redwine, "The Distribution of Endometriosis in the Pelvis by Age Groups and Fertility," *Fertility and Sterility* 47 (1987): 173.
33. S. Kenney, "What Is Important to the Patient with Endometriosis? Discussion," *British Journal of Clinical Practice* 45, no. 3, Supplement 72 (Autumn 1991): 11.
34. M. L. Ballweg, "A Few Comparative Findings: Endometriosis Association, British Endometriosis Society and Australian Endometriosis Association," *Overcoming Endometriosis: New Help from the Endometriosis Association,* 297.
35. G. F. Rosen, "Treatment of Endometriosis-Associated Infertility," *Infertility and Reproductive Medicine Clinics of North America: Endometriosis* 3, no. 3 (1992): 721.
36. A. F. Haney, "The Pathogenesis and Aetiology of Endometriosis," *Modern Approaches to Endometriosis,* 4.

37. A. L. Yap, "Endometriosis and the Urinary Tract: Endometriosis of the Bladder, Bladder and Urinary Tract Symptoms, New Directions in Understanding and Treatment, and Related Problems," *Endometriosis Association Newsletter* 13, no. 1, (1992): 2–3.

38. M. L. Ballweg, "Endometriosis and the Intestines: Endometriosis of the Bowel, Intestinal Symptoms, New Directions in Understanding and Treatment," *Endometriosis Association Newsletter* 9, no. 1 (1988): 5.

39. D. A. Grimes, S. A. LeBolt, K. R. T. Grimes, and P. A. Wingo, "Two-Fold Risk of Endometriosis in Hospitalized Patients with Lupus," *American Journal of Obstetrics and Gynecology* 153 (1985): 179.

40. M. G. Brush, "Increased Incident of Thyroid Autoimmune Problems in Women with Endometriosis," *Endometriosis: A Collection of Papers Written by PGs, Researchers, Specialists and Sufferers About Endometriosis,* compiled by the Coventry Branch of the Endometriosis Society (March 1987).

41. M. L. Ballweg, *Overcoming Endometriosis,* 228–31.

42. N. Fletcher, "Mitral Valve Prolapse," *Endometriosis Association Newsletter* 13, no. 2 (1992): 1–2.

43. C. Jessop, "Clinical Features and Possible Etiology of CFIDS, Chronic Fatigue and Immune Dysfunction Syndrome: Unravelling the Mystery," conference (Charlotte, North Carolina, November 18, 1990). *Summary: The CFIDS Chronicle 1991* (spring): 70–73.

44. M. L. Ballweg, "Fibromyalgia/Endo Link?" *Endometriosis Association Newsletter* 12, no. 3 (1991): 6–8.

45. M. L. Ballweg, *Overcoming Endometriosis,* 205.

46. Gibbons, Ann, "Dioxin Tied to Endometriosis," *Science* (January 1985).

47. M. L. Ballweg, *Overcoming Endometriosis,* 219.

48. J. Campbell, "Is Simian Endometriosis an Effect of Immunotoxicity?" Ontario Association of Pathologists (October 1985).

49. S. E. Rier, D. C. Martin, R. E. Bowman, W. P. Dmowksi, and J. L. Becker, "Endometriosis in Rhesus Monkeys (*Macaca mulatta*) Following Chronic Exposure to 2,3,7,8-Tetrachlorodibenzo-p-Dioxin," *Fundamental and Applied Toxicology* 21, no. 4 (1993): 433–41.

50. S. E. Rier, "Research News—Immunological Findings in Dioxin Monkey Colony," *Endometriosis Association Newsletter* 13, no. 4 (1992): 1, 6.

51. D. C. Martin, S. E. Rier, R. E. Bowman, W. P. Dmowksi, and J. L. Becker, "Dioxin-Induced Endometriosis in Rhesus Monkeys (*Macaca mulatta*)," *Abstracts,* Annual Meeting of the Society for Gynecologic Investigation (Toronto, April 1993): 330.

52. S. E. Rier, B. L. Spangel, D. C. Martin, R. E. Bowman, and J. L. Becker, "Production of IL-6 and TNF by Peripheral Blood Mononuclear Cells from Rhesus Monkeys with Endometriosis," American Association of Immunology (Denver, May 1993).

53. Consensus Statement, "Chemically Induced Alterations in Sexual Development: The Wildlife/Human Connection." Wingspread Conference (Racine, Wisconsin, July 26–28, 1991).

54. R. Hong, K. Taylor, and R. Abonour, "Immune Abnormalities Associated with Chronic TCDD Exposure in Rhesus," *Chemosphere* 18, no. 1–6 (1989): 313–20.

55. A. F. Haney, "The Pathogenesis and Aetiology of Endometriosis," *Modern Approaches to Endometriosis,* 14.

56. L. Halstead, P. Pepping, and W. P. Dmowski, "The Woman with Endometriosis: Ignored, Dismissed and Devalued," Second International Symposium on Endometriosis (Houston, Texas, May 1989).

57. L. Halstead, P. Pepping, L. Haile, and W. P. Dmowski, "Women's Experiences with Endometriosis: Delay and Disbelief," *Abstracts,* Third World Congress on Endometriosis (Brussels, June 1992).

58. M. L. Ballweg, "Endometriosis: The Patient's Perspective," *Infertility and Reproductive Medicine Clinics of North America: Endometriosis,* 747–61.

59. K. J. Armitage, L. J. Schneiderman, and B. A. Bass, "Response of Physicians to Medical Complaints in Men and Women," *Journal of the American Medical Association* 241 (1979): 2186–87.

60. J. Delaney, M. J. Lupton, and E. Toth, *The Curse: A Cultural History of Menstruation* (Urbana and Chicago: University of Illinois Press, 1988).

61. E. Martin, *The Woman in the Body: A Cultural Analysis of Reproduction* (Boston: Beacon Press, 1987).

62. *Hysterectomies in the United States, 1965–1984.* Vital and Health Statistics, U.S. Department of Health and Human Services, Public Health Service, Centers for Disease Control, National Center for Health Statistics, series 13, no. 92 (1987).

63. A. M. Rosenthal, "Female Genital Torture," *New York Times* (December 29, 1992).

64. P. J. Donoghue and M. E. Siegel, *Sick and Tired of Feeling Sick and Tired: Living with Invisible Chronic Illness* (New York: W. W. Norton, 1992).

65. K. Lamb, L. Breitkopf, K. Hamilton, et al., "Does Total Hysterectomy Offer a Cure for Endometriosis?" *Endometriosis Association Newsletter* 12, no. 3 (1991): 1–5.

66. J. Delaney, M. J. Lupton, and E. Toth, *The Curse: A Cultural History of Menstruation*, 62.

■ *An earlier version of this article was written in 1993 for the medical textbook* Endometriosis, Advanced Management and Surgical Techniques *by Drs. Camran Nezhat, Gary Berger, Farr Nezhat, Veasy Buttram, and Ceana Nezhat, Springer-Verlag, 1995.*

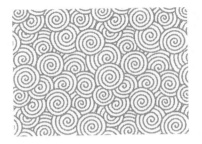

PART V

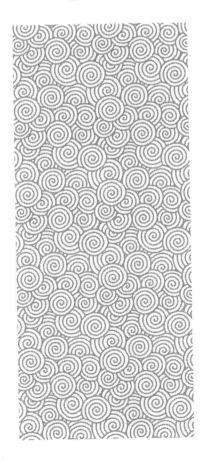

Working Toward Conquering Endometriosis

17

⚛⚛

Working Together Worldwide to Conquer Endometriosis

By Nicole Denison

"*Y*our book was a revelation and truly opened my eyes, not only about the links between endometriosis and several of my health problems (ranging from low blood sugar to allergies to low blood pressure), but it also made me aware of millions of other women all over the world who share the same pain and sufferings. I want to express my thanks and gratitude to Mary Lou Ballweg for her courage and her efforts to found the first endometriosis association in the world and writing a book about her fight coping with endo, sharing her insights and information with women not only in the English-speaking countries.*"

Angelika Stephani, Augsburg, Germany

"*D*ear Sisters,
    "Thank you very much for your letter of May 15. I really appreciate your kindness, especially Japanese brochures were wonderful! Actually it was the first time to receive any information in Japanese from a foreign group or organization. I was really impressed by seeing your work.*"

Sumie Uno, Osaka, Japan

"*I* was diagnosed with endometriosis in December of 1988 during an operation called a laparotomy. At that time I was put on six months of drug therapy and was told nothing about the disease or the medication I was to take, nor given other options for treatment. I went to the library and bookstores to try to find something about endometriosis but found almost nothing. . . .
    "I felt very frustrated, depressed, helpless, and alone, as almost nobody else I talked to had ever heard [of] the disease. I suffered from constant fatigue, had missed a lot of work because of doctor's appointments and operations, and the people around me were acting as if

433

I were a hypochondriac or imagining the whole thing because nobody had ever heard of it or knew anything about it. I chose to do nothing for another year and suffered in silence.

"Finally, in the fall of 1992, I found a book on endometriosis. It was the most information I had ever seen on a subject, and it was information about the Endometriosis Association. I called them, became a member immediately, and ordered all the information they had, which included two books and many back editions of the newsletters. It was the best money I have ever spent. They saved my sanity and gave me hope. Through the Endometriosis Association I was able to educate myself about the disease, its symptoms, every type of surgery and medication available, their possible side effects and success rates, treating infertility, and the ability to go to my doctor with confidence and become a partner in the treatment of the disease.

"In December I contacted the Endometriosis Association to find out if they had an office in Brazil as I am now living in São Paulo and was told that one was being started. They gave me the name and address of Eleuze Mendonça, whom I contacted and have been happily working with ever since. My greatest concern is that women are needlessly suffering and are frequently unable to find the help they need because they don't know who or where to turn to. Self-education, communication, and persistence are the keys to overcoming this disease and regaining some control over your life. Their support groups and telephone hot lines have been invaluable to me as well as thousands of other women by just being able to talk to other women with the disease. . . .

"The medical information alone on the disease and its various treatments that the Endometriosis Association has compiled is astounding. . . .

"One of the most important functions they have fulfilled has been to get the information out to the doctors and the public, and to put pressure on the government for acknowledgment of the disease and its seriousness, research into its causes, medications and operations for its treatment, and the search for a cure. This has been very successful, which has been shown by the great increase in public knowledge, not just in the United States but all over the world, doctor information, government funding, and the increase in the number of types of treatments and medications that are now on the market. Thanks to them, many women today are receiving the help they need and regaining control of their lives, including I."

Keely Acosta, São Paulo, Brazil

As word about the Endometriosis Association and association brochures in 13 languages have reached the far corners of the globe, international interest has continued to grow. Along with that has come a greater demand for support groups, prompting the association to help women around the world network with each other and begin formal organizing. As a result, a spate of new support groups is forming.

Whether these groups have been initiated and run by doctors or by the women themselves, women in the association's international network are finding the help that evaded them when they thought they were all alone. It's exciting to see them awakening to the fact that they have a right to inform themselves, a right to be treated with dignity, and a right to have a say in what form of treatment to pursue.

Nevertheless, at times our overseas members face greater obstacles and very different cultural and social factors from women in the United States and Canada. For various reasons women with endo in many countries do not enjoy the same degree of access to the health care community and its resources (and, as we know all too well, we in North America lack much in *our* medical care for endometriosis). And they may also have fewer resources, whether financial, educational, or otherwise, that would facilitate taking charge of their own health care.

For many of these women simply receiving the Endometriosis Association's initial information package and reading the "yellow" brochure (*What Is Endometriosis?*), often in their own language, has proven to be a turning point in their lives. The impact of the revelation that there is someplace they can turn to for help cannot be overestimated. As the women share this basic information with physicians, family and friends, school groups, clinics, and so on, they're repeating a familiar pattern begun 15 years ago in the United States and followed by many start-up groups the world over.

The groups profiled here offer examples of what women are accomplishing in a diverse group of countries. The list is by no means all-inclusive. Support groups are constantly evolving, and at the time of this writing, for instance, a chapter in Singapore was getting off to a promising start. We now have contacts and networks in most areas of the world, a wonderful testimony to the inspiring determination of women with endometriosis. The following highlights serve to give a sense of the worldwide momentum mustered by millions of women who refuse to remain passive victims of endometriosis.

United States and Canada

Women from all walks of life have come together to form the more than 150 support groups and chapters across the United States and Canada. Through sharing common experiences and exchanging information about various treatments, doctors, and local and national resources, group members realize they are not alone. By helping each other, they help themselves cope with this often frustrating and confusing disease.

The support groups encourage members to be proactive in taking charge of their personal health care decisions and by actively working with their physicians to determine the best course of treatment available. Members have access to the most comprehensive, current information on endometriosis in the field today. Their families can also benefit by learning more about the issues related to living with someone with the disease, helping to create a supportive and nurturing environment.

Some of the support groups' myriad activities include displaying educational materials at health fairs and promoting endometriosis coverage in the media. They also bring in speakers who focus on alternative therapies, coping strategies, pain management, the latest surgical techniques, and other topics of vital interest. They distribute literature to the local health care community, find sponsorship for the group, participate in membership drives, and organize fund-raisers to help support the Endometriosis Association or to provide much-needed dollars for research.

Fund-raising activities may vary from the fashion shows put on by the Jacksonville, Florida, chapter, to selling entertainment books as the Northwest Ohio Support Group has done, to a raffle and drawing for a beautiful handmade quilt put on by the Kitchener/ Waterloo, Ontario, group during Endometriosis Awareness Week 1995. In addition to raising money, these types of activities serve to raise awareness of endometriosis in the community. The Los Angeles chapter has furthered community outreach by purchasing copies of the association's first book, *Overcoming Endometriosis,* and donating them to the local library system. The Merrimack Valley, Massachusetts, support group targeted area high schools to include association brochures in the health packets given out to all girls in health classes.

Several groups have also held successful conferences. A one-day statewide conference organized by the San Antonio, Texas, group in 1994 brought together support group leaders from all over the state with nationally renowned physicians. The Honolulu Support Group organized a statewide conference in 1995 and lobbied the governor's office to officially proclaim Endometriosis Awareness Week for the state of Hawaii. (Endometriosis Awareness Week is held worldwide the last full week of March each year.) Such events promote membership as well as providing a forum for the exchange of ideas and information.

All these efforts and more serve to bring women together for mutual support and encouragement, helping to make endometriosis a more manageable disease as well as increase public awareness.

Brazil

The Brazilian support group, which refers to itself as ABEN (Associação Brasileira Endometriose), was started in 1993 in São Paulo by law student Eleuze Mendonça, who serves as president. Together with another member, Keely Acosta, and Dr. Reginaldo Lopes, Eleuze has formed a very active group with several branches in various locations.

Infertility is an especially great preoccupation for the woman with endometriosis in Brazil, where the culture places tremendous emphasis on motherhood. Strong family ties can work in support of afflicted women here, too. Mendonça reports that members were accompanied to one conference by husbands, sisters, brothers, and other relatives who wanted to learn more about the disease. One of ABEN's main objectives is to form additional support groups so as to reach more women in this vast nation, and, as of this writing, they've initiated affiliate groups in seven states around Brazil.

The Brazilian group has been very active in education about endometriosis. They distribute educational materials and often feature knowledgeable speakers at their meetings from an affiliated medical and scientific commission. Media outreach is also a big priority, as is giving talks on endometriosis at various schools, clubs, and associations. When Mendonça and Dr. Lopes presented a lecture at a São Paulo Rotary Club meeting, they were encouraged when the club offered ABEN a donation. Mendonça was also interviewed on television in late 1994, prompting many telephone calls, including one from a grateful woman aged 70.

This group's energy and enthusiasm are much needed to support Brazil's estimated two million women—out of a total population of 160 million—who have endometriosis.

Germany

Despite Germany's progressive social welfare system and tradition of free medical care, until recently there has been a surprising lack of awareness about endometriosis. Women are usually diagnosed by chance—for instance, because of infertility. Self-help books do not mention the disease, and German-language information is all but impossible to find.

Because Germans have tended to rely on the "social net" without getting involved themselves, innovations can be difficult. Compounding the dilemma for German women, they must also fight myths such as endometriosis as the career woman's disease or the result of an unresolved conflict between the demands of a highly industrialized society and traditional female roles.

Angelika Stephani had suffered from misdiagnosed endometriosis for three decades before she happened to stumble on the association's book *Overcoming Endometriosis* while browsing in a bookstore during a visit to the United States. She and Petra Muck together began groups in Munich, and Augsburg in 1994. In Munich a newspaper article and brief mention on a television broadcast attracted some 150 inquiries, and the monthly meetings began drawing women ranging in age from their early twenties to their midsixties who were eager to get involved.

In 1995 the Augsburg and Munich groups took a major step forward by organizing the first German Endometriosis Conference in Augsburg, inviting five German experts in the field and association headquarters staff to lecture about the latest research. The program also included traditional Chinese and Indian medicine as well as other alternative approaches.

Although group members wish efforts had begun earlier in Germany, they're excited about the information and assistance provided by their peers overseas and are more than determined to make up for lost time.

Japan

In contrast to physicians in many other countries, Japanese doctors are quick to diagnose endometriosis and readily prescribe hormones, often danazol and buserelin acetate. (Japanese physicians believe a laparoscopy is unnecessary to diagnose the disease, and in fact, laparoscopy is rarely used.) Even any evidence of dysmenorrhea can be diagnosed as endometriosis.

Because doctors are held in such high authority in Japan, it is difficult for Japanese women to obtain information about the disease and exercise a say in what kind of treatment they prefer. Women also suffer from a basic lack of privacy in the doctor's office due to the layout of clinics and hospitals, and other patients in the waiting room can easily hear what is going on in the examination room.

The newly formed Japan Endometriosis Association is well equipped to begin confronting these problems. The group traces its origins to the Osaka Women's Center, which held seminars and published a booklet on endometriosis in response to increasing calls about the disease on its women's hot line. The Women's Center held a symposium with Endometriosis Association president Mary Lou Ballweg in 1994, and at that point the Osaka Support Group was officially formed. Headed by members Sumie Uno and Masumi Inui, the Osaka group now has about 350 members and has set up 10 self-help groups throughout the country. It publishes a newsletter three times a year and holds seminars with invited doctors.

The group has adopted the Endometriosis Association formula of education, support, and research as its model and is greatly encouraged by the accomplishments of similar groups in other countries.

South Africa

This fledgling group is closely tied with the South African Fertility Society, which has pledged to provide computer facilities, secretarial support, and meeting space for the South African Support Group at its meetings throughout the country. Assistance has also been offered by the company that owns the private clinics throughout South Africa, as well as the manufacturer of Synarel.

Endometriosis has never been studied in South Africa before. Because the nation has a very diverse population spanning first, second, and third worlds, the South African group expects to provide critical information, particularly in regard to the incidence of endometriosis in different racial groups. Led by gynecologist Dr. Johan Van Der Wat and organizer Joy Margolis, the new group shares the mission of its sister chapters around the world to change attitudes about endometriosis and to provide better care for sufferers.

Taiwan

Formed in 1991 because Dr. Kiu-Kwong Chu felt his patients needed more help with endo, the Taiwan chapter faces several special challenges. According to Dr. Chu, women in Taiwan may be unwilling or afraid to seek help, especially if they are teenagers or are single. In addition, they tend to keep silent about their pain at work for fear of losing their jobs and are warned not to use the disease as an excuse for a break from work. They also may face disbelief on the part of elders in the extended Chinese family who have never heard of the disease and are skeptical that it can cause so much pain and suffering.

Obviously, there is a great need for basic information, and the Taiwan group has wisely chosen education as its initial primary focus. As with many young groups, volunteers are limited and now include one full-time leader and a few others who offer part-time help. Nevertheless, the Taiwan support group has managed to hold symposiums every three months in south and central Taiwan and also has a monthly get-together for new members.

The chapter's greatest coup since its formation was getting six members who had various problems related to endometriosis, as well as the group's chairman, Dr. Yu-Chen Wu, on a national television program to discuss the disease.

Sister Groups

Our sister groups in Australia and Great Britain share long-standing relationships with the association as well as common goals and struggles. As we exchange newsletters with them and maintain regular contact, we rejoice in each other's victories, identify with our mutual challenges, and continue to draw mutual inspiration from knowing we are not alone.

Australia

The Endometriosis Association (Victoria) was established in 1984. Although it is based in the state of Victoria, its 850 members come from all over Australia, with about 20 affiliated groups around the country.

For its first eight years the association operated on an informal, voluntary basis out of the home of one of its founding members. Now with its own office and two paid workers for a few hours a week, the group is run by a management collective of eight women.

A large proportion of resources goes into providing a popular telephone hot line that receives more than 2,000 calls annually. But perhaps the group's most innovative activity is an Endometriosis Clinic it established in 1991. Staffed by a team of gynecologists and members of the association, the clinic also maintains close contact with a small team of alternative health practitioners.

One of the chief aims of the clinic is to provide women with information and enable them to make well-informed decisions about the management of their endometriosis. Each woman has a 30-minute consultation with the gynecologist, who makes a thorough assessment of her condition before discussing the range of treatments available. She then has a consultation with a member of the association to discuss the options proposed by the gynecologist, as well as any further questions she may have.

The group also has several research projects in the works, but because of a shortage of staff, progress has been slow. Their main interest has been in documenting the delay between the onset of endometriosis and diagnosis. A 1989 survey revealed that 43 percent of women surveyed had first experienced their symptoms as teenagers and that many had experienced a long and tortuous pathway to diagnosis that lasted an average of 6.1 years. The association is now working on building a more detailed picture of what happens to women with endometriosis before they're diagnosed.

The group has also begun another study documenting the reasons why women have hysterectomies to treat their endometriosis and whether the operations are helpful in controlling symptoms. They hope to use the results to make the medical profession more aware of the fact that hysterectomy is often not a "cure" for women with endometriosis.

This extremely active organization from down under is enthusiastic about staying in touch with us and possibly arranging for members of both organizations to meet from time to time to share ideas.

Great Britain

Ailsa Irving founded the British Endometriosis Society in 1982 after meeting a fellow sufferer at a hospital and then advertising for others to help form a support group. The society now has 3,235 members and more than 60 support groups throughout the British Isles. The women gain tremendously from meeting with others and often find new confidence and skills they did not realize they possessed.

The group focuses on support, education, and research and is administered by a board of trustees who have all experienced the disease. The society produces a member newsletter four times a year, strives to provide other inexpensive publications, and vigorously promotes publicity about endometriosis in the national media. The group usually holds two conferences per year that bring in conventional and alternative practitioners who speak about their treatment or research.

The British Endometriosis Society keeps a separate fund for research donations and is currently trying to raise £50,000 for a project to be chosen by a panel of gynecological experts. Members have often been recruited for clinical trials of new drugs or complementary therapies, meaning that sometimes their knowledge about treatments gets ahead of their physicians'.

The society has a tiny paid staff in its London office with an urgent need for volunteers. Like groups around the world, they've experienced the tremendous relief women feel at discovering the society and realizing they are not alone.

In a recent association newsletter, Dian Mills, former trustee of the society, wrote: "Perhaps together we can form a powerful force around the world to help educate the public and increase medical understanding of endometriosis. . . . The more that we as individuals can spread the word, the better it will be. To our sisters across the Atlantic, we send our mutual greeting—together we make a difference."

The tremendous relief and empowerment women feel at finally connecting with fellow sufferers creates an instantaneous bond—a bond that renders cultural and language barriers virtually inconsequential. And it's a good thing. With the discovery of the potential link between endometriosis and chemicals such as dioxin and PCBs that know no national boundaries, worldwide cooperation to fight endometriosis has taken on a new sense of urgency.

There is still much more to be done—but there's no telling what we can accomplish as we continue to marshal the remarkable power of women working together around the world. As the motto of the association states: Together We Make a Difference!

■ *Nicole Denison is the associate editor for* On Wisconsin *magazine, the alumni magazine for the University of Wisconsin–Madison, and a member of the Endometriosis Association.*

Additional Resources

Following is a list of self-help and resource organizations, some of which may prove useful to readers. Be advised that because some of these groups have little funding and rely on volunteer power, they may change addresses and phone numbers if their coordinators relocate. The information included in this list is current as of our printing. Should readers have difficulty contacting any of these organizations, they may want to get in touch with one of the national self-help clearinghouses, or call directory assistance, 800-555-1212, in the cities in which these groups are based.

For all aspects of endometriosis:

Endometriosis Association

International Headquarters

8585 N. 76th Place, Milwaukee, WI 53223-2600, U.S.A.

414-355-6065 fax

800-992-3636 (North America)

First-time callers may leave name and address to receive an introductory packet.

For women with endometriosis in the British Isles:

The Endometriosis Society

35 Belgrave Square, London SW1X 8QB, England

071-235-4137

For women with endometriosis in Australia:

Endometriosis Association (Victoria) Inc.

37 Andrew Crescent, South Croydon, Victoria 3136, Australia

03-879-1276

For women with endometriosis in New Zealand:

New Zealand Endometriosis Foundation

PO Box 1683, Palmerston North, New Zealand

0800-733-277

For women with endometriosis in other countries:

Contact Endometriosis Association International Headquarters (first listing)

Acupuncture:
American Association of Acupuncture and Oriental Medicine
    433 Front St., Catasauqua, PA 18032-2506
    610-433-2448
California Association of Acupuncture and Oriental Medicine
    2180 Garnet Ave., Ste. 361, San Diego, CA 92109
    619-270-1005
Institute for Traditional Medicine and Preventive Health Care
    2442 S.E. Sherman, Portland, OR 97214
    800-544-7504
    or, in Europe
    I.T.M., v.z.w., Laaglandlaan 23, B-2060 Merksem, Belgium
    This is a tax-exempt organization that gathers information about Chinese
    medicine through a range of resources and methods, including visits to China
    and translation of Chinese medical research, and prepares fact sheets based on
    these resources for practitioners.
National Commission for the Certification of Acupuncturists
    1424 16th St., NW, Ste. 105, Washington, DC 20036
    202-232-1404

Adoption:
National Adoption Center
    1500 Walnut St., Ste. 701, Philadelphia, PA 19102
    800-TO-ADOPT

Candida:
Candida and Dysbiosis Information Foundation
    PO Box JF, College Station, TX 77841-5146
    409-694-8687

Chronic Fatigue Syndrome:
CFIDS Association of America
    PO Box 220398, Charlotte, NC 28222-0398
    800-442-3437
    CFIDS information line: 900-896-2343
National Chronic Fatigue Syndrome and Fibromyalgia Association
    33521 Broadway #222, Kansas City, KS 66111
    816-931-4777
The Nightingale Research Foundation
    383 Danforth Ave., Ottawa, ON Canada K2A OE1
    613-728-9643

DES:
 DES Action USA
  2845 24th Street, San Francisco, CA 94110
  415-826-5060

Fibromyalgia:
 American Fibromyalgia Syndrome Association, Inc.
  PO Box 9699, Bakersfield, CA 93389-9699
  805-633-1137
 Fibromyalgia Network
  PO Box 31750, Tuscon, AZ 85751-1750
  602-290-5508

Headaches:
 American Council for Headache Education (A.C.H.E.)
  875 Kings Highway, Ste. 200, Woodbury, NJ 08096
  800-255-2245
 National Headache Foundation
  5252 N. Western Ave., Chicago, IL 60625
  800-843-2256

Health and Health Care:
 American College of Obstetricians & Gynecologists
  409 12th St., SW, Washington, DC 20024-2188
  202-638-5577
 National Health Information Center
  PO Box 1133, Washington, DC 20013-1133
  800-336-4797
 National Women's Health Network
  514 10th St., NW, Ste. 400, Washington, DC 20005
  202-347-1140

Holistic Health Care:
 American Holistic Medical Association
  4101 Lake Boone Trail #201, Raleigh, NC 27607
  919-787-5146
 The Holistic Health Hotline
  PO Box 25717, Seattle, WA 98125
  206-481-4445

Homeopathy:
 International Foundation for Homeopathy
  2366 Eastlake Ave. East #329, Seattle, WA 98102
  206-324-8230

Ileitis/Colitis:
Crohn's & Colitis Foundation of America, Inc.
386 Park Ave. South, 17th Floor, New York, NY 10016
212-685-3440

Incontinence:
Simon Foundation
PO Box 835, Wilmette, IL 60091
800-23-SIMON

Infertility Issues:
Infertility Awareness Association of Canada, Inc.
396 Cooper Street, Ste. 201, Ottawa, Ontario, Canada K2P 2H7
613-234-8585
800-263-2929 (Canada)
Resolve
National Headquarters
1310 Broadway, Somerville, MA 02144-1731
main office: 617-623-1156
national Helpline M–F: 9–12, 1–4 EST: 617-623-0744

Interstitial Cystitis:
Interstitial Cystitis Association
PO Box 1553 Madison Square Station, New York, NY 10159
212-979-6057

Loss: For Parents Grieving Miscarriage, Stillbirth, and Infant Death:
Unite, Inc.
Jeanes Hospital, 7600 Central Ave., Philadelphia, PA 19111
215-728-3777

Lupus:
The American Lupus Society
260 Maple Court, Ste. 123, Ventura, CA 93003
805-339-0443 or 800-331-1802
Lupus Foundation of America
4 Research Place, Ste. 180, Rockville, MD 20850-3226
800-558-0121 or 301-670-9292, or, for Spanish, 800-558-0231

Medical Records:
Medical Information Bureau
Consumer Information Office, PO Box 105, Essex Station, Boston, MA 02112
617-426-3660

People's Medical Society
    462 Walnut St., Lower Level, Allentown, PA 18102
    610-770-1670
Public Citizen's Health Research Group
    2000 P St., NW, Ste. 700, Washington, DC 20036
    202-833-3000

Naturopathy:
American Association of Naturopathic Physicians
    2366 Eastlake Ave. East #322, Seattle, WA 98102
    206-323-7610

Osteoporosis:
National Osteoporosis Foundation
    1150 17th St., NW, Ste. 500, Washington, DC 20036
    202-223-2226

Pain:
American Chronic Pain Association
    PO Box 850, Rocklin, CA 95677
    916-632-0922
National Chronic Pain Outreach Association
    822 Wycliffe Court, Manassas, VA 22110
    703-368-8884

Pesticides:
National Pesticide Telecommunications Network
    800-858-7378
U.S. Environmental Protection Agency
    Office of Pesticide Programs (7506C), 401 M St., SW, Washington, DC 20460
    703-305-5805

Physicians: To Verify Board Certification:
American Board of Medical Specialties
    47 Perimeter Center East, Ste. 500, Atlanta, GA 30346
    800-776-CERT

Premenstrual Syndrome (PMS):
PMS Access
    PO Box 9326, Madison, WI 53715
    800-222-4PMS or 608-833-4PMS

Self-Help Organizations:
  National Self-Help Clearinghouse
      City University of New York, Graduate Center, Room 620
      25 W. 43rd St., New York, NY 10036
      212-642-2944
  New Jersey Self-Help Clearinghouse
      Northwest Covenant Medical Center, 25 Pocono Rd., Denville, NJ 07834
      201-625-9053

Urinary Tract Disorders, Including Interstitial Cystitis:
  American Urogynecologic Society
      401 N. Michigan Ave., Chicago, IL 60611
      312-644-6610

Vulvodynia:
  National Vulvodynia Association
      PO Box 19283, Sarasota, FL 34276-2288
      813-927-8503
  The Vulvar Pain Foundation (VPF)
      PO Drawer 177, Graham, NC 27253
      910-226-0704

Well-Spouse Support:
  The Well Spouse Foundation
      PO Box 28876, San Diego, CA 92198
      619-673-9043

Glossary

Acupuncture—"Chinese medicine views the body as a complex system of interconnected energy pathways known as *meridians*. Good health depends on the smooth, harmonious flow of energy and blood through these meridians. The energy, referred to as *chi*, collects at distinct places (points) on these meridians. Very fine needles are inserted at these points to open the healing pathways." (Yo San University Clinic brochure.)

Acute pain—severe pain over a short time.

Adenomyosis—a disease in which the endometrium, the lining of the uterus, seems to grow into the muscular part of the uterus.

Adhesions—bands of scar tissue that bind together normally separate surfaces and organs.

Anabolic—stimulates growth.

Anaphylaxis—an allergic hypersensitivity reaction of the body to a protein or foreign substance, including drugs. Systemic anaphylaxis involves cells throughout the body; if severe, this reaction can be fatal.

Androgen—male sex hormone, such as testosterone.

Antagonizing—exerting an opposite effect.

Anticoagulant—a substance that prevents or delays clotting of the blood, such as heparin.

Anus—the canal (1½ inches long) from the rectum, through a ring of muscles, and including an opening to the outside of the body through which solid wastes are moved as bowel movements.

Aspiration of cyst—surgical puncture of a cyst and suctioning out of the old blood and other material inside it.

Autoantibody—an antibody against one's own cells or their components.

Autoimmune disease—one caused by autoantibodies or lymphocytes that attack one's own tissues or cells.

Autoimmunity—a condition in which immune cells mistakenly see the body's own tissues or cells as foreign and attack them, resulting in inflammation and autoimmune diseases such as rheumatoid arthritis and lupus.

Avascular—lacking in blood vessels; having a poor blood supply.

Barium enema—lower bowel x-ray in which barium, used to provide contrast, is inserted into the colon through the rectum and x-rays are taken.

Bilateral salpingo-oophorectomy—removal of both ovaries and fallopian tubes.

Biopsy—removal and examination of a sample of tissue to make a diagnosis.

Bladder—the membranous sac that collects and stores urine until it is eliminated.

Bowel obstruction—partial or complete blockage of the intestine.

Broad ligaments—folds of peritoneum attached to the sides of the uterus.

Candidiasis—a condition of both allergy to and overgrowth of the yeast *Candida albicans* in the body, causing illness and allergic manifestations. See *Overcoming Endometriosis* for more information.

Cauterize—to burn so as to destroy tissue.

Cecum—the pouch where the small intestine ends and the large intestine begins in the human body.

Centimeter (cm)—part of the metric system of measurement. 1 cm = .39 inch (U.S.).

Cephalopelvic disproportion—situation in pregnancy and labor in which the fetus's head is too large for the mother's pelvis.

Cholecystitis—acute or chronic inflammation of the gallbladder.

Chronic pain—pain that persists for a long time, showing little change.

Clomid—the most commonly used fertility drug. Stimulates ovulation.

Coagulate, coagulation—clotting; the process of changing a liquid into a solid, especially of the blood. This term is frequently used instead of *desiccation*. See desiccation.

Colon—the major tubular part of the large intestine from the cecum to the rectum.

Colonoscopy—a procedure to study the condition of the colon from the inside of the colon. A colonoscope, a long, flexible tube with a fiberoptic lighting system like a laparoscope, is inserted into the colon through the rectum.

Colostomy—surgical creation of an opening in the abdominal wall for drainage of bowel contents. In temporary colostomy the opening is closed after healing of the cut parts of the intestines and the person returns to normal bowel movements. In permanent colostomy the person uses a bag at the site of the surgical opening or uses a pad over the opening and needs a bag only at the time of bowel movement. (Permanent colostomy is not used for endometriosis of the bowel.)

Colpotomy—surgical procedure in which an incision is made in the vagina just behind the cervix.

Compromised immune system—an immune system that is injured, impaired, unable to function completely normally.

Constipation—infrequent or difficult passage of dry, hardened feces.

Correlation—"the extent to which one of a pair of characteristics affects the other in a series of individuals" (*Bantam Medical Dictionary*, rev. ed. 1990). Example: there is a positive correlation between cigarette smoking and lung cancer.

Crohn's disease—a chronic inflammatory bowel disease.

Cul-de-sac—the space between the uterus and rectum that forms a pouch.

Cyst—a closed cavity or sac, epithelium-lined, usually containing liquid or semi-solid material.

Cystectomy—surgical removal of all or part of the bladder.

Cystitis—inflammation of the bladder.

Cystoscopy—a procedure in which a scopelike device is inserted through the urethra while the patient is anesthetized, allowing the physician to see the inside of the bladder.

Cytotoxic—toxic to cells.

D & C— abbreviation for *dilation and curettage*, a procedure in which the cervix, the opening of the uterus at the top of the vagina, is dilated, widened or stretched with a dilator, and the endometrium, the inside lining of the uterus, is scraped and examined under a microscope. D & Cs are frequently done to determine the cause of and to treat unusual bleeding but are also used for other gynecological reasons.

Dermal—referring to the skin.

DES—diethylstilbestrol (DES), a synthetic estrogen, was given to pregnant women to prevent miscarriage between 1941 and 1971. Subsequent research showed that the drug did not prevent miscarriage. DES has since been linked to breast cancer in the mothers, pregnancy complications and a rare form of vaginal cancer in exposed daughters, and fertility problems in both daughters and sons.

Desiccate, desiccation—the drying of tissue with cellular destruction. This is the tissue effect of using a bipolar or thermal coagulator.

Diarrhea—abnormally frequent passage of loose, watery stools. The American Medical Association *Family Medical Guide* notes, on the topic of constipation and diarrhea, "there is no 'normal' pattern for bowel movements. Most people have about one a day, but some have as many as three. At the other extreme there are people who regularly have only three bowel movements a week. . . . Consider yourself constipated only if your normal pattern changes and you begin to have irregular, unusually infrequent, and/or difficult movements. Similarly, you have diarrhea only if you have unusually frequent and particularly loose bowel movements."

Dysfunction—disturbance in the functioning of an organ or system.

Dysmenorrhea—painful periods.

Dyspareunia—painful intercourse.

Dysuria—painful urination.

Ectopic pregnancy—implantation of a fertilized egg in any location other than the uterus; a very dangerous condition that can lead to rupture, internal bleeding, and sometimes even death.

Electrocautery—method for destroying endo by burning it with a wire heated by electric current.

Electrosurgery—the use of electric current to burn (cauterize), desiccate (coagulate), fulgurate, or excise endometriosis.

Endocrine system—the network of glands and other structures that produce hormones. Glands of the endocrine system include the thyroid, pituitary, pancreas, ovaries, and testicles.

Endometrioma—a mass containing endometrial tissue, often described as a *chocolate cyst* because of its color.

Endometrium, endometrial—tissue that lines the inside of the uterus and builds up and sheds each month in the menstrual cycle.

Endorphins and enkephalins—substances produced by the body to lower the perception of pain.

Epithelium—the covering of the internal and the external organs of the body, including the lining of vessels. It consists of cells bound together by connective material and varies in the number of layers and the kinds of cells. The plural is "epithelia."

Estradiol—the major estrogen of the menstruating years. Estradiol in menstruating women varies enormously from individual to individual, as well as fluctuating from day to day within the cycle and even within the day. Levels of 40 to 350 picograms per milliliter have been shown in large groups of healthy menstruating women, with an average of 125 to 200 picograms per milliliter over the cycle. Other estrogens are estriol and estrone.

Et al.—the abbreviation for *et alia*, a Latin phrase meaning "and others." Used, for example, in research papers to show that there were other researchers besides the names listed, as in "R.W. Kistner, M.R. Cohen, R.L. Friedlander, et al."

Excise, excision—to cut out.

Feces—stool.

Femoral neck—the middle portion of the femur, or thigh bone—the longest and strongest bone in the body. Doctors studying bone strength may also look at the spine, the forearm, and the wrist.

Fibroid—noncancerous, nonendometriotic tumor of the uterus.

Fibromyalgia—a painful condition of the fibrous connective tissue that sometimes affects women with endo.

Flank—the fleshy part of the back and side of the body between the ribs and hip. The back area over the kidneys.

Follicles—balls of cells in the ovary with an immature egg in the center.

Fulguration—burning of tissue to destroy it by means of electrical sparks.

Functional deficits—defects or errors in the way the organism works in its metabolic processes.

Gallbladder—a pear-shaped organ about 4 inches long, located under the liver in the right upper corner of the abdomen, which stores the bile manufactured by the liver. Bile is a substance that aids in the digestion and absorption of fats.

Gastric—pertaining to the stomach.

Gastritis—acute or chronic inflammation of the lining of the stomach.

Gastrointestinal—relating to the stomach and intestine.

Gestalt—a school of psychology that originated in Germany; noted for emphasis on looking at a whole situation rather than just parts.

Growths—another word, along with *nodules* and *lesions*, to describe endometriosis.

Heliocobacter—a type of bacteria.

Hematuria—abnormal presence of blood in the urine.

Hemostasis—arrest of bleeding.

Heparin—a drug that prevents blood from clotting.

Histamine—a substance found in all body tissues, histamine dilates small blood vessels and contracts smooth muscles; it may also be a neurotransmitter. Excess amounts of histamine are released during allergic reactions or shock.

Holistic—an approach to health care that considers the whole person, including physical, social, emotional, economic, and spiritual needs, rather than simply symptoms and disease.

Homeopathy—the theory or system of curing diseases with very minute doses of medicine which in a healthy person and in large doses would produce a condition like that being treated. See *Overcoming Endometriosis*, 97–98.

Hymen—The membranous fold that partially or wholly occludes the external opening of the vagina.

Hyperparathyroidism—abnormally increased activity of the parathyroid glands, causing loss of calcium from the bones and excessive secretion of calcium and phosphorus by the kidney. Symptoms include kidney stones, back and joint pains, thirst, nausea, and vomiting.

Hypothalamus—attached to pituitary gland; controls production and release of hormones in the pituitary.

Hysterectomy—surgical removal of the uterus.

Hysterosalpingogram—x-ray test in which a dye is injected into the uterus and tubes to determine their condition.

Incontinence—the inability to control urination; unintentional loss of urine.

Inguinal—pertaining to the groin.

Intestines, bowel, gut—the tubular part of the digestive tract that extends from the stomach to the anus. The small intestine is about 20 feet long and is the section from the stomach to a part of the intestine called the *cecum*; it is smaller in diameter than the large intestine. The large intestine is about 5 feet long and includes the cecum, colon, rectum, and anal canal.

Irritable bowel syndrome—a poorly understood, loosely defined bowel problem characterized by irregular and uncoordinated contractions of the intestines.

Keloid—elevated, irregularly shaped scar tissue.

Kidneys—the two bean-shaped organs located in the lower back, each to one side of the spine, that clean the blood. The wastes and excess water from this process is urine.

Lactated Ringer's—a fluid and electrolyte replenisher.

Laparoscopy—surgical procedure, generally done on an outpatient basis under general anesthesia. A small incision is made near the naval, and a lighted, thin tube is inserted, through which the surgeon can view organs in the abdomen. Additional small incisions may be made to introduce other instruments into the abdomen for removing endo growths and adhesions or performing other surgical procedures. A diagnostic laparoscopy is a laparoscopy done to diagnose the problem. An operative laparoscopy means that surgical procedures besides diagnosis are carried out during the laparoscopy. Most endo specialists now do operative laparoscopies even at the time of first diagnosis.

Laparotomy—major surgery done through an incision in the abdominal wall.

Laser—extremely concentrated beam of light that can be directed precisely to destroy diseased tissue or to excise it.

Lesion—word used in endometriosis to describe the patches, colonies, or growths of endometrial tissue outside the uterus. In general, *lesion* refers to any abnormal patch of tissue.

Lipids—fatty substances, insoluble in water. Lipids are important sources of fuel to the body and in maintaining cell membranes. Ratios of certain lipids are thought to predict cardiovascular disease.

Lupus (systemic lupus erythematosus)—an inflammatory disease, generally occurring in young women, that causes deterioration of the connective tissues and may attack soft internal organs as well as bones and muscle. Symptoms vary widely but may include fever, rash, abdominal pains, weakness, fatigue, and pain in joints and muscles.

Lymphocyte—a lymph cell; part of the body's system that filters bacteria from the bloodstream.

Lyse, Lysis—to cut, break up, divide, separate; cutting or dividing or separating surgically.

Macrophages—immune cells that destroy bacteria and other foreign material by surrounding them and gobbling them up.

Metabolic—relating to metabolism, the chemical processes of a living organism that result in energy production, growth, elimination of wastes, and other bodily functions related to distribution of nutrients after digestion.

Microsurgery—surgery using magnification, tiny sutures, and very gentle handling of tissues.

Millimeter (mm)—part of the metric system of measurement. 1 mm = .04 inch (U.S.).

Mitral valve prolapse—a defect in which a valve on the left side of the heart flaps up instead of closing tightly, allowing some blood to backflow.

Morbidity—the condition of being unhealthy or diseased.

Moxibustion—*moxa* is an herb used in traditional Chinese medicine that is burned over the point of the energy meridians, stimulating the flow of *chi* (energy). (Yo San University Clinic brochure.)

Mucous colitis—another term for irritable bowel syndrome.

Multiple sclerosis (MS)—a chronic disease, generally occurring in young adults, characterized by hardened patches scattered randomly throughout the brain and spinal cord, interfering with the nerves in those areas. Can cause visual disturbances, balance impairment, unsteady walk, loss of bladder and bowel control, and paralysis.

Myofascial release massage—a type of physical therapy, or massage, that slowly stretches the fascia, or connective tissue, releasing restrictions occurring in the connective tissue that may be causing pain, stiffness, and/or other problems.

Myomectomy—Surgical removal of a myoma (fibroid).

Myometrial, Myometrium—having to do with the myometrium, the outer lining, layer/muscular coat of the uterus.

Narcotics (legal definition)—habit-forming drugs.

Narcotics (medical definition)—drugs that produce narcosis, depression of the central nervous system.

Necrosis—localized tissue death that occurs in groups of cells in response to disease or injury.

Nocturia—urinary frequency at night.

Nodule—a small, firm lump of tissue.

Oophorectomy—surgical removal of the ovaries.

Opiate—a narcotic that contains opium or its derivatives.

Opioid—a synthetic narcotic that acts like an opiate but is not derived from opium.

Osseous—bonelike.

Osteopathy—osteopathy is, according to *Stedman's Concise Medical Dictionary*, "a school of medicine based upon the idea that the normal body when in 'correct adjustment' is a vital machine capable of making its own remedies against infections and other toxic conditions; employs the diagnostic and therapeutic measures of ordinary medicine in addition to manipulative measures."

Osteoporosis—disease of the bones in which the bones become thin and porous and break easily.

Ovarian remnant syndrome—the presence of ovarian tissue in the pelvis after the ovaries have been removed; more common when adhesions and inflammation made the surgery difficult.

Pain receptors—(also called *nociceptors*) free nerve endings distributed abundantly in the superficial layers of the skin and in certain deeper tissues. Pain receptors are the first to respond to injury.

Pain threshold—the least stimulus at which a person perceives pain. The pain threshold may be lowered or raised by changes in temperature, the presence of certain chemicals, or other factors.

Palpate—to feel with the hands.

Papillar—small, nipple-shaped elevation.

Pelvic congestion—abnormal accumulation of blood in the pelvis.

Pelvic inflammatory disease—an infection in the pelvic area that can be caused by a variety of bacteria and can attack various pelvic organs; often abbreviated *PID*.

Pergonal—fertility drug usually used when Clomid is not effective. Pergonal is sometimes responsible for multiple births.

Peritoneal, Peritoneal fluid—pertaining to the peritoneum or the fluid surrounding the abdominal organs.

Peritoneum—the thin membrane covering the walls of the abdomen and pelvis and the organs contained within them.

Peritonitis—inflammation of the peritoneum; may be caused by internal bleeding or irritating substances from a ruptured cyst, gallbladder, or gastric ulcer.

Permeability—condition whereby fluids and other substances can pass through.

Petechial—minute, non-raised, purplish red spots.

Phospholipids—molecules containing phosphate groups, glycerol, and fatty acids that are major components of the membranes of cells.

Physiological—relating to physiology, the physical and chemical processes involved in the functioning of living organisms.

Pituitary gland—located at the base of the brain; secretes, regulates, and stores a number of different hormones that affect the thyroid, reproductive organs, and other areas of the body.

Polycystic ovarian disease—simultaneous formation of many cysts on both ovaries; also called Stein–Leventhal syndrome. Symptoms include infrequent or no periods, failure to ovulate, and abnormal hairiness.

Porphyria—a genetic disorder characterized by a disturbance in porphyrin metabolism; an increase in the formation and excretion of porphyrins (components of hemoglobin); gastrointestinal, neurologic, and psychologic symptoms; sensitivity to light; pigmentation of the face; and anemia with enlargement of the spleen.

Postpartum—occurring after childbirth, with reference to the mother.

Precocious puberty—precocious puberty is unusually early sexual maturation. It is sometimes caused by endocrine disease or, as in a well-known series of cases in Puerto Rico, by hormones in meat, or may be of unknown origin.

Preeclampsia—a metabolic disturbance of late pregnancy characterized by high blood pressure, edema, and excess protein in the urine.

Premature menopause—before natural menopause would occur.

Prenatal, perinatal, and antenatal—*natal* refers to birth. *Pre* means "preceding"; *Peri* means "the period shortly before and after birth." (It's the time period from the 29th week of pregnancy to 1 to 4 weeks after birth.) *Ante* means "before." All of the three prefixes mean much the same thing connected to other terms (*peri* would mean around or surrounding).

Presacral neurectomy—a procedure severing the nerves at the back of the uterus to help provide pain relief.

Primary dysmenorrhea—painful periods and other symptoms due to an imbalance in prostaglandins.

Proctoscopy—direct examination of the interior of the rectum using a proctoscope, a short lighted scope or speculum, to allow the physician to see abnormalities.

Progesterone—a hormone that prepares the uterus for reception and development of the fertilized egg.

Prognosis—prospect for recovery.

Prophylactic—any regimen or agent that contributes to the prevention of infection and disease.

Prostaglandins—substances found in semen, menstrual fluid, and various body tissues. Stimulate contractions of the uterus (responsible for some cramping) and of other smooth muscles. Also can lower blood pressure and affect the action of certain hormones.

Psychosomatic—having physical symptoms stemming from emotional or mental origins.

Pyloric—adjective form of pylorus, which is the part of the stomach that leads to the duodenum.

Rectosigmoid colon—the part of the colon from the sigmoid colon to the rectum.

Rectovaginal septum—a septum is a partition or dividing wall; the rectovaginal septum is the wall separating the rectum and vagina.

Rectum—the end portion of the large intestine.

Resect—to excise (remove by cutting) part of an organ or other structure.

Resection—excision (removal by cutting) of a portion of an organ or other structure.

Retroperitoneal—behind the peritoneum.

Sacral—pertaining to the sacrum, which is the triangular bone at the base of the spine.

Sex-hormone binding globulin—a protein that binds sex hormones in blood.

Shiatsu massage—the Japanese equivalent of acupressure. Similar to acupuncture except the points on the meridians are stimulated by fingertip pressure rather than needles.

Sigmoid colon—the part of the left colon located in the pelvis and extending to the rectum.

Sigmoidoscopy—direct examination of the interior of the sigmoid colon using an instrument called a *sigmoidoscope*, a tube with lighting to allow the physician to see abnormalities.

Spastic colon—another term for irritable bowel syndrome.

Steroids—a group of molecules based on a common structure that includes the sex hormones (estrogens, testosterone, progestins), cholesterol, bile acids, and many other biologically active compounds.

Stool—bowel movement; the waste matter discharged in a bowel movement; feces.

Surgical menopause—menopause brought on by surgical removal of the ovaries.

Surgically castrated—removal of the ovaries. (*Castration* medically means "removal of the testicles or ovaries.")

Suture—a surgical stitch taken to repair an incision, tear, or wound; material used for surgical stitches, such as absorbable or nonabsorbable silk, catgut, wire, or synthetic material.

Synergism—joint action or cooperation by two or more structures or drugs; the simultaneous action of separate entities which together have greater total effect than the sum of their individual effects.

Synthesis—the production of a substance by the combination of parts or elements to form a whole.

Systemic—pertaining to the body as a whole.

Systemic immunity—the part of the immune system involving the immune cells that circulate throughout the whole body.

Taoism—a way of living and understanding based on universal principles observed by some ancient Chinese. Emphasizes living harmoniously with nature, maintaining health, balanced living, and spiritual cultivation.

T cells—a type of lymphocyte (white blood cells) responsible for immune recognition (determining what is self and what is foreign tissue or an invader). They coordinate the immune response.

Teratogen—an agent that causes defects in a developing fetus.

Testosterone—part of a group of male hormones know as *androgens*.

TNF (tumor necrosis factor)—an important substance produced by cells of the immune system that helps in fighting infection. It was originally named because it was first discovered by its ability to kill tumor cells. However, we now know that it performs many necessary functions in the body.

Trigone—a triangular area at the base of the bladder.

Umbilicus—navel.

Ureters—two small tubes carrying urine from the kidney to the bladder. The ureters run from the kidneys behind the peritoneum, which is the thin membrane covering the walls of the abdomen and pelvis. Surgeons must be careful to find the ureter on each side of the pelvis and abdomen when doing surgery to be sure not to cut it.

Urethra—a small tube that drains urine from the bladder to the outside of the body. The opening of the urethra is above the vagina and below the clitoris.

Urgency—the feeling of the need to void urine immediately.

Urinary tract/urinary system—all the organs involved in the formation and elimination of urine, including the kidneys, ureters, bladder, and urethra.

Urination—the act of passing urine.

Urine—the fluid secreted by the kidneys, carried by the ureters to the bladder, and stored until elimination through the urethra.

Urology—the branch of medicine that studies and treats the urinary system.

Uteri—plural form of the word *uterus*.

Uterosacral ligaments—tough bands of tissue supporting the uterus.

Vaporization—destruction of tissue by instant boiling of the cellular water with a high-power-density laser or high-power-density electrosurgical knife.

Vascularized—pertaining to or composed of blood vessels.

Videolaseroscopy—laser laparoscopy augmented by video equipment, including video camera, video recorder, and high-resolution video monitor. This increases magnification of the operating field, allows the surgeon to work in an upright, comfortable posture (watching the video monitor rather than bent over the laparoscope), and provides a permanent record of the extent of disease and of the procedure. Operating with video equipment has become standard with operative laparoscopy.

Visceral pain—pain in the viscera (the internal organs, such as the bladder, colon, and ureter).

Index

Acknowledgment of Permissions

⊚⊘

The editor gratefully acknowledges permission from the following to reprint material in this book:

Selected excerpts from two chapters from *Overcoming Bladder Disorders* by Rebecca Chalker and Kristene Whitmore, M.D. Copyright © 1990 by Rebecca Chalker. Reprinted by permission of HarperCollins Publishers, Inc.

Infertility and Reproductive Medicine Clinics of North America: Endometriosis, 3:3, July 1992, David L. Olive, M.D., guest editor, for material from "Foreword" by Michael P. Diamond, M.D., and Alan H. DeCherney, M.D., "Treatment Options for Endometriosis—Medical Therapies" by B. S. Hurst, M.D., and W. D. Schlaff, M.D., "Treatment Options for Endometriosis: Surgical Therapies" by A. A. Luciano, M.D., and D. Manzi, M.D., "Treatment of Endometriosis-Associated Infertility" by G. F. Rosen, M.D., M.S., and "Future Directions for Endometriosis Research" by D. L. Olive, M.D. Copyright © 1992 by W. B. Saunders Company. Reprinted by permission of W. B. Saunders Company.

Selected excerpts from *No More Hot Flashes and Other Good News* by Penny Wise Budoff, M.D. Copyright © 1983 by Penny Wise Budoff, M.D. Reprinted by permission of G. P. Putnam's Sons.

Selected excerpts from *No More Menstrual Cramps and Other Good News* by Penny Wise Budoff, M.D. Copyright © 1980 by Penny Wise Budoff, M.D. Reprinted by permission of G. P. Putnam's Sons.

Endometriosis: Contemporary Concepts in Clinical Management by Robert S. Schenken, M.D., editor, for material from "Preface" by Robert S. Schenken, M.D., "Conservative Surgery: Goals of Conservative Surgery" by David L. Olive, M.D., and "Extrapelvic Endometriosis: Urinary Endometriosis" by G. W. Mitchell, M.D. Copyright © 1989 by J. B. Lippincott Company. Reprinted by permission of Robert S. Schenken, M.D.

Selected excerpts from *Womancare* by Lynda Madaras and Jane Patterson, M.D., F.A.C.O.G. Copyright © 1981 by Lynda Madaras. Reprinted by permission of Lynda Madaras. A revised and updated edition of *Womancare* will be available in 1997.

Science Vol. 262, 26 November 1993, for material from "Dioxin Tied to Endometriosis" by Ann Gibbons. Copyright © 1993 by American Association for the Advancement of Science. Reprinted by permission of American Association for the Advancement of Science.

Hydrodissection drawing from Camran Nezhat and Farr R. Nezhat: "Safe Laser Endoscopic Excision or Vaporization of Peritoneal Endometriosis." *Fertility and Sterility* 1989, 59:149–51. Reproduced with permission of the publisher, the American Society for Reproductive Medicine (The American Fertility Society).

THE **UGLY TRUTH** ABOUT **ENDOMETRIOSIS**

We asked women suffering from endometriosis to draw a picture showing what the disease felt like to them. The illustration you see here was created by one of those women.

For her and millions like her, endometriosis is an ongoing struggle with chronic pain, frustration, and fatigue. There is no cure. But there is hope.

The Endometriosis Association is a nonprofit organization for women with endometriosis and others interested in exchanging information and promoting research on the disease. The organization provides sufferers with invaluable emotional support and understanding through support groups, crisis call help, books and brochures, a newsletter, educational programs, and an information clearinghouse.

Above all, we let women know they are not alone. For more information about endometriosis, including how to order a diagnostic kit, write or call today!

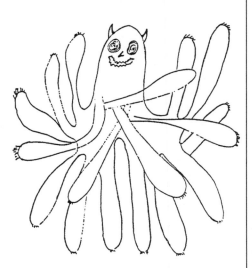

ENDOMETRIOSIS **A**SSOCIATION

8585 North 76th Place, Milwaukee, WI 53223   (800) 992-3636 U.S. (North America)

Endometriosis Association Membership/Donation Form

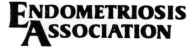

| (Last) | NAME | (First) |

Street — Apt #

City — State/Province

Zip/Postal Code — Country

Phone

CHARGE TO: ☐ VISA   ☐ MASTERCARD

Card No.

Exp. Date

Make checks payable to:
ENDOMETRIOSIS ASSOCIATION
8585 N. 76th Pl., Milwaukee, WI 53223 U.S.A.
Call or fax your membership:
(414) 355-2200   Fax (414) 355-6065

☐ I am interested in helping to start a chapter in my area if one does not exist. Please send me guidelines. (Local listings will be sent when you join.)

☐ I am willing to serve as a Contact Person—women with endometriosis may call me to share information and support.

Please check: ☐ I have/had endometriosis.
☐ I have not had endometriosis.

MEMBER (For those who have or have had endometriosis.)
☐ 1 Year dues. $25.00 U.S./35.00 Canadian
☐ 2 Year dues. $40.00 U.S./55.00 Canadian
☐ 3 Year dues. $75.00 U.S./104.00 Canadian
    (Includes FREE book, *Overcoming Endometriosis*)
☐ 5 Year dues. $100 U.S./138.00 Canadian $ _____

ASSOCIATE (For those who have not had endometriosis—Physicians, Women's Ctrs., Institutions, and interested individuals.)
☐ 1 Year dues. $30.00 U.S./41.50 Canadian
☐ 2 Year dues. $50.00 U.S./69.00 Canadian
☐ 3 Year dues. $90.00 U.S./124.50 Canadian
    (Includes FREE book, *Overcoming Endometriosis*)
☐ 5 Year dues. $120 U.S./166.00 Canadian $ _____

Donation (optional).
I have enclosed an additional $ _____

ADDITIONAL POSTAGE
Canadian members add: $5.00
Other foreign countries add: $10.00 $ _____
TOTAL $ _____